CLINICAL
FOOT
ROENTGENOLOGY

SECOND EDITION

FELTON O. GAMBLE, D.P.M., F.A.C.P.R., Ed.D. (Hon.)
    Professor Emeritus of Roentgenology, Temple University, School of Chiropody.
    Past President and Fellow, American College of Podiatric Radiologists.
    Past President, American Podiatry Association.
    Formerly, Chief of Foot Clinic, Metabolic Department, Presbyterian Hospital, Philadelphia.
    Author, *Applied Foot Roentgenology.*

IRVING YALE, D.P.M., F.A.C.P.R., Ed.D. (Hon.)
    Past President, American Podiatry Association
    Past President and Fellow, American College of Podiatric Radiologists.
    Formerly, Lecturer in Roentgenology, Long Island University, College of Podiatry
    Formerly, Chief of Podiatry Service, Orthopedic Section, Department of Surgery, Yale-New Haven Community
        Hospital
    Associate Fellow, American College of Foot Surgeons.
    Fellow, American Public Health Association.
    Author, *Clinical and Roentgenological Interpretations in the Lower Extremities, Podiatric Medicine.*

CLINICAL
FOOT
ROENTGENOLOGY

SECOND EDITION

by **FELTON O. GAMBLE** and **IRVING YALE**

ROBERT E. KRIEGER PUBLISHING COMPANY, INC.
HUNTINGTON, NEW YORK

Origional Edition 1966
Second Edition 1975

Printed and Published by
Robert E. Krieger Publishing Co., Inc.
645 New York Avenue
Huntington, New York 11743

Library of Congress Card Number 74-15632
ISBN 0-88275-102-6

Printed in the United States of America

DEDICATED TO OUR DEVOTED WIVES,
Romaine Gamble and Bernice Yale

PREFACE

This second edition of *Clinical Foot Roentgenology* is a continuance of the previously published works of the authors: *Clinical and Roentgenological Interpretations in the Lower Extremities* by Irving Yale (1952), *Applied Foot Roentgenology* by Felton O. Gamble (1957), and *Clinical Foot Roentgenology,* a joint effort by Gamble and Yale (1966). Science is not static. The authors consider it a privilege to revise this text because the opportunity is afforded to advance new concepts, to revise old ones, and to discard some that are obsolete. A great responsibility is engendered in producing a text that is to be used by the college student and by the practitioner at large. Basic facts are needed on one hand and practicality on the other. We seek to achieve a blend of both facets.

The present edition of *Clinical Foot Roentgenology* includes the results of our continuing research and development and additional references from an assiduous search of pertinent literature. Four new chapters have been added: "Hereditary and Congenital Anomalies," "Roentgenology and Biomechanics," "Radiation Hazards and Protection," and "Charting in Foot Roentgenology." We have included new trends in the clinical application of foot roentgenology to biomechanics and foot surgery. Care has been exercised to avoid elaboration on orthopedic and surgical procedures, which more appropriately belong in texts for those disciplines. Among the innovations presented is a chart that clarifies and compares biomechanical, roentgenologic, and traditional terms, descriptions, and sequelae of foot deformities. Several methods of charting roentgenograms are illustrated and some of the pitfalls and fallacies as well as advantages are discussed. A new type of instant positive X-ray paper is introduced. A simultaneous exposure of film and paper provides a film roentgenogram and a paper duplicate of many uses. Recently developed devices and technics are presented. Roentgenograms of dissected anatomical specimens demonstrate important features unattainable in conventional roentgenologic studies.

The new book is a larger size and is completely redesigned in typo and layout. Many new illustrations and drawings and an expanded bibliography are offered.

Although unidentified in these pages, every roentgenogram in this book represents a patient who has received clinical consideration. We are cognizant of this doctor-patient relationship and are grateful to all patients who have unwittingly contributed to the body of knowledge in this book.

Felton O. Gamble, D.P.M.　　　　　　　　　　Irving Yale, D.P.M.
Tucson, Arizona　　　　　　　　　　　　　　Ansonia, Connecticut

January 1975

ACKNOWLEDGMENTS

The authors extend profound thanks and appreciation to Helen R. Hauck for editing, proofreading, and providing literary expertise to help this book become a reality. Alan K. Whitney, D.P.M. has provided anatomical drawings and tracings. We are grateful for his fine contributions. A. Clifford Pollack, chief medical photographer, Medical Audiovisual Services, Arizona Medical Center, The University of Arizona, has photographed new technics and devices, reproduced roentgenograms, and willingly assisted with graphic chores, for which the authors are most appreciative. We have credited colleagues for all newly contributed roentgenograms where shown, acknowledged communications in the bibliographies, and made mention of those associated with special projects included in this text. Our thanks to all who have helped in any way, especially to any we may have inadvertently failed to name.

Dr. Yale extends special thanks to Elizabeth Maciecki for compiling material from the additional references and to the reference library staff of Yale University Medical Library for their generous assistance. Dr. Yale's son, Jeffrey F. Yale, D.P.M. was most helpful in editing new illustrations and bibliographic material, which is very much appreciated. Mr. Eugene Kone of the Rockefeller University staff has rendered advice for which sincere thanks are offered.

Dr. Gamble is grateful to Charles E. Krausz, D.P.M., Stewart E. Reed, D.P.M., J. Colin Dagnall, M.Ch.S., S.R.Ch., and Dr. Shanker H. Vyas for assistance in obtaining special bibliographic material. Many courtesies have been extended by Miriam E. Miller, acquisitions librarian, Arizona Medical Center Library, The University of Arizona, for which due thanks are offered. Personal conferences with James V. Ganley, D.P.M. concerning pediatric roentgenology, the late Charles M. Hammonds, D.P.M. and Richard M. Stess, D.P.M. about tri-plane scanography, and Harry F. Hlavac, D.P.M., Merton L. Root, D.P.M., John H. Weed, D.P.M., Roy O. Kroeker, D.P.M., Fritz Moller, D.P.M. and Richard O. Schuster, D.P.M. about biomechanics have been invaluable and their cooperation is greatly appreciated. G. Elmer Harford, D.P.M. expertly performed the dissection work of the anatomical specimen roentgenographed by Leon H. Kehr, D.P.M. and thanks are extended for taking care of this assignment.

The authors wish to thank The Williams and Wilkins Co. for referring our work to Robert E. Krieger Publishing Co., Inc., who is publishing the present edition. The authors acknowledge with much appreciation the kind cooperation of Robert E. Krieger and his competent staff in bringing this edition to fruition. Special credit is extended to Beverly E. Beyer for designing the book from type style and page layout to final cover design.

CONTENTS

SECTION TWO • Roentgenologic Diagnosis of Foot Pathoanatomy

SECTION THREE • Foot Roentgenographic Technic

SECTION ONE
ROENTGENOLOGIC DIAGNOSIS OF FOOT DISEASE

1 NORMAL BONE

A critical assessment of the development, growth, histology, and gross structure of bone is essential to the analytical study of bone roentgenograms. The roentgenologic features of normal bone from infancy to adulthood should be so well mastered that any alteration will be immediately recognized.

Bone is living tissue with active chemophysiologic processes taking place constantly. The normal changes of mineral content, osseous and other cellular elements contribute to the total roentgenologic appearance of normal bone. Body metabolism and endocrine function affect the chemical balance of bone.

Bone functions. It is hematopoietic. Bone is highly vascularized and bleeds easily when traumatized. Much more is to be inferred in the roentgenogram of bone than its function as a skeletal framework.

The reader must appraise alterations in the bones of the feet as being physiologic, within the bounds of normalcy, or as pathologic and secondary to trauma, abnormal physiologic reactions to stress, faulty genetic patterns, and a myriad of intrinsic and extrinsic influences. The astute diagnostician will consider all bodily functions and structure together with laboratory studies in evaluating normal bone.

DEVELOPMENT

The foot consists of tubular long bones and small irregular bones which develop endochondrally. Bone shapes formed in cartilage are present at birth with some primary centers of ossification (Fig. 1).

Phases of Development

1. Centers for *ossification* of the diaphysis and of the epiphysis develop from cartilage which is replaced by bone.

2. The diaphyseal bone and epiphyseal bone unite at a predictable skeletal age in the process of *maturation,* female before male.

3. In the process of growth, bone is *remodeled* in shape.

4. There is *subperiosteal* bone formation in long bones.

5. The small irregular bones develop to maturity from one center of ossification.

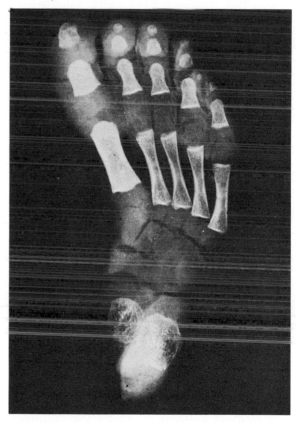

Fig. 1. Bone shape pattern at birth, *dorsoplantar view.* Nine-month stillborn specimen, skin integument removed. Note outlines of cartilaginous bones. Also, observe the relationship of mineralized zones of talus and calcaneus to the entire bone shape.

Histology of Endochondral Bone Development

1. Condensation of the mesenchyme to precartilage tissue occurs.

2. Precartilage tissue differentiates into chondrocytes with a hyaline ground substance forming the shape of a skeletal part.

3. Trabeculae are laid down, and a perichondral splinting supports the shaft.

4. The cartilage degenerates and the intercellular matrix distends in preparation for removal of the cartilage.

5. The intercellular substance calcifies and connective tissue invades the substance from the periosteum.

6. The periosteum covers the perichondral splint in the diaphysis.

7. The vascular tissue enters into and destroys the cartilage cells. The cells are removed by macrophages and chondroclasts, which are multinucleated giant cells.

8. An early marrow cavity is formed following resorption of the cartilage cells.

9. The remaining bonelike calcified cartilage becomes condensed and mineralized. Calcification of the osteoid matrix takes place. "Completion of mineralization once it has begun normally seems to be able to occur in the absence of active osteoblast cells" (Frost, 1963).

10. Before calcification of the cartilage ground substance, the cartilaginous longitudinal growth proceeds by interstitial development.

11. The new bone grows in thickness by accretion or appositional growth on its outer surface.

12. With advancement of growth, one or more centers of ossification may develop at the site of the future epiphysis.

13. The developmental cartilage calcifies, degenerates, and then ossifies, forming an epiphysis.

14. Wanken and Eyring (1972) used strontium-87m as a tracer to study the epiphyses of the lower extremity and their contribution to skeletal growth. The study demonstrated that there is a variation in the metabolic activity of the different epiphyses with respect to time. Varying rates of uptake of radiostrontium correspond to the well-known spurts of growth occurring in children. The rate of bone

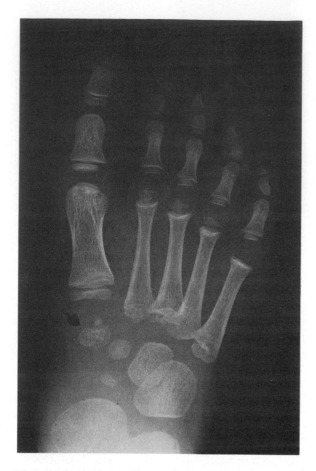

Fig. 2. Immature foot bones. Multiple nuclei for ossification of cuneiform.

salt deposition also varied with age.

15. Ham (1953) noted that epiphyseal bone forms when channels invade the cartilaginous model of the epiphysis from the metaphyseal side of the growth plate. The growth-plate cartilage is protected from ossification by perichondral cells lining these channels. However, Kalayjian and Cooper (1972) consistently noted epiphyseal penetration by perichondrial vessels. The investigators conclude from their studies that "once the bony center appears, ossification along the articular side is different from that along the metaphyseal side. Enchondral ossification beneath the articular surface accounts for most expansion of the bony epiphysis." As the cartilage becomes mineralized, growth gradually ceases and the chondrocytes survive but the articular cartilage remains unmineralized. Some chondrocytes entrapped in the mineralized matrix appear as osteocytes.

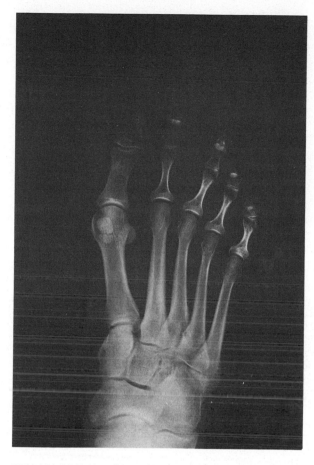

Fig. 3. Mature foot bones. Note remodeled shape of metatarsal bones.

ROENTGENOLOGIC FEATURES OF IMMATURE FOOT BONES (Fig. 2)

LONG BONES.

1. *Diaphysis* — shaft. Cortex of increased density. Medullary cavity of decreased density.

2. *Metaphysis* — flared end of shaft and the growing part of the bone.

3. *Preparatory zone of calcification* — area of increased density at end of metaphysis.

4. *Epiphyseal disk* — cartilage zone. Area of decreased density.

5. *Center of ossification for the epiphysis* — center of increased density.

6. *Articular cartilage* — covers the articular end of bone. Of soft-tissue density. Seldom defined but always present.

IRREGULAR BONES.

Only the mineralized center of ossification is visible.

GROWTH OF FOOT BONES

1. The calcaneus has a secondary ossification center, shell-like in shape, called the apophysis, and this irregular bone matures in a manner similar to tubular long bones.

2. All other small irregular bones of the feet grow through a continuation of endochondral bone development. One secondary ossification center is present, although more than one nucleus may constitute this locus.

3. The metatarsal bones and phalanges are the tubular long bones of the foot, and they normally have only one secondary center of ossification.

4. Tubular long bones grow in the following pattern:

a. The *diaphysis* is formed by the primary ossification into a shaft with cortex bounded on its endosteal surface by medullary bone of the medullary cavity, containing bone marrow, and on its periosteal surface by the soft tissues.

b. The *metaphysis* is the end of the diaphysis that flares out in shape through interstitial growth.

c. Lengthening of the diaphysis occurs as the metaphysis creates new bone at its ends. Trauma or stress can influence this growth.

d. Normal remodeling of the diaphysis by constriction narrows the shaft.

e. At the distal end of the metaphysis, there is a zone of provisional calcification where bone cells replace cartilage cells.

f. The *epiphysis* is the secondary nucleus of ossification at the end of the bone beyond the metaphysis that enlarges by interstitial growth and undergoes calcification, degeneration, resorption, and then ossification.

g. The area of cartilage between the metaphysis and epiphysis is referred to as the *epiphyseal disk.*

h. When bone growth unites metaphysis and epiphysis, fusion occurs and the bone is fundamentally mature.

5. Articular cartilage provides the protective covering over the ends of the bones entering a joint. The bone ends of diarthrodial joints are covered by cartilage that varies with the age of the patient. The cartilage is essentially white with a slight bluish tinge in the child. In the young adult, cartilage is generally white, glossy, and compressible. In the

middle aged to the elderly, one may note color changes in the cartilage varying from yellowish white to a yellow brown. Cartilage is generally thicker in the larger and more active joints. Thus, the activity of middle age increases the thickness of the cartilage in contradistinction to the inactivity of the older person which decreases the thickness.

6. A nutrient foramen carrying blood vessels enters the diaphysis almost parallel to its long axis. The course of the nutrient foramen is away from the growing metaphysis of the bone.

Remodeling of Bone

1. As tubular long bone develops, a basic remodeling of its shape takes place with the diaphysis becoming narrower and the terminal metaphysis flaring.

2. Frost (1963) states, "Bone remodelling is the sum of the formative (osteoblastic) and resorptive (osteoclastic) activities occurring over time."

3. Remodeling may occur at the surface or internally within the cortex.

4. The replacement of old bone by Haversian systems takes place within the cortex during internal remodeling.

5. Remodeling activity of osteoblastic and osteoclastic function is not even. One phase may work more rapidly than the other. However, the final result of remodeling is the sum total of both functions.

6. Remodeling may occur in mature bone in the repair of fractures and under stress reactions (Wolff's law).

7. Bone regenerates following trauma and does not repair by forming scar tissue as do other tissues.

ROENTGENOLOGIC FEATURES OF MATURE FOOT BONES (Fig. 3)

LONG BONES.

1. *Diaphysis* — shaft. More constricted and narrow than immature bone. Cortex of increased density. Medullary cavity of decreased density.

2. *Metaphysis* — the flared end of the shaft. Less flared than in immature bone. More trabecular pattern than shaft. Decreased cortical density.

3. *Epiphysis* — the end of the bone that has formed from a center of ossification. Usually loosely trabeculated of decreased density with

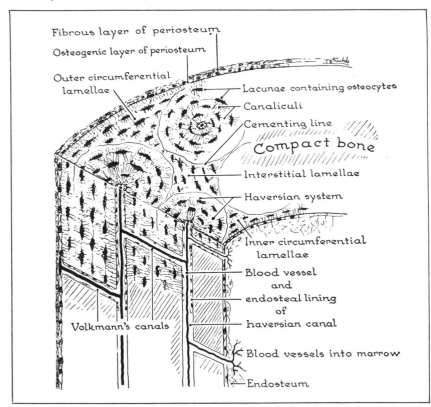

Fig. 4. Three-dimensional diagram of a typical long bone composition. (Reproduced with permission from *Histology*, ed. 5, A.W. Ham and T.S. Leeson. Philadelphia: J.B. Lippincott, 1965.)

a marginal layer of cortex of increased density.

4. *Site of epiphyseal-metaphyseal fusion* — a fairly constant finding consisting of a line of increased density where fusion occurred.

HISTOLOGY OF BONE
Bone Composition (Fig. 4)

1. Periosteum covers all bones. It consists of the following:
   a. The outer fibrous layer.
   b. The inner cellular layer of a lighter connective tissue known as the cambium or osteogenetic layer.
2. Muscles are attached to bone through the periosteum by means of Sharpey's fibers.

3. Ground substance contains the permanent tissue of bone.

4. Osteoblasts are responsible for the formation and calcification of bone matrix. Following this process, some osteoblasts differentiate into osteocytes.

5. Osteocytes are bone cells in lacunae within Haversian systems. They send their processes out into the canaliculae which unite one bone cell with another.

Resorption (Absorption) of Bone

1. Resorption not only occurs during endochondral bone development but may oc-

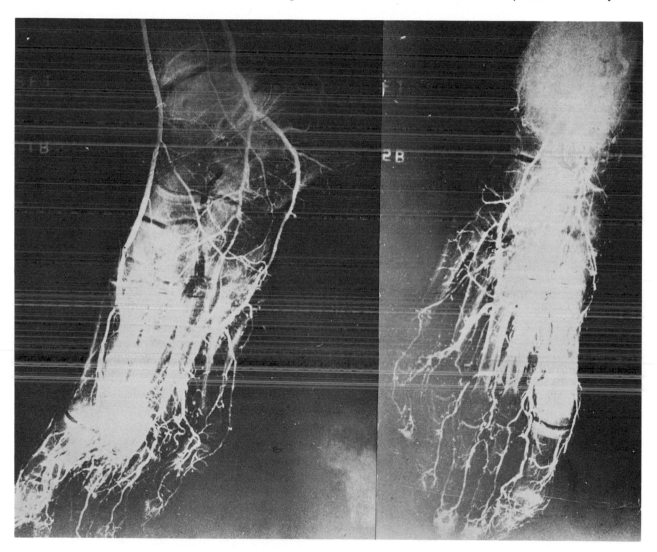

Fig. 5. Arteriograms of the foot. Note the intricate arterial anastomoses.

cur continuously throughout life.

2. Resorption commences with the removal of organic components from intercellular substance by a proteolytic action of the osteoclasts.

3. Calcium salts are liberated, enter the tissue fluid, and are believed to be carried away by the macrophages.

4. Osteocytes may be digested by proteolytic activity or even be differentiated into osteoblasts or osteoclasts.

5. Osteoclasts are believed to develop under the following conditions (after Weinmann and Sicher, 1955):

a. Chemical changes take place in the ground substance with aging and necrosis of bone cells (osteocytes). Cells of the adjacent connective tissue are stimulated by this chemical change to form osteoclasts.

b. A second theory suggests that increased pressure is the cause of bone resorption; e.g., a circulatory stasis and edema in the periosteum or bone marrow lead to a rise in pressure. The pressure in this case would stimulate osteoclasis.

c. Another theory implicates the enzymes, chemical constituents of blood, and the hormones as factors in the differentiation of osteoclasts; e.g., low blood calcium and overproduction of parathyroid hormone.

6. Death of osteocytes before absorption may be shown as an increase in density in the roentgenogram.

7. Removal of calcium from the bone entails removal of the ground substance as well. This is demonstrated as a decrease in bone density in the roentgenogram.

Metabolic and Endocrine Effects on Bone

1. Vitamin D intake is essential for calcium and phosphorus absorption from the intestinal tract.

2. Deficiency of vitamin D results in lower absorption of calcium and stimulates a hyperfunction of the parathyroid glands. Thus, the blood calcium is restored by the parathyroid hormones which deplete the osseous matrix of calcium.

3. Hyperfunction of the parathyroids increases excretion of phosphorus and mobilization of calcium from the matrix to maintain the blood ratio of calcium to phosphorus at 2:1. Excretion of phosphorus may lower the blood phosphorus from 3 to 0.6 mg/100 ml. This creates a drop in serum calcium below 8 or 9 mg/100 ml to maintain a 2:1 ratio of calcium to phosphorus.

4. As the calcium is removed from the ossified skeletal tissue, the blood alkaline phosphatase will rise and the osteoblasts are stimulated to form new bone to resupply the deficit.

5. Adequate amounts of vitamin D diminish excretion of phosphorus and decrease the phosphatase. The need for calcium mobilization from the bone to maintain proper serum level is thus unnecessary and the parathyroids return to normal.

6. Inadequate supply of calcium causes a low serum calcium, as seen in rickets.

7. Vitamin D in substantial amounts increases absorption of calcium and phosphorus. Abundant sunshine ensures endogenous synthesis of large amounts of vitamin D, and this improves absorption of calcium. Parathyroid hormone is also thought to promote intestinal absorption of vitamin D. Small quantities of fat ingested daily may create an acid intestinal medium to promote calcium absorption. When fats are increased, the opposite effect may result in fatty stools and faulty calcium metabolism with diminished absorption of calcium. Sometimes increased amounts of calcium and a normal phosphorus intake may not be absorbed in the lower intestines in adequate amounts due to the combination of these substances into a relatively insoluble calcium phosphate. However, if the calcium-phosphorus intake ratio is changed to a low calcium and high phosphorus, most of the calcium is absorbed higher up in the small intestine and very little remains to combine with the phosphorus in the lower intestine.

8. Termine (1972) states that bone mineral is an integral part of bone tissue, having individual physical and chemical properties that affect tissue as a whole. The mineral in bone tissue is the least inert fraction of all the structural constituents of bone. From Termine's studies it is postulated that the major inorganic chemical steps involved in bone mineral formation are an initial deposition of labile amorphous calcium phosphate, the

change of noncrystalline salt into minute crystals of carbonate-bearing apatite, and crystal development and growth into bone mineral formation. Complex molecular changes and matrix-mineral interactions result in direct cellular action involving mineral deposition in bone.

HISTOLOGY OF BLOOD SUPPLY TO BONE

1. Blood vessels in compact bone are found in the network of the longitudinal Haversian system and Volkmann's canals. A free anastomosis is developed with the periosteum and the marrow.

2. Volkmann's canals contain arterioles, prearterioles, and venules that anastomose with the periosteal and medullary blood vessels. Veins in the bone accompany the arteries and do not have valves.

3. Arteries perforate the outer compact bone and ramify in the bone marrow and in the spongy bone.

4. If complete union has not taken place and the epiphyseal disk separates the diaphysis from the epiphysis, each part receives a separate arterial supply.

5. The shaft is supplied from three sources:

a. Nutrient artery enters through a canal in the compact bone in an oblique course. It anastomoses with the periosteal vessels, Volkmann's canals, the Haversian systems, and sends ascending and descending anastomotic branches through the marrow to the ends of the bone.

b. Metaphyseal vessels from the surrounding ligaments and muscles anastomose with the terminal vessels in the marrow.

c. The periosteal vessels enter Volkmann's canals to supply the compact bone and anastomose with the metaphyseal vessels.

6. The epiphysis is supplied by vessels derived from the capsular structures.

ROENTGENOLOGIC FEATURES OF THE CIRCULATORY NETWORK (Fig. 5)

BIBLIOGRAPHY

Caffey, J.P.: *Pediatric X-ray Diagnosis.* Chicago: The Year Book Publishers, Inc., 1946.
Calcification in Biological Systems, A.A.A.S., 1960.
Engfeldt, B., and Strandh, T.: Microchemical and Biophysical Studies of Normal Human Compact Bone Tissue, Clin. Orthop. 17:63, 1960.
Enlow, D.H.: Functions of the Haversian System, Amer. J. Anat. 110:269, 1962.
Enlow, D.H.: *Bone Remodelling.* Springfield, Ill.: Charles C Thomas, 1963.
Evans, F.G.: *Stress and Strain in Bones.* Springfield, Ill.: Charles C Thomas, 1957.
Frost, H.M.: *Bone Remodelling Dynamics.* Springfield, Ill.: Charles C Thomas, 1963.
Frost, H.M., Roth, H., and Villaneuva, A.R.: A Qualitative Method for Measuring Osteoclastic Activity, Henry Ford Med. Bull. 10:217, 1962.
Frost, H.M., and Villaneuva, A.R.: Measurement of Osteoblastic Activity in Diaphyseal Bone, Stain Techn. 35:179, 1960.
Fourman, L.P.R.: *Calcium Metabolism and the Bone.* Oxford: Blackwell, 1960.
Ham, A.W.: *Histology,* ed. 2. Philadelphia: J.B. Lippincott, 1953.
Ham, A.W., and Leeson, T.S.: *Histology,* ed. 4. Philadelphia: J.B. Lippincott Co., 1961.

Irving, J.T.: Histochemical Changes in the Early Stages of Calcification, Clin. Orthop. 17:92, 1960.
Jaffe, H.L.: *Metabolic, Degenerative, and Inflammatory Diseases of Bones and Joints.* Philadelphia: Lea & Febiger, 1972.
Kalayjian, D.B., and Cooper, R.R.: Osteogenesis of the Epiphysis, Clin. Orthop. 85:156, 1972.
Kemler, N.F.: Cell Division in Enchondral Ossification, J. Bone Joint. Surg. 42-B:824, 1960.
Maksimov, A.A., and Bloom, W.: *A Textbook of Histology.* ed. 6. Philadelphia: W.B. Saunders Co., 1952.
Neuman, W.F., and Neuman, N.W.: *The Chemical Dynamics of Bone Mineral.* Chicago: University of Chicago Press, 1958.
Rodahl, K., Nicholson, J.T., and Brown, C.J., Jr.: *Bone as a Tissue.* New York: Blakiston Div., McGraw-Hill Book Co., Inc., 1960.
Sevastikoglou, J.A., Larsson, S-E.: Osteoporosis and Parathyroid Glands, from the Department of Orthopedic Surgery, Umeå University, Sweden, supported by Grant K 68-12 × - 69 - 04, Swedish Medical Research Council, 1972.
Termine, J.D.: Mineral Chemistry and Skeletal Biology, Clin. Orthop. 85:151, 1972.
Wanken, J.J., and Eyring, E.J.: Changes in Metabolic Activity of Various Epiphyses with Age. Clin. Orthop. 85: 156, 1972.
Weinmann, J.P., and Sicher, H.: *Bone and Bones,* ed. 2. St. Louis, C.V. Mosby Co., 1955.

2 PHYSIOLOGIC AND PATHOLOGIC CHANGES

It is a clinical circumstance that initiates the need for roentgenologic examination. The diagnostician must correlate his clinical and laboratory criteria with his roentgenologic impressions in arriving at a diagnosis. A basic knowledge of pathology is fundamental.

Identification of the outstanding physiopathologic features visualized on the roent-

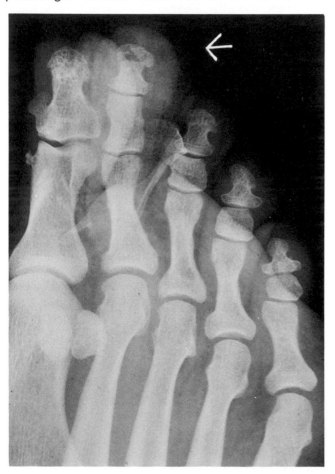

genogram is the first phase in roentgenologic interpretation. It is the basic pathologic process that is shown by the roentgenogram that classifies the disease. Additional roentgenologic features that are characteristic of a specific disease provide the evidence to make a roentgenologic diagnosis.

Outstanding roentgenologic features and the tissues with which they are associated will be discussed in this chapter. Roentgenologic interpretation tells what is happening to bone and to its adjacent tissues.

SOFT-TISSUE CHANGES

Soft-tissue changes adjacent to bone are indicative of pathology.

Swelling in Soft Tissue

CLINICAL ORIENTATION

1. Diffuse swelling may have local conges-

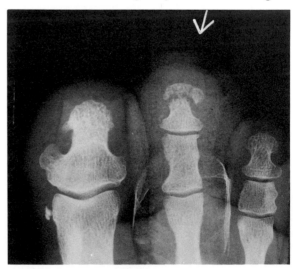

Fig. 6. Posttraumatic swelling, transverse fracture, hemorrhage in soft tissue.
  1. Complete transverse fracture, head of distal phalanx second toe.
  2. Marked increase in density of soft tissue due to hemorrhagic extravasation.

tive or systemic etiology.

2. Localized swelling occurs with trauma, inflammation, or infection.

3. Swelling may be pitting or nonpitting.

4. Deformity with a loss of normal anatomic contour is common.

5. The discoloration is dependent on the etiology.

6. A temperature increase is local or systemic.

7. There is usually a limitation of function with diffuse swelling.

8. Pain is dependent on the extent of swelling and the etiology. A dull ache and a sensation of fullness are the usual complaint.

9. Cardinal signs of infection are noted if swelling is secondary to infection.

10. Jackson and Kinmonth (1970) describe a family history of both pes cavus and lymphedema. The edema was pitting and further investigation confirmed a hypoplastic variety of lymphedema.

11. Venous and lymphatic obstruction due to pressure from a mass, constriction, or vascular disease, or faulty fluid exchange due to hematologic disease and metabolic disorders may cause swelling in the soft tissues.

ROENTGENOLOGIC INTERPRETATION

STATIC OR POSTTRAUMATIC SWELLING (Fig. 6).

1. There is an increased thickening of soft tissue from the bone outline to the skin margin.

2. Fascial planes are visible in posttraumatic swelling.

3. The increased density of the soft tissue is clear rather than hazy.

4. The swelling is diffuse and not confined or delineated.

5. This swelling is visible following trauma or is secondary to stasis.

6. If trauma involves a joint or encapsulated tissue, the soft-tissue swelling may be confined and sharply delineated.

INFECTIOUS OR REACTIVE SWELLING (Figs. 7 and 8).

1. An increased thickening of soft tissues is noted.

2. Obliteration of the fascial planes is usually present with reactive swelling.

3. A hazy and indistinct increase in density of the soft tissues is consistent with reactive swelling.

4. Reactive swelling is usually adjacent to an infectious process in bone or soft tissue.

5. The increased thickening of the soft tissues is confluent with adjacent tissue.

Soft-tissue Mass

CLINICAL ORIENTATION

1. Definitive thickening of the soft tissues may be freely movable or adherent depending on the extent of pathology.

2. A deformity, tumor, cyst, or bursa may distort the anatomy.

3. Acute bursitis may present an increase in local temperature with redness and the presence of a palpable mass.

4. Compression on blood vessels may present a decrease in local temperature with pallor or cyanosis.

5. Active and passive motion may be limited if muscle or joints are involved.

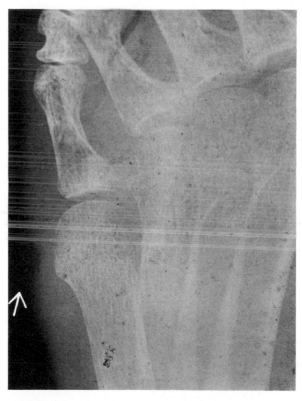

Fig. 7. Soft-tissue ulcer. A loss of continuity and a lack of substance in the soft tissues.

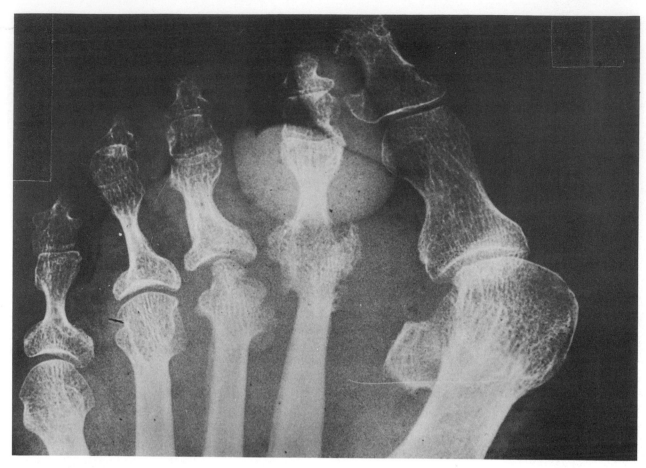

Fig. 8. Infectious or reactive swelling
    1. Pyogenic arthritis secondary to infection of second toe.
    2. Infectious type of soft-tissue swelling.
    3. Active destruction of second and third metatarsophalangeal joints.
    4. Irregular subperiosteal calcification confluent with cortex at head and base, second and third metatarsophalangeal joints.

6. The pain from compression of a soft-tissue mass on adjacent tissues may be characterized as a burning, tingling, aching, or a sensation of fullness.

7. A localized abscess may show evidence of a cellulitis, heat, redness, swelling, and lymphadenopathy.

ROENTGENOLOGIC INTERPRETATION

1. A clear, circumscribed, or elongate increase in density of soft tissues suggests the presence of a mass.

2. There is a definite outline of increased density differentiated in texture from the adjacent soft tissue. Delineation and demarcation are obvious (Fig. 9).

3. A deformity is noted when a mass is present.

4. A soft-tissue mass is extraosseous (Fig. 10).

5. A mass may undergo degenerative calcification and calcinosis (as described in this chapter).

6. A mass may be present in any tissue developed from the mesenchyme.

CALCIFICATIONS IN SOFT TISSUE

A comparison to the density of the cortex of bone, commonly described as calcareous density, is used in the roentgenologic description of tissue density. Thus, a density less than that of the cortex is called soft-tissue density, decrease in density, or lesser bone density, and a greater density than that of the cortex is metallic density. An increase in soft-tissue density outlining the course of a muscle is called muscle density and is less than calcareous density (bone density).

Calcification is an extraosseous, dense, irregular, calcareous density that appears amorphous, presents no evidence of a trabecular pattern, and is blotchy and flocculent (Fig. 11).

.Calcifications occur in arteries, veins, muscle, fibrous connective tissue, ligaments, fat, bursae, sinus tracts, cysts, and any tissue developed from the mesenchyme. Periarticular calcifications may occur as a manifestation of vitamin D intoxication. A serum calcium value of 14 mg/100 ml and a nonprotein nitrogen value of 63 mg/100 ml were noted by Jaffe (1972).

Calcifications are often referred to as the following:

a. *Calcinosis circumscripta,* which is usually a localized calcinosis.

b. *Calcinosis universalis,* which affects the deeper tissues, may be more extensive and is often disabling.

Calcified Arteries

CLINICAL ORIENTATION

1. Swelling of the feet may be a consequence of arteriosclerosis.

2. Onychauxis, onychatrophia, and dystrophic alterations in the toenails may be secondary to a decrease in circulation.

3. In arteriosclerosis, one may note a rubor on dependency and pallor on elevation.

4. The skin is cool to touch and the temperature is usually decreased.

5. Bodily activity may be limited by affected calcified arteries.

6. Cramps, intermittent claudication, burning, and tingling are some of the symptoms of this disease.

7. Pulsations may be feeble or absent in the presence of arteriosclerosis.

8. The skin is dry, scaly, and pigmented.

9. Pallor and cyanosis may be pathognomonic.

ROENTGENOLOGIC INTERPRETATION
(Fig. 12)

1. The calcified artery appears as calcareous lines of increase in soft-tissue density, broken at intervals, outlining a tubelike structure.

2. These calcareous lines follow the anatomic course of the arteries.

3. Lateral views may show early evidence of calcification of the medial calcaneal branch of the posterior tibial artery in age group 20-40 (Yale, 1957).

4. The communicating branch at the base of the first intermetatarsal space is calcified early. This must be differentiated from the os intermetatarseum. In the dorsoplantar view, the examiner may note that he is viewing the calcified lumen of the communicating vessel and not an accessory ossicle.

5. Arteriosclerosis is commonly accompanied by degenerative joint pathology in the feet.

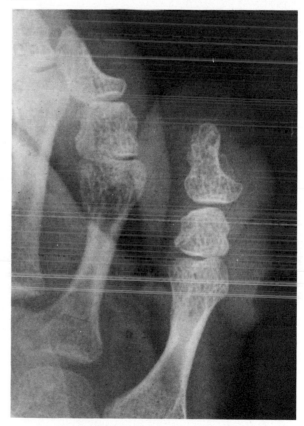

Fig. 9. Soft-tissue mass
1. Acute bursitis beneath heloma dura.
2. Circumscribed, clearly delineated and demarcated increase in soft-tissue density.

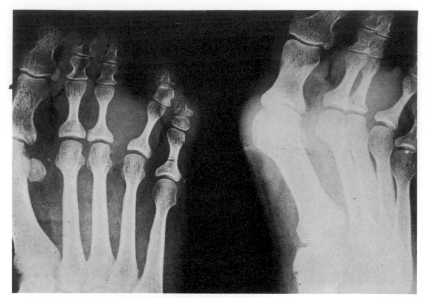

Fig. 10. Soft-tissue mass — secondary subluxation of third and fourth toes

1. Sharply circumscribed area of increase in density forcing apart the third and fourth toes.

2. On operation, excision of a fibroma with strands of fibrous connective tissue enveloping the flexor and extensor tendons to the third and fourth toes.

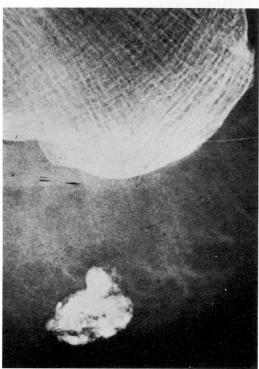

Fig. 11. Calcification *vs.* ossification

1. Irregular calcareous deposits in soft tissues, plantar surface calcaneus.

2. No evidence of a cortex or internal trabecular pattern.

3. Appears flocculent and uneven in density (calcification).

4. In contrast, the calcaneus above has a cortical outline and trabecular pattern (ossification).

Calcified Veins

CLINICAL ORIENTATION

1. There is nonpitting swelling of feet and ankles in the latter part of the day.

2. Superficial varicose veins are tortuous, dilated, and distended.

3. There is often a bluish discoloration with mild rubor and brownish pigmentation of the skin.

4. A cordlike structure at the site of phlebitis may cause indurated swelling.

5. Local increase in temperature with inflammation in phlebitic lesions is noted.

6. There may sometimes be ulceration.

7. Occasional cramps in legs due to circulatory stasis may be noted.

8. There may be a heavy feeling of limbs after prolonged weight bearing.

ROENTGENOLOGIC INTERPRETATION
(Fig. 13)

1. The calcareous deposits in vein wall appear as streaks.

2. Phleboliths are rounded calcareous deposits with an eccentric area of decrease in density found in the vein.

Calcification of Muscles (Myositis Calcificans, Myositis Ossificans, Calcinosis)

CLINICAL ORIENTATION

1. Hypertrophy of muscle substance is evident on palpation.

2. There is an indurated swelling about the affected part.

3. Deformity may occur in extensive calcification of the muscles.

4. Mild rubor is present in acute phases.

5. There may be pallor in extensive lesions due to pressure on surrounding tissue.

6. Local temperature is increased with the activity of calcification.

7. Active, passive, and resistive functions are limited.

8. The patient complains of a dull ache.

ROENTGENOLOGIC INTERPRETATION
(Figs. 14-18)

1. Calcareous deposits in a muscle belly or

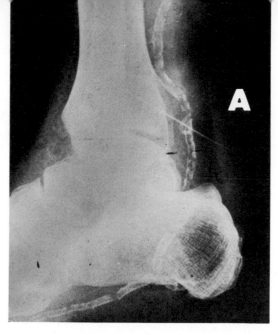

Fig. 12. Arteriosclerosis

A. Arteriosclerosis of posterior tibial and plantar arteries. Note tubelike structure composed of parallel lines of increase in density. Lines appear to lose continuity at intervals.

B. Arteriosclerosis of intermetatarsal arteries.

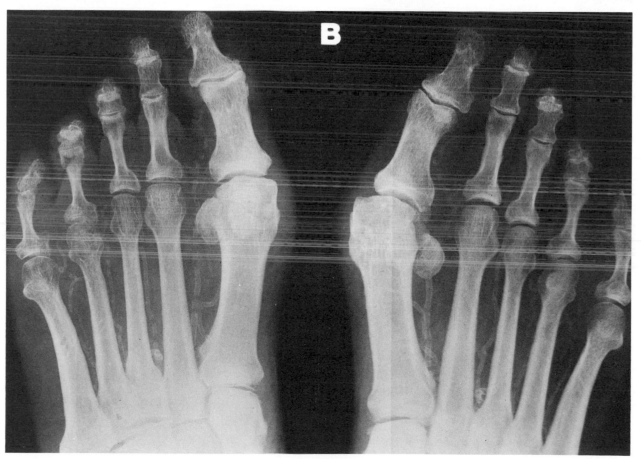

tendon occur as streaks or flakes. They follow the anatomic contour of affected muscle.

2. Calcifications in the tendo achillis appear to develop an ossific reticular pattern and cortical outline.

3. Extensive calcifications have been known to differentiate into malignant lesions.

4. Extensive lesions overlapping bone may alter the appearance of the bone by virtue of a compounding of densities.

Calcification of Bursae

CLINICAL ORIENTATION

1. Bursitis may develop at a site of trauma.

2. It commonly occurs over bony prominences and at sites of stress between tendons and bones.

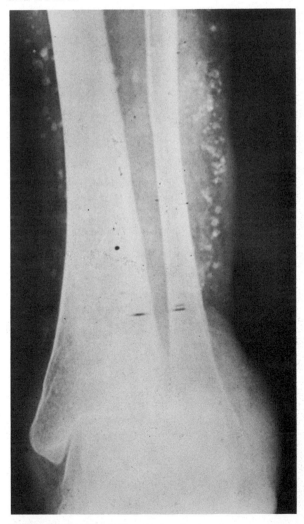

Fig. 13. Phleboliths. Rounded calcareous deposits in the vein wall.

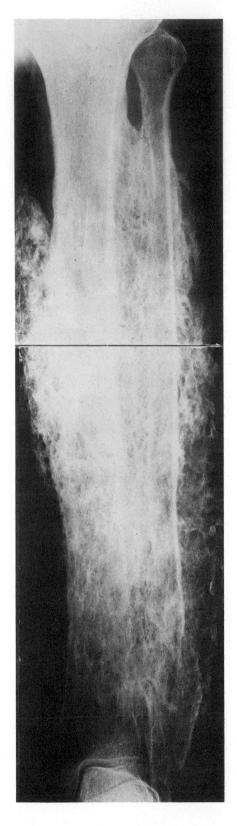

Fig. 14. Myositis calcificans

3. Calcification of bursae may occur under chronic helomata or tylomata.

4. All bursae are capable of undergoing degenerative calcification.

5. An indurated localized swelling is usually present.

6. Mild rubor or cyanosis is circumscribed and clearly demarcated as in a mass.

7. Increase in local temperature is not uncommon.

8. Function is often limited.

9. A burning pain is present at the site of the lesion.

10. Compression of the metatarsals causes pain when an intermetatarsal bursitis is present.

11. Aspiration may deliver a pasty fluid or calcium flakes in early calcification of a bursa.

ROENTGENOLOGIC INTERPRETATION
(Figs. 19-23)

1. A blotchy, flocculent, irregular, calcareous deposit is usually present in the soft tissues.

2. Occasional increase in soft-tissue density is circumscribed, clearly delineated, and appears flat in density.

3. There is no evidence of a cortical outline.

4. Underlying bone appears decreased in density due to local hyperemia.

Calcified Sinus Tract

CLINICAL ORIENTATION

1. A sinus tract is usually secondary to infection.

2. A tract is continuous with the bursa or joint and may be serpentine.

3. It develops readily in heloma or bursa following injudicious cutting and laceration of the skin.

4. The part is swollen with rubor or cyanosis.

5. The lining of a sinus tract is fibrous, cordlike, and bony.

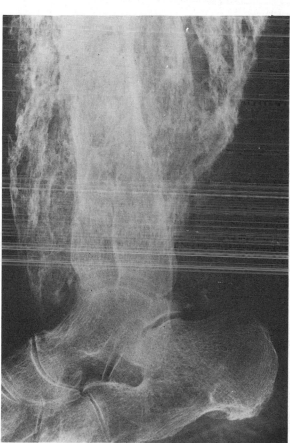

Fig. 15. Myositis calcificans

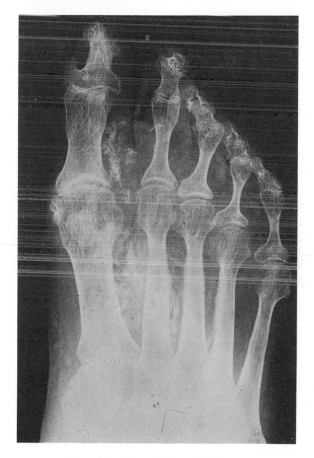

Fig. 16. Myositis calcificans

6. Sinus tracts are common in peripheral vascular disease or diabetes.

7. Serous, serosanguineous, or seropurulent exudate oozing out of the sinus tract is common.

8. A congenital dermal sinus tract leading nowhere has been reported (Lusskin, 1961).

9. Sequestra may extrude through a sinus tract.

ROENTGENOLOGIC INTERPRETATION
(Figs. 24-28)

1. Calcification of a sinus tract is visualized on the roentgenogram as an elongate calcareous deposit which may be continuous with underlying infected bursa or joint space.

2. Osteomyelitis of the toe phalanges is not uncommon.

3. Occasional sequestra may be lodged in a tract.

4. A serpentine sinus tract that leads nowhere can be visualized by the injection of contrast medium.

5. Radiopaque material injected into a sinus tract must not be confused with calcification of the tract.

6. Dilute solutions of meglumine iothalamate (Conray) may be injected into a chronic sinus tract in the absence of infection for visualization of the extent of the tract.

PERIOSTEUM

Periosteum is not visible on the roentgenogram unless physiologic or pathologic changes take place beneath it.

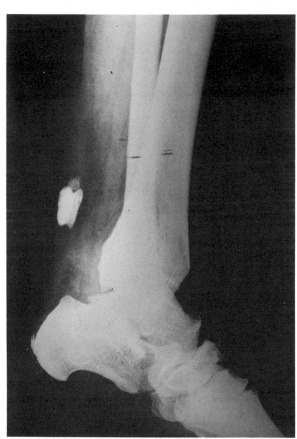

Fig. 17. Calcification of the tendo achillis
1. Two elongate, dense, smoothly outlined calcareous deposits with a light ossific pattern located on their proximal ends.
2. An infiltrative swelling fills the posterior triangle.

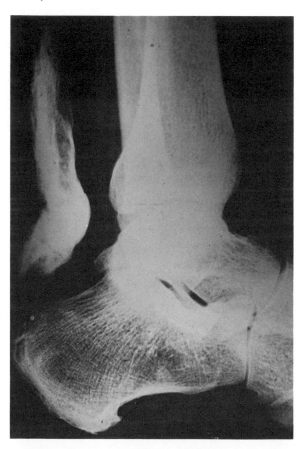

Fig. 18. Calcifying tendonitis. It is interesting to note that calcifications of the tendo achillis usually show evidence of an ossific pattern with cortical outline as noted in the upper one third of this calcareous deposit.

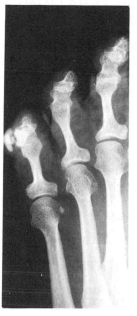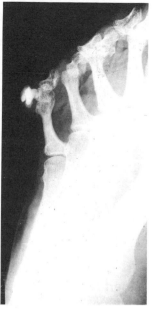

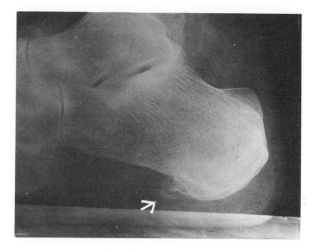

Fig. 21. Calcaneal spur — calcified bursa. Calcareous deposit in soft tissue at tip of spur.

Fig. 19. Calcified bursa
1. Heloma dura (chronic), dorsum distal interphalangeal joint.
2. Underlying blotchy, flocculent, irregular calcareous deposit.
3. No evidence of a central trabecular pattern or cortical outline.

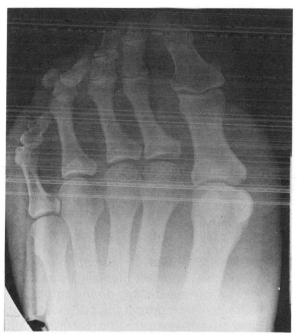

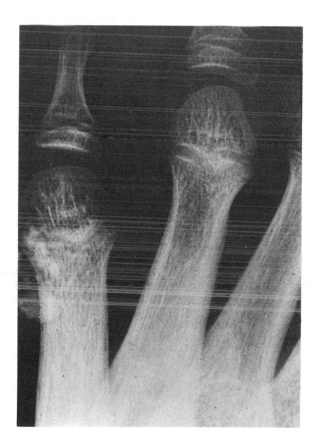

Fig. 20. Osteochondroma, fourth toe
1. Heloma dura developed over deformity.
2. Note cortical outline and trabecular pattern.

Fig. 22. Calcified bursa, plantar surface, fifth metatarsal head in talipes equinus varus. Fifth metatarsal serves as a fulcrum.

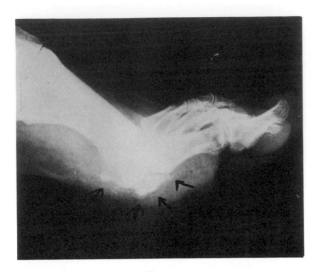

Fig. 27. Acute bursitis with calcification and resorption. Lateral views show evidence of a rudimentary tibial sesamoid and an irregular calcareous deposit, plantar surface of first metatarsophalangeal joint, with marked swelling.

Posttraumatic Subperiosteal Alterations

CLINICAL ORIENTATION

1. There is a history of trauma.
2. Contusion in the soft tissues is seen early with its bluish-red discoloration.
3. A slight increase in temperature is dependent on the degree of trauma.
4. The swelling is usually indurated and with severe injury often causes deformity.
5. Active and passive function may be limited and motion is painful.
6. Pain on palpation at the site of injury may range from tenderness through sharp discomfort. A dull ache is noted at rest.
7. Laboratory findings are negative.

ROENTGENOLOGIC INTERPRETATION
(Figs. 29-32)

1. There is usually a thickening of the soft tissues with an increase in density. The fascial planes are visible.

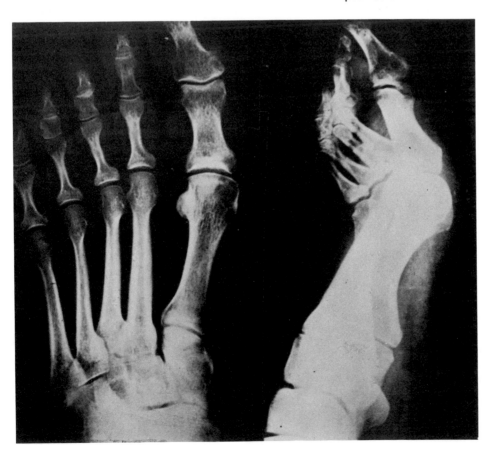

Fig. 28. Acute bursitis with calcification and resorption. Views several months later present a normal-appearing joint, loss of swelling, and resorption of calcareous deposit. Pain has subsided and objective signs have disappeared without treatment. Note resorption of tibial sesamoid.

2. The periosteum is visualized as being smooth in outline, uniform in density, fusiform, and separated from the cortex.

a. A rupture of the periosteum may take on a bizarre appearance with hemorrhagic extravasation into the soft tissue. Subsequent absorption and calcification are the rule.

b. When the periosteum is stripped or torn, it may later calcify and extend out into the soft tissues as an irregular calcareous deposit, an exostosis, spur, or osteophyte.

3. An increase in the density of soft tissue is noted beneath the periosteum. This may be hemorrhage, fibrosis, or a subperiosteal calcification between the periosteum and cortex.

a. Seen early following trauma, the subperiosteal area may be hemorrhagic and appear light in density.

b. Later, this density increases to almost that of the cortex.

Infectious Subperiosteal Alterations

CLINICAL ORIENTATION

1. Cardinal signs of infection may or may not be present.

2. A sinus tract or infected soft-tissue ulcer may be present.

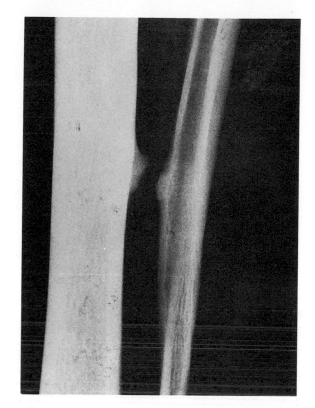

Fig. 29. Posttraumatic subperiosteal calcification. Note fusiform shape, smooth outline, and uniform density.

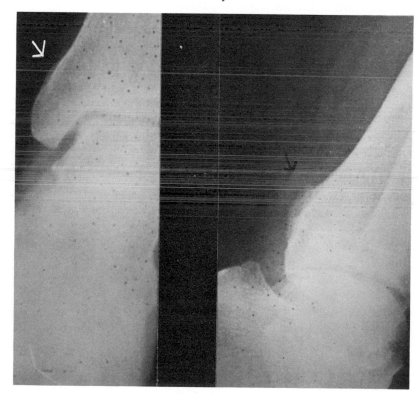

Fig. 30. Posttraumatic subperiosteal calcifications. Subperiosteal calcification following trauma presents smooth outline, fusiform shape, uniform density, and separation from cortex.

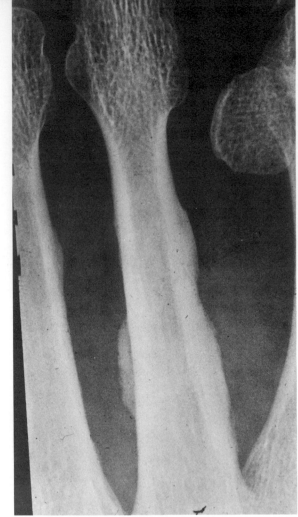

Fig. 31. Subperiosteal calcification of post-traumatic type

3. In the chronic stage, the part may be indurated and cyanotic.

4. Pain on palpation and on motion is common when the condition is acute.

5. Pain may be present at rest and manifest itself as a dull, thumping ache.

6. Cellulitis, lymphangitis, and lymphadenopathy may or may not be present.

7. Bacteria may be cultured from material obtained by biopsy.

8. The bone changes may be due to an extension of a primary local infection in the adjacent soft tissues or may be a localized manifestation of a systemic infectious process.

9. Pyogenic periostitis, tuberculous periostitis, and bone abscess may cause infectious subperiosteal alterations in bone.

ROENTGENOLOGIC INTERPRETATION
(Figs. 33-34)

1. The subperiosteal deposit appears hazy

and indistinct. It has an irregular, indefinite outline and is confluent with the cortex.

2. In pyogenic infections, the density approaches that of cortex but is flat looking and is not as great as the density of the cortex.

3. The density of a subperiosteal lesion caused by a tuberculous infection appears very light, although the other features of infectious alterations, such as an indistinct outline and a hazy, flat-looking density, are present.

4. If the lesion is superficial, it is an infectious periostitis. When circumscribed within bone with an infectious subperiosteal overlay, it may be a bone abscess.

5. Infectious subperiosteal calcification may be an objective finding together with other signs of an osteomyelitis, such as active

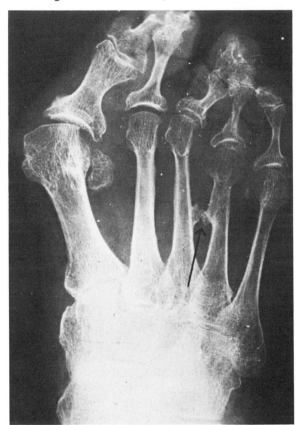

Fig. 32. Posttraumatic subperiosteal calcification

1. Reparative calcification.

2. Attempt to remodel a fracture of the fourth metatarsal with posttraumatic subperiosteal calcification, lateral aspect, third metatarsal shaft.

3. Table-top exostosis.

destruction, reaction area, and condensation of bone.

6. The soft tissue appears thick and indistinct with a loss in fascial planes. Soft-tissue swelling may accompany infectious subperiosteal alterations in bone.

Reactive Subperiosteal Alterations

CLINICAL ORIENTATION

1. Thorough history and evaluation of systemic disorders are essential for diagnosis.

2. Swelling, hypertrophy, atrophy, and deformity are the symptoms representative of the cause.

3. The patient is usually ill.

4. Pain varies with the extent of the pathologic process.

5. Redness, pallor, or cyanosis may be noted and is related to the acuteness or chronicity of the disease.

6. Increase or decrease in temperature must be correlated with other findings.

7. Atrophy of the musculature is seen more commonly than is hypertrophy.

8. The cause of the reactive subperiosteal alterations may be anemia, neoplasia, hypertrophic pulmonary osteoarthropathy, syphilis, or ossifying periostitis.

9. Bone lesion may develop 2-15 weeks after a primary chancre in syphilis.

10. Periosteal arteritis in lupus erythematosis may be the cause of reactive subperiosteal alterations (Ball and Grazzel, 1964).

ROENTGENOLOGIC INTERPRETATION
(Figs. 35-36)

1. Reactive subperiosteal alterations will vary in appearance with the cause.

2. Basically, the outline is irregular and appears indistinct.

3. The density will vary with the pathologic process.

4. The subperiosteal calcification is confluent with the cortex.

5. Alterations in the cortex and medullary bone may give a further clue to the possible cause of the process.

6. In sickle cell anemia, the periosteal change may appear as dense perpendicular streaks off an atrophic cortex.

7. A sunburst effect with invasive destruc-

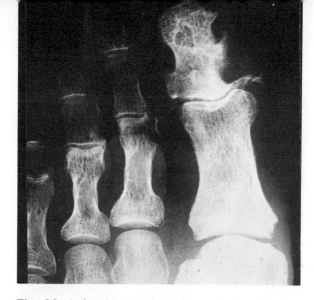

Fig. 33. Infectious subperiosteal alterations

1. Medial aspect of distal phalanx presents an irregularly outlined, hazy, indistinct subperiosteal calcification indicative of infection.

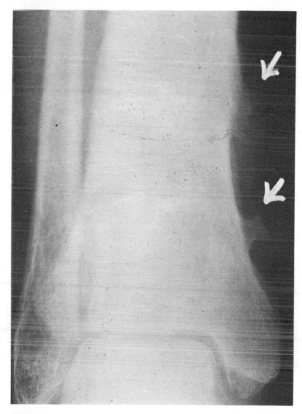

Fig. 34. Infectious subperiosteal alteration in bone — osteomyelitis

1. Note the upper medial margin of the tibia with its hazy, indistinct subperiosteal calcification.

2. The outline is irregular, flat looking, and confluent with the cortex.

3. Below the infectious change is a table-top exostosis.

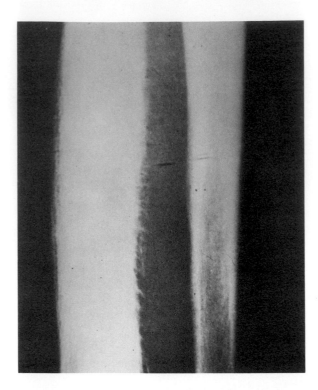

Fig. 35. Reactive subperiosteal alterations — malignancy. Note the periosteal reaction manifest by perpendicular calcareous strands radiating from the cortical margin.

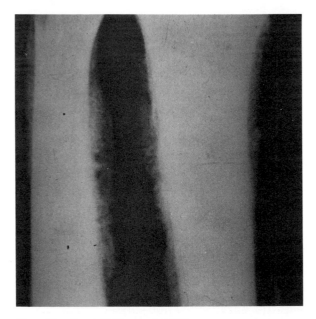

Fig. 36. Syphilitic periostitis
1. A bumpy, lacework type of periosteal reaction.
2. Must be differentiated from hypertrophic pulmonary osteoarthropathy.

tion may suggest a malignant neoplastic disease.

8. A subperiosteal calcification with lacework-type outline, confluency with the cortex, and indistinct density as great or greater than the cortex may be due to syphilis. Bumps or rounded projections on the shaft of the bone are seen in tertiary syphilis.

9. In hypertrophic pulmonary osteoarthropathy the cortical outline presents a wavy appearance that may have to be differentiated from that of syphilis by history and clinical findings.

10. Ossifying periostitis may slowly develop an abscess with sequestration and must be differentiated from Ewing's sarcoma and syphilis.

CORTEX

The cortex is that dense homogeneous tissue in bone that is bounded on its endosteal surface by the medullary bone and on its periosteal surface by the soft tissues. It is confined within the periosteal-endosteal envelope. The density of the cortex is used as a basis for determining the varying densities viewed on the roentgenogram. The cortex is thicker at the center of a diaphysis and tapers proximally and distally as it approaches the ends of the bone. Haversian systems in the cortex contain the osteocytes and the canaliculi which serve as vehicles for transporting nourishment necessary for maintenance of healthy bone.

Hypertrophy

CLINICAL ORIENTATION

1. There is usually a history of either direct trauma or multiple minimal traumata.

2. Callositas at a site of stress indicates abnormal gravitational stress.

3. Swelling in the soft tissues is uncommon.

4. Mild rubor in adjacent soft tissues is common.

5. Mild discomfort and often a dull ache are common complaints.

6. Systemic disease must be considered where hypertrophy exists.

   a. Metabolic and endocrine disorders must be considered where hypertrophy exists.

   b. Hypertrophic pulmonary osteoarthropathy may be present.

   c. Osteitis deformans (Paget's disease) may be considered.

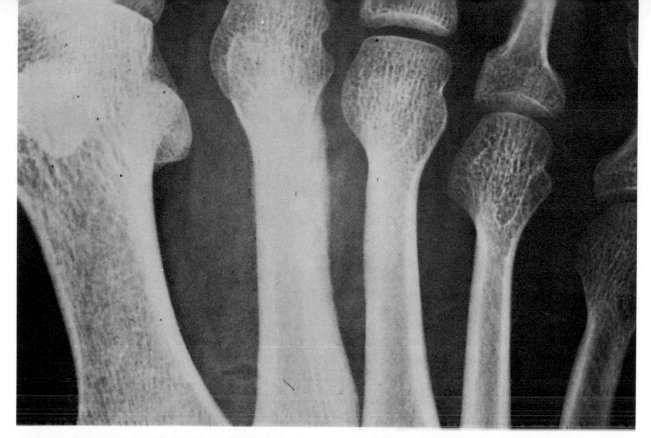

Fig. 37. Stress fracture, second metatarsal

1. Increase in soft-tissue density and thickness of part.

2. A posttraumatic, fusiform, smoothly outlined subperiosteal calcification representative of hemorrhagic extravasation and reparative calcification at the lateral aspect, distal one third of shaft of second metatarsal.

3. This must be differentiated from the hypertrophy of bone.

d. Melorheostosis (Leri's hyperostosis) is a familial disorder that presents hypertrophic changes.

7. If heat is present overlying hypertrophic changes, further clinical and laboratory study is indicated.

ROENTGENOLOGIC INTERPRETATION

(Fig. 37)

1. Thickening of otherwise normal cortex is *hypertrophy* of bone.

2. Recent activity in bone is represented by an irregularity of cortical outline.

3. Soft-tissue swelling may be seen about the site of hypertrophy.

4. Sites receiving stress in any bone of the foot, such as the second metatarsal shaft in Morton's syndrome, become hypertrophied.

5. The cortex is thickened following repair of a fracture.

6. Hypertrophy of the cortex is seen in mel-

orheostosis (Leri's hyperostosis) as an irregular thickening on one side of long bones. A melted-wax appearance of the cortex may be noted in the bones on one side of the body.

7. In osteitis deformans (Paget's disease), the cortex is thickened, medullary bone is narrowed, and the cortex is decreased in density.

8. A wavy but thickened cortex with enlargement of the ends of fingers and toes may suggest hypertrophic pulmonary osteoarthropathy.

9. Hypertrophy of the cortex is noted on the concave surface of a long bone bowed by rickets.

10. A deformity may be present if hypertrophy is extensive.

Atrophy

Atrophy is a thinning of otherwise normal cortex. Atrophy must not confused with deossification, decrease in density, development, or underdevelopment of bone.

CLINICAL ORIENTATION

1. Atrophy may occur in the following:
   a. Rheumatoid arthritis.
   b. Scleroderma.
   c. Disuse of a part, such as occurs with prolonged bed rest or immobilization in a cast or brace.
   d. Post trauma, such as Sudeck's atrophy.
   e. Neurotrophic disorders.
   f. Aging.
   g. Enchondroma.

2. Swelling of the proximal interphalangeal joints, effusion in the metacarpophalangeal joints, and a decrease in density at the ends of long bones with thinning of the cortex (atrophy) may be seen in rheumatoid arthritis.

3. In Sudeck's atrophy, a causalgic state may be associated with redness, cyanosis, and

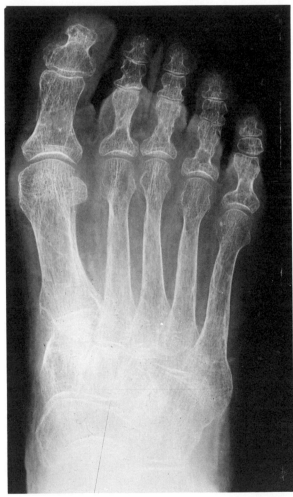

Fig. 38. Atrophy. Note thinning of cortices and concomitant deossification.

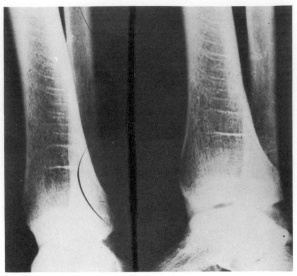

Fig. 39. Sclerosis

1. Transverse sclerotic lines are often referred to as "growth lines."

2. Note the increase in density without loss of trabecular pattern at the talocrural articulations.

trophic changes in the affected parts.

4. Atrophy of the musculature often accompanies bone atrophy.

5. Temperature alterations in atrophy depend on the pathologic process.

6. Function is limited where atrophy exists.

ROENTGENOLOGIC INTERPRETATION
(Fig. 38)

1. Thinning of the cortex of the involved bone varies with the degree of involvement.

2. Atrophy often occurs with demineralization, especially in old age.

3. Sudeck's atrophy consists of multiple and minute spotty areas of decrease in density in the bone with thinning of the cortex. It is often accompanied by soft-tissue swelling.

4. In enchondroma, the bone is expanded with atrophy of the cortices.

5. Other pathologic processes may be present to complicate the atrophic changes.

6. Atrophy must be considered as an objective roentgenologic sign of a greater pathologic entity.

Nutrient Foramen

The nutrient foramen is viewed as an infrequent smooth line of decrease in density seen on roentgenograms of the foot. In the typical long bone the nutrient foramen enters the cortex rather subtly and extends obliquely away from the growth center through the cortex into the marrow.

CLINICAL ORIENTATION

1. Damage to the nutrient foramen may result in death of bone due to disturbance of circulation.

2. Bacteria entering a foramen may result in infection and engorgement of the canaliculi with destruction of osteocytes and bone substance.

ROENTGENOLOGIC INTERPRETATION

1. In endochondral bone development, the nutrient foramen is found midshaft.

2. The line of decrease in density is smooth and even and must be differentiated from a fracture line which is irregular and spiculated.

3. The nutrient foramen slips into the cortex without disruption, displacement, irregularity, or angulation of the cortical margins. The foramen can be followed into the medullary portion of the bone.

4. It may be seen in the metatarsal bones or in the calcaneus, although it is not readily visible on the roentgenogram.

Sclerosis (Eburnation)

Sclerosis is a physiologic alteration in bone. It is a normal reaction to stress within physiologic limits. It must be differentiated from true pathologic bone changes.

CLINICAL ORIENTATION

1. Abnormal weight distribution creates stress on bones and joints within physiologic limits.

2. No characteristic clinical findings are present with sclerosis.

3. Sclerosis is normal in the fetus and premature and mature infant.

ROENTGENOLOGIC INTERPRETATION

1. There is an increase in bone density with no loss of trabeculations. An intermingling of trabeculae with adjacent bone is noted at the periphery of the sclerotic bone.

2. A subarticular sclerosis is common at the base of the proximal phalanx of the hallux, the concave posterior surface of the navicular, and the posterior plantar angle of the calcaneus.

3. Sclerotic bone does not completely obliterate soft-tissue elements in bone.

Transverse Sclerotic Lines ("Growth Lines")

CLINICAL ORIENTATION

1. These lines may form in the healthy or ill and persist from fetal through adult life.

2. Transient disturbances in bone formation from maternal illness during pregnancy may be a cause.

3. Malnutrition causing a retardation of development for a short time may produce bone changes with sclerosis.

4. Paralysis during the developmental years may result in sclerotic lines.

5. Trauma may be the cause when severe enough to retard bone growth; e.g., following surgical trauma during development of the bone.

ROENTGENOLOGIC INTERPRETATION
(Fig. 39)

1. Irregular sclerotic lines are usually visualized at the ends of bones, proximal to and subjacent to the metaphysis.

2. These may be multiple, with the thickest line closest to the epiphyseal line.

3. As the bone grows, the sclerotic lines are seen deeper into the shaft and they become thinner.

4. When seen on a flat plane, the line is irregular and the ends are uneven, spiculated, and fail to touch the cortex.

5. Growth lines are not necessarily the result of arrest of growth but may be the manifestation of faulty bone physiology at the time of serious trauma or illness during growth and development.

Nonreticulated Areas in Bone — Compact Islands

CLINICAL ORIENTATION

1. A compact island is a dense structureless

bone of no clinical significance.

2. It is believed that compact islands are accumulations of cancelled bone that have not been absorbed in the development of bone.

ROENTGENOLOGIC INTERPRETATION
(Figs. 40-41)

1. A compact island manifests itself as an abrupt transition from the normal reticulation of the bone in which it exists.

2. There is no central reticulation or trabeculation in the calcareous deposit to suggest a new bone growth.

3. It often occurs in spongy bone, usually at the ends of long bones and commonly occurs in the calcaneus, matatarsal shafts, and phalanges, less commonly in the other bones of the feet.

DECREASE IN BONE DENSITY

(Demineralization, Deossification, Decalcification, Osteoporosis)

Deossification is a loss of bone density with some evidence of trabeculation in bone. A thinning of the spongy trabeculations not associated with osteoclastic resorption together with thinning and porosity of the cortices of the affected bones is pathognomonic in osteoporosis. Removal of chemicals from the bone entails removal of the bone substance itself. Defects in osteoblastic activity influenced by steroid hormones, stresses, and strains may cause a decrease in density. There is a decrease in the amount of osseous tissue per unit of bone volume.

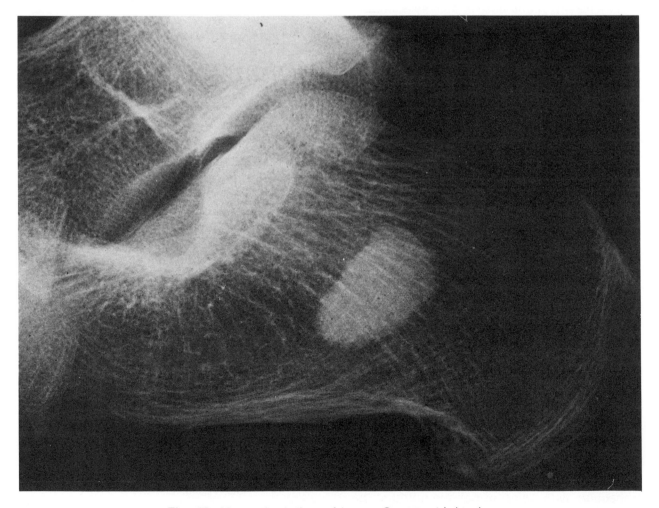

Fig. 40. Nonreticulation of bone. Compact island.

Systemic Decrease in Density

A decrease in density may affect many bones and be found in all parts of the body.

CLINICAL ORIENTATION

1. Extensive paralysis, old age, starvation, anemia, endocrine disturbances, rheumatoid arthritis, metabolic dysfunctions, and long-standing infections may cause systemic deossification.

2. An increased metabolic rate with a negative protein balance due to digestive disturbances and depletion of serum albumen interferes with adequate nutrition causing dysfunction of the osteoblasts in laying down a bone matrix.

3. Hyperplasia of reticuloendothelial marrow produces pressure against the cortex causing atrophy and demineralization in thalassemia (Cooley's anemia).

4. A diminished intake and inadequate utilization of proteins and vitamin C occur in most deossifications.

5. Lack of vitamin D may decrease absorption of calcium and phosphorus in the intestines thus causing a systemic loss of density in bone.

6. Hyperparathyroidism stimulates renal excretion of calcium and phosphorus with resultant resorption of minerals from bone and decrease in density. Osteoclasis is stimulated resulting in osteoporosis.

7. Inadequate estrogen and corticoadrenal osteoblastic-stimulating hormone diminish osteoblastic function and bone matrix formation. Menopause makes women more susceptible to osteoporosis.

8. Stress is necessary to stimulate and maintain proper osteoblastic function. Conversely, lack of stress and disuse disturb bone formation (Wolff's law), as in osteoporosis.

9. It is a natural physiologic function for bone to add to itself when the need arises and to resorb those tissues which are unnecessary.

10. Nervousness, weakness, and easy fatigue are often noted with osteoporosis.

11. Bones are tender to touch when osteoporosis takes place. Fractures are common.

12. Osteoporosis develops with stimulation of osteoclasis. Rickets or osteomalacia results

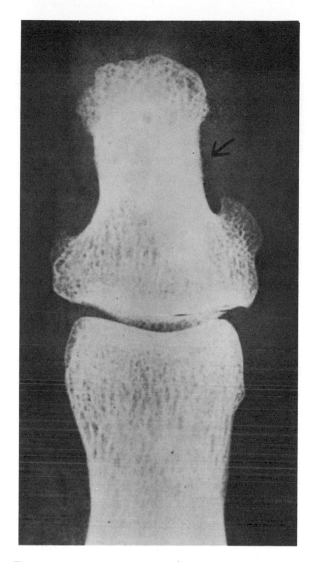

Fig. 41. Nonreticulation of bone. Compact island. Definitively outlined compact bone in distal phalanx with no evidence of trabecular pattern.

from a failure of calcium deposition by the osteoblasts.

ROENTGENOLOGIC INTERPRETATION
(Fig. 42)

1. All or most of the bones of the body are affected by systemic deossification with evidence of decrease in density and no loss of trabeculation.

2. In anemia, the marrow may be widened and the cortex narrowed and decreased in density. The trabeculations are coarse.

3. One of the early signs of rheumatoid arthritis is a decrease in density at the ends of long bones at their chondro-osseous surfaces.

4. In avitaminosis C, the significant signs of scurvy, including systemic demineralization, are noted.

5. In avitaminosis D, a significant systemic decrease in density and other signs of rickets are in evidence.

6. With demineralization, the nutrient foramina may be clearly differentiated on the roentgenogram. Bone may be atrophic with thinning of the cortices.

7. Fragility may predispose to fracture.

8. Osteoporosis may also be noted in hypervitaminosis D.

9. Vertebral column is generally affected in women after menopause.

General Decrease in Density (General Deossification, General Demineralization)

This decrease in density affects a general area, such as the forefoot, hindfoot, or one leg, but not all bones of the body as in the systemic type. More than one bone in the area may be affected.

CLINICAL ORIENTATION

1. A generalized decrease in density may be seen in patients with a paralysis of a single extremity, trauma, or local circulatory dysfunction.

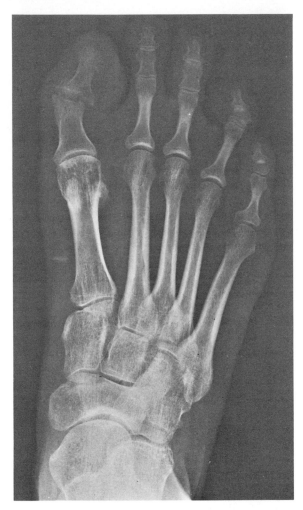

Fig. 42. Systemic deossification, demineralization (polyarthritis of unknown cause)

1. Loss of density in bone with atrophy.

2. Trabecular pattern is present, but density is lacking.

3. Bone resorption, interphalangeal joint, great toe.

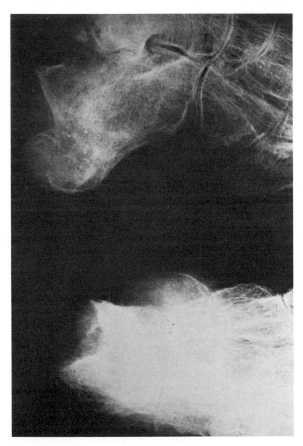

Fig. 43. General deossification

1. Triangular loss of substance due to tear of tendo achillis at posterior surface of calcaneus.

2. Prolonged casting results in a generalized decrease in density involving entire foot.

2. Swelling and deformity may exist with loss of density in bone.

3. Redness, cyanosis, and pain may be present in causalgic states that are seen with trophic osteitis or spotty, general deossification.

4. The temperature may be increased or decreased depending on the pathologic process.

5. Active and passive function may be limited in severe generalized deossification.

6. Burning and tingling pain are the rule in causalgia or vasospastic disorders accompanied by a general decrease in density of bone.

ROENTGENOLOGIC INTERPRETATION
(Fig. 43)

1. Decrease in density may affect those bones that have been immobilized by plaster or braces.

2. Bones distal to a fracture are demineralized and decreased in density.

3. Sudeck's atrophy is a spotty generalized decrease in density due to resorption secondary to congestion.

4. Soft-tissue swelling very often accompanies general deossification of the bones of the feet.

Local Decrease in Density (Local Deossification, Local Demineralization, Local Decalcification).

This demineralization is a decrease in density usually localized to a part of a bone from which the bone matrix and its minerals have been absorbed.

CLINICAL ORIENTATION

1. Local decrease in density may occur under a site of soft-tissue inflammation, cellulitis, or hyperemia.

2. Acute bursitis may cause a local decrease in density, such as found beneath an inflamed heloma, tyloma, or in an acute bunion.

3. Pressure in tissue adjacent to bone stimulates osteoclasis and subsequent resorption. A bone tumor may cause sufficient pressure to stimulate osteoclasis and resorption of bone.

4. A theoretical concept relative to decrease in density revolves about the differentiation of osteoclasts from loose connective tissue.

 a. Multinucleated giant cell osteoclasts are said to originate from fusion of osteocytes.

 b. Aging and death of osteoclasts cause chemical changes in the tissue fluid of the adjacent ground substance.

 c. Loose connective tissue may be activated by the alterations in chemistry to stimulate differentiation of osteoclasts.

ROENTGENOLOGIC INTERPRETATION
(Fig. 44)

1. A local decrease in density is a loss of

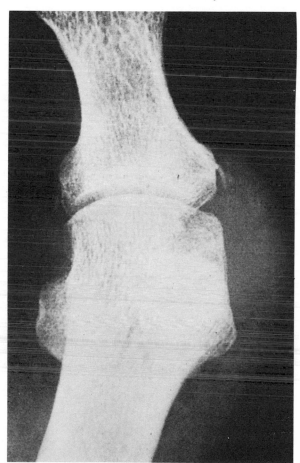

Fig. 44. Local deossification
1. Acute bursitis with a local demineralization of bone at the medial aspect of the hallux joint.
2. Hyperemia aids in resorption and deossification.

density localized to a part of a bone.

2. An inflamed soft-tissue mass or swelling may overlie a localized area of decreased bone density.

3. A localized decrease in density is common at chondro-osseous margins of bone.

Posttraumatic Decrease in Density (Syn: Sudeck's atrophy, trophic osteitis, posttraumatic causalgic osteoporosis.)

CLINICAL ORIENTATION

1. The symptoms of pain and loss of function are out of proportion to the extent of injury.

2. Vasomotor changes are evident and may be secondary to a vasospastic disorder.

3. Slight trauma to periarticular tissues may be the cause of pain and immobility out of proportion to the extent of the injury

4. Following an acute onset, the condition progresses to become more severe in about 4 weeks after injury.

5. It may develop following fractures or injury to articular structures.

6. Some degree of osteoporosis exists after pain subsides.

7. Prolonged physical therapy which stimulates hyperemia aggravates symptoms of pain and decreases the density of the bone.

8. Swelling and inflammation of the soft tissues are usual.

9. Atrophy and spasm of musculature may be present.

10. Rubor or often cyanosis is present with Sudeck's atrophy.

11. Temperature is usually increased while active and passive functions are limited.

12. Burning and aching pain persist during activity and while at rest.

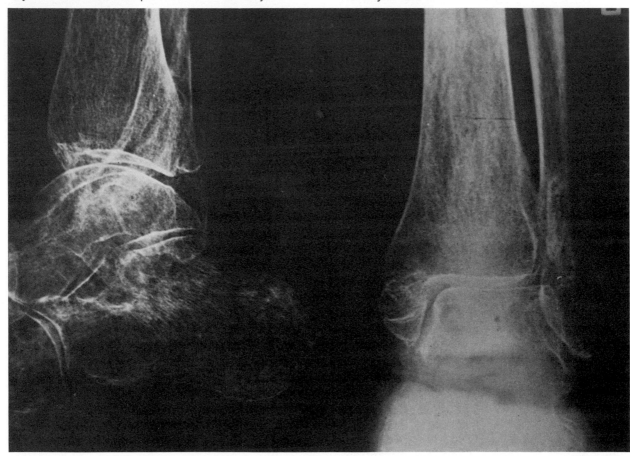

Fig. 45. Sudeck's atrophy. Multiple small spots of deossification, lower one third of tibia, fibula, and tarsus following immobilization and strenuous physical therapy.

13. With activity, the osteoporosis repairs and pain subsides.

14. In some acute causalgic states, the pulse may be strong and bounding.

ROENTGENOLOGIC INTERPRETATION
(Figs. 45-47)

1. Minute, abundant, spotty areas of decrease in density are visualized, usually distal to a site of trauma. These may develop distal to a fracture or site of vasospastic disorder.

2. Tarsal and metatarsal bones are often affected by mottling accompanied by a hazy, indistinct, spotty demineralization.

3. The cortex is thin and the trabecular pattern appears indistinct.

4. Soft-tissue swelling is usually apparent and the joint spaces are often widened by effusion in the acute atrophy of Sudeck.

ALTERATIONS IN BONE (TRANSFORMATIONS)

An alteration in bone is considered as a change in the normal physiologic development and viability of the bone as represented by changes in bone substance and structure due to noxious agents. These transformations are in direct proportion to the extent of the pathologic process. Sudden alterations in the structure or texture of bone are abnormal.

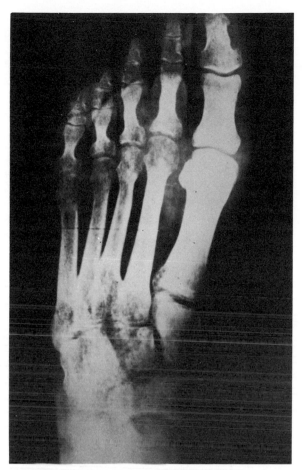

Fig. 46. Sudeck's atrophy. Multiple, minute, spotty demineralization of bone.

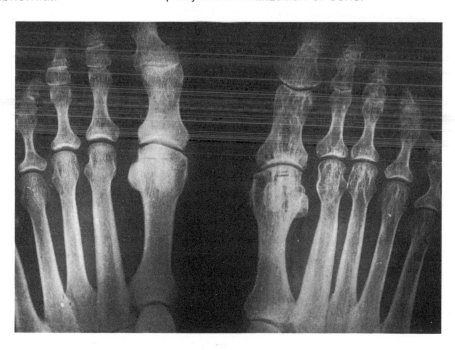

Fig. 47. Sudeck's atrophy, causalgia, and unilateral trophic osteitis. Spotty demineralization of bone found in unilateral vasospastic disorder.

1. Bizarre calcifications protruding out into the soft tissues may develop following rupture of the periosteum.

2. Hemorrhagic extravasations into the soft tissues with subsequent calcification may develop following injury.

3. Bone is constantly undergoing solution, absorption, and accretion.

4. Decreased stress on bone may limit accretion.

5. Sclerosis is an increase in bone density without a loss of visible trabecular density. The soft-tissue elements in bone decrease in size when circulation to the bone is decreased.

6. Transformations are to be differentiated from formation and development of bone from fibrous and chondral tissue, bone growth, tumor formation, and destruction and repair of bone.

Lack of Bone Substance

CLINICAL ORIENTATION

1. Lack of bone substance may be present with agenesis of bone or an anatomic part.

2. If lack of bone substance is extensive, an atrophy of musculature may result from limitation of function.

3. There are no color changes or temperature alterations.

4. There is no pain associated with lack of substance.

ROENTGENOLOGIC INTERPRETATION

1. No soft-tissue swelling is evident.

2. There may be no roentgenologic evidence of any previous calcareous elements in the area of the lesion.

3. The remaining bone is normal in density, texture, and structure.

4. Lack of bone substance usually involves the margin and surface of a bone.

Loss of Substance

Atrophic loss of substance is a slow transformation process in the areas of bone from which minerals have been removed, with the bones then adapting themselves to this loss.

CLINICAL ORIENTATION

1. A nonspecific inflammation of soft tissues may exist.

2. Atrophic loss of substance occurs in gout, rheumatoid arthritis, neurotrophic degenerations, and metabolic disorders of various causes.

3. Swelling is common.

4. Marked rubor or cyanosis with severe pain and increase in temperature is common in acute gout, and the blood uric acid is high.

5. Pain may be sharp or a dull ache depending on the disease process present.

6. There is generally a limitation of function due to joint damage.

7. The sedimentation rate is increased in rheumatoid arthritis.

8. Neurotrophic changes are noted in diabetes, extensive paralysis, pernicious anemia, and disease of the spinal cord.

ROENTGENOLOGIC INTERPRETATION
(Fig. 48)

1. Punched-out areas of loss of substance at chondro-osseous margins of bone represent a loss of substance. The margins are smooth, but the bone substance is absent.

2. Gout presents large areas of atrophic loss of substance, soft-tissue swelling, and effusion. Biurate crystals are often deposited in soft tissues.

3. Neurotrophic lesions show evidence of loss of substance transverse to the long axis of the bone with marked, indurated soft-tissue swelling.

4. Rheumatoid arthritis presents atrophic loss of substance, systemic decrease in density, and narrowed joint spaces.

5. A deformity of bone is secondary to atrophic loss of substance.

Active Destruction (Loss of Substance *en Masse*)

Active destruction may be seen in infections and malignant neoplasias.

CLINICAL ORIENTATION

1. Cardinal signs are local heat, redness,

swelling, and pain where infection exists.

2. Body temperature may be increased.

3. Function is often limited.

4. A throbbing ache is common.

5. Sinus tract or ulceration in the soft tissues may be a primary focus.

6. Systemic infection with localized focus of active destruction is not uncommon.

7. Cellulitis, lymphangitis, and lymphadenopathy are notable.

8. Sedimentation rate may be increased, and the white count is high.

ROENTGENOLOGIC INTERPRETATION
(Fig. 49)

1. Eroded and spiculated margins are seen at the sites of loss of substance.

2. A heavy, irregular, indistinct subperiosteal calcification and condensation are often evident in bone adjacent to the active destruction.

3. Active destruction of bone can be compared with gangrene of the soft tissues.

4. Adjacent bone may appear hazy, indistinct, and flat looking as the destructive process progresses with loss of substance *en masse.*

5. Loss of substance *en masse* with metastasis and invasion of adjacent bone may suggest a malignant lesion.

Lack of Structure in Bone

CLINICAL ORIENTATION

1. Swelling in the soft tissues adjacent to the pathologic process obliterates fascial planes.

2. Expansion of the bone often produces hypertrophic changes or bone deformity which may be visible and/or palpable.

3. Mild rubor may be present overlying the lesion.

4. Function may be limited if lack of structure is great.

5. Pain will vary with the extent of expansion of bone and its concomitant pressure.

6. Thickening of soft tissues and often an

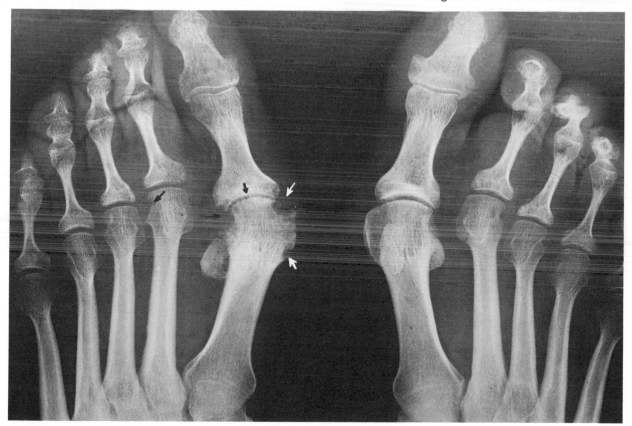

Fig. 48. Atrophic loss of substance. Smoothly outlined, punched-out areas of bone at the chondroosseous margins of hallux and second metatarsophalangeal joints.

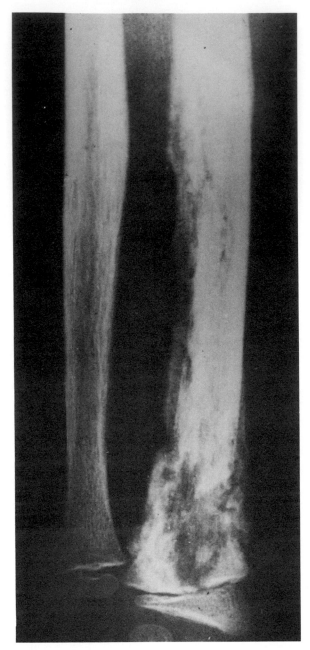

Fig. 49. Osteomyelitis with active destruction and loss of substance *en masse*

1. Active destruction evidenced by irregular loss of substance with condensation.

2. An irregular, hazy, indistinct subperiosteal alteration in bone.

3. Destruction progresses away from joint.

oval or spheroid mass in the soft tissues suggest the presence of a pathologic process.

7. An obscure bone lesion with lack of structure may be found adjacent to a soft-tissue pathologic process.

ROENTGENOLOGIC INTERPRETATION
(Fig. 50)

1. Areas of lack of structure show an actual loss of trabeculations (trabeculations are visible in areas of decreased density).

2. These areas in bone may be ovoid or spheroid.

3. No active destruction is visible about the areas of lack of structure.

4. These areas in bone may be composed of osteoid, cystic, fibrous, fat, or cartilaginous tissue.

5. With expansion, the cortex is often thinned.

6. Lack of structure is commonly seen in the phalanges, metatarsals, and calcaneus.

CIRCULATORY DISTURBANCES IN BONE

CLINICAL ORIENTATION

1. Circulatory disturbances in bone may be secondary to peripheral vascular or neurologic disorders with all their symptoms.

2. Local disturbance of circulation in bone may be secondary to trauma, infection, spreading inflammatory lesions, or metastatic tumor.

3. Swelling may develop in circulatory stasis.

4. Atrophied limbs develop in severe circulatory and neuropathologic conditions.

5. Rubor, cyanosis, and swelling with acute pain are present in causalgic states.

6. There is rubor on dependency and pallor on elevation in circulatory disease.

7. Pulsations may be feeble or absent.

8. The skin temperature may be either elevated or lowered.

9. Burning, tingling, and numbness are common.

10. With infection, local heat, redness, swelling, fever, pain, cellulitis, lymphangitis, and often lymphadenopathy are present.

ROENTGENOLOGIC INTERPRETATION

1. Active destruction of bone is demon-

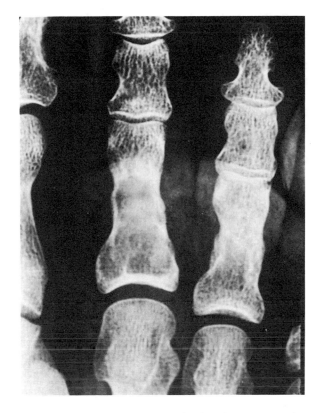

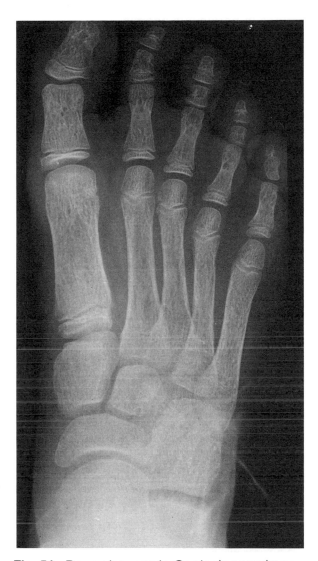

Fig. 50. Enchondroma — lack of structure in bone

1. Proximal two thirds of proximal phalanx presents an expansion of bone and multilocular areas of lack of structure.

2. Cortex is thinned.

strated at the site of loss of circulation.

2. There is a decrease in the density of bone where hyperemia exists.

3. Active destruction occurs where the Volkmann's, Haversian, and canalicular canals become plugged with debris, bacteria, phagocytes, or leucocytes.

4. Other roentgenologic findings will be discussed where specific disorders are considered; *e.g.,* arteriosclerosis, calcified veins, causalgia, etc.

Anemias and the Feet

Neurologic and circulatory disturbances occurring with anemias may produce symptoms in the foot.

CLINICAL ORIENTATION

1. In chronic secondary anemia, there is a diminution in red blood cells and hemoglobin

Fig. 51. Bone changes in Cooley's anemia

1. Demineralization of metatarsals and phalanges.

2. Wide medullary bone and thinning of cortex in phalanges.

3. Alteration of normal trabecular pattern.

(which may be secondary to some chronic infection), inability to digest and absorb food, or frequent hemorrhages.

2. Faintness with a complaint of a "swimming head," loss of appetite, pallor, dyspnea, and a soft, rapid pulse are subjective symptoms.

3. A nonpitting edema of feet and ankles may be noted in pernicious anemia.

4. Neurologic changes may result in sensory disturbances and alterations in reflex re-

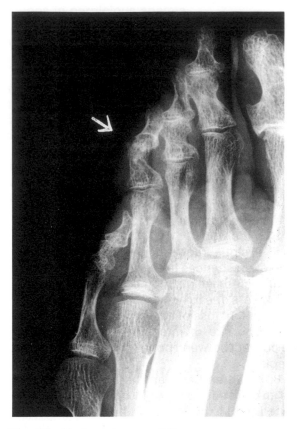

Fig. 53. Early osteomyelitis

1. Sinus tract, dorsum fourth toe over distal interphalangeal joint.

2. Active destruction, loss of normal trabecular pattern and shape of middle phalanx with increased thickness of the soft tissue.

10. An osteomyelitis may be acute, subacute, or chronic.

11. Severe, throbbing pain with increase in temperature over the infected part is often the earliest symptom of osteomyelitis.

12. Only slight redness and pain occur in the soft tissues.

13. A brawny swelling results when drainage is inadequate.

ROENTGENOLOGIC INTERPRETATION
(Figs. 52-60)

1. Early osteomyelitis presents a diffuse, *reactive swelling* surrounding the bone.

2. A *reaction area* is present and is evidenced by a hazy, flat-looking, indistinct, soft-tissue density in bone.

3. *Subperiosteal* abscess is noted in the acute hematogenous type of osteomyelitis. Periosteum is often stripped for some distance by pus. An *infectious subperiosteal calcification* is often an early sign of an osteomyelitis.

4. A *sequestrum*, a portion of bone demarcated from the body of the bone, may be seen at the site of reaction.

a. Sequestra may be longer than broad, increased in density, irregular in outline, and are often spiculate at the ends.

b. They may be passed out through an abscess sinus tract or be absorbed or removed. They may also remain united to bone and become reossified.

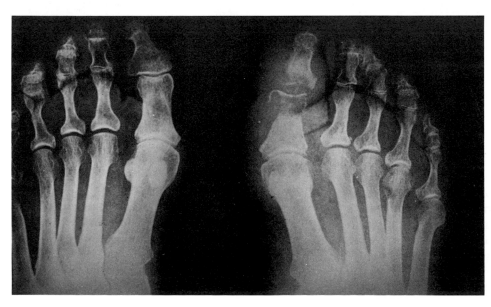

Fig. 54. Diabetic osteomyelitis. Reactive soft-tissue swelling with active destruction of bone, right hallux.

c. In osteomyelitis variolosa, sequestra remain uniform in density (Davidson and Palmer, 1963).

5. *An involucrum,* reparative calcification and sclerosis creating a bone shell, may entirely encapsulate and surround the sequestra.

6. The area of involvement in osteomyelitis is generally triangular with the base toward the epiphysis and necrotic areas sloping away toward the midshaft and toward the periosteum.

7. Smallpox osteomyelitis often presents an unevenly distributed patchy destruction.

8. *Pathologic fractures* may occur in osteomyelitis.

9. Separation of the epiphysis of a long bone may develop with extensive infection.

10. Repair.
   a. An involucrum may be laid down.
   b. Bone is clear and transparent.
   c. Some increase in density remains after repair.

11. Haziness, decrease in density, and soft-tissue swelling indicate continued activity of infection.

12. Bone infection rarely spreads across a joint.

Brodie's Abscess

CLINICAL ORIENTATION

1. Brodie's abscess originates from a septicemia.

2. The abscess develops in patients with low resistance to infection following a systemic illness or trauma.

3. Pain manifests itself as a dull, throbbing ache.

4. A palpable, indurated swelling in the soft tissues is common.

5. An increased body temperature is a common finding.

6. Regional lymph nodes may be inflamed and tender.

7. Soft, granular, infected tissue may be found in the abscess on incision and drainage or at biopsy.

8. Laboratory studies corroborate the clinical and roentgenologic impression.

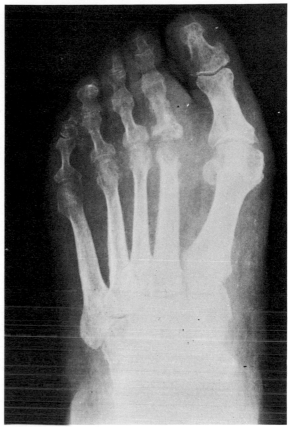

Fig. 55. Osteomyelitis — ulcer
1. Active destruction of the second metatarsophalangeal joint.

2. Infectious subperiosteal alteration in bone.

3. Reactive soft-tissue swelling that is hazy and indistinct with loss of fascial planes.

ROENTGENOLOGIC INTERPRETATION

1. Brodie's abscess is characterized by a central, circular area of decreased density at the metaphyseal region of long bone.

2. The area of rarefaction is flat looking, indistinct, hazy, and translucent.

3. Cortical bone is expanded and the margins are increased in density with condensation of surrounding bone.

4. As the cortex is expanded and thickened, the periosteum develops an irregularity which is confluent and increased in density.

5. Increased soft-tissue density and thickening of the soft tissues are apparent.

6. A Brodie's abscess may be differentiated from a bone cyst by the following:

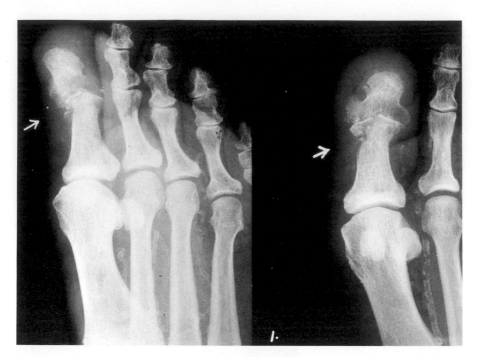

Fig. 56. Arteriosclerotic ulcer (osteomyelitis)

1. *Early* evidence of active destruction at interphalangeal joint of hallux.

2. Calcification of intermetatarsal arteries.

a. Size, which is smaller than that of a cyst.

b. Evidence of infection, which is lacking in a cyst.

c. Cortical shell, which is thinner in a cyst.

d. Cortical expansion, which is greater in a cyst.

Syphilitic Lesions in Bone

CLINICAL ORIENTATION

1. Bone lesions are usually recognized late in the disease.

2. The femur and tibia are often affected late in childhood. The feet are rarely affected.

3. Epiphyses are involved in the first 6

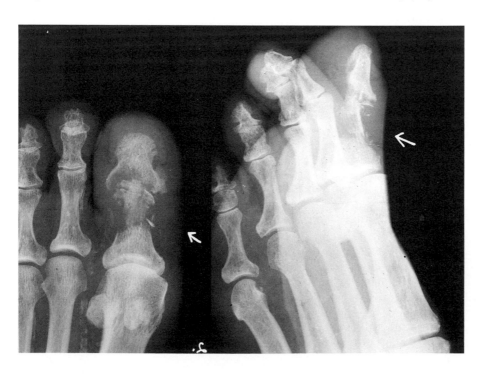

Fig. 57. Arteriosclerotic ulcer (osteomyelitis)

1. Advanced osteomyelitis with active destruction spreading back from joint and destroying the proximal phalanx.

2. Ulceration healed at this stage with loss of pain and vibratory sensation.

Fig. 58. Pyogenic osteomyelitis

1. Destruction of interphalangeal joint secondary to soft-tissue infection.

2. Irregular spiculation at the proximal interphalangeal joint.

3. Reactive soft-tissue swelling.

4. Indistinct, flat-looking trabecular pattern.

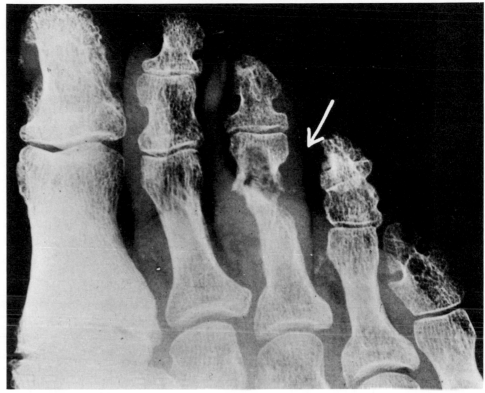

months of infection.

4. The history, clinical findings, and serologic examinations are necessary to establish a diagnosis and to differentiate lesions simulating those caused by syphilis.

5. Osseous lesions develop in 50% of patients with congenital syphilis.

ROENTGENOLOGIC INTERPRETATION

EARLY CONGENITAL SYPHILIS.

1. The metaphysis is broadened and the epiphyseal line is irregular.

2. Areas of loss of substance in bone are often characteristic.

Fig. 59. Osteomyelitis

1. Condensation.

2. Active destruction.

3. Infectious subperiosteal alterations.

4. Hazy, irregular, indistinct bone density.

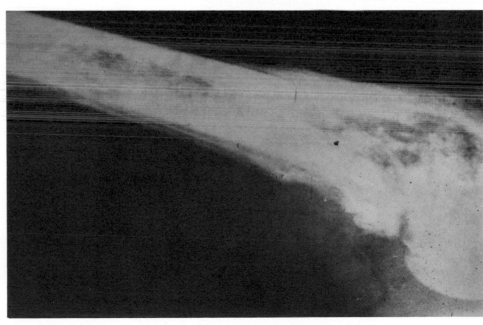

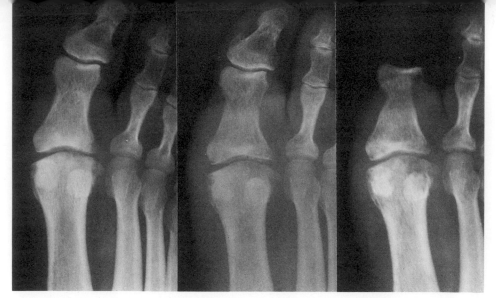

Fig. 60. Progressive diabetic osteomyelitis, distal phalanx hallux

3. Dense, harsh cortical thickening along the shaft of the tibia is common.

4. Syphilitic dactylitis of the hands and feet may be seen from the sixth month through the fourth year in patients with congenital syphilis.

a. It is manifested by expansion of the phalanges by accretion.

b. There is dense sclerotic bone production with almost complete loss of the cortex due to resorption from the endosteal surface.

LATE CONGENITAL AND ACQUIRED SYPHILIS (Figs. 61-62).

1. A combined active destruction and hypertrophic reaction is noted.

2. The cortex may become thick and irregular due to syphilitic subperiosteal calcifications.

3. A bumpy lacework type of periostitis may develop, or the cortex may appear hypertrophied due to a reactive density of bone condensation.

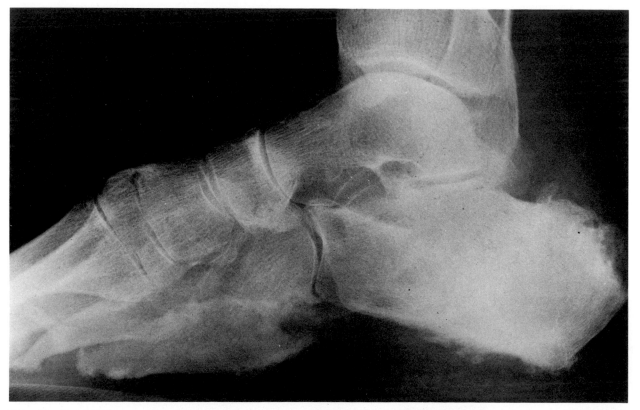

Fig. 61. Syphilitic periosteal reaction. Bumpy, lacework type of reactive subperiosteal calcification with dense condensation of bone.

4. The density of the subperiosteal alterations is usually as great or greater than the densities of cortex.

5. In congenital syphilis, a saber shin with anterior bowing of the tibia may develop as a delayed manifestation.

Tuberculosis in Bone

CLINICAL ORIENTATION

1. Tuberculosis in bone is common in childhood and adolescence and is usually secondary to a latent focus elsewhere in the body.

2. It may be disseminated through the circulatory system or it may extend from adjacent infected tissue.

3. Tubercle bacilli may spread from a primary pulmonary lesion to the bronchopulmonary lymph nodes, thence by metastasis of the organisms to bone or directly to the synovial fluid.

4. Tuberculous Negroes are especially susceptible to bone involvement.

5. The epiphysis of long bones and the cancellous tissues of small bones are invaded.

The Haversian canals are involved through the many vascular anastomoses.

7. In youngsters, there usually is a sharply defined, fusiform swelling of the fingers.

ROENTGENOLOGIC INTERPRETATION
(Fig. 63)

1. Local deossification develops slowly in the infected bone.

2. Bone may slowly and insidiously become hazy and indistinct, developing a single area of destruction and sequestration.

3. The joint cartilage and joint cavity may be invaded from the bone infection.

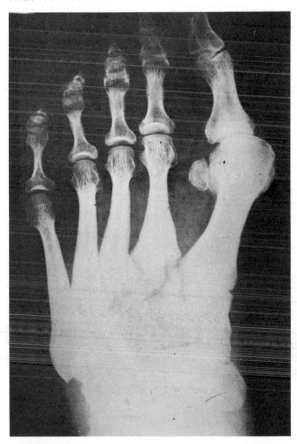

Fig. 62. Syphilitic arthritis
1. Woman, age 28, known syphilitic.
2. Marked destruction, base of second metatarsal, transverse to long axis of bone.
3. Hypertrophy of shaft of second metatarsal with marked thickening of cortex.
4. Note the obliteration of tarsometatarsal and intertarsal articulations.

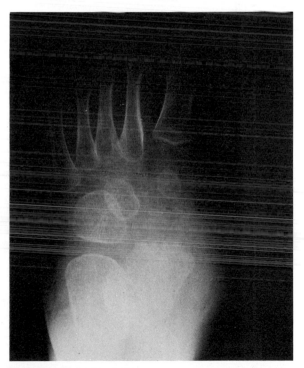

Fig. 63. Tuberculosis
1. Slow, chronic, insidious destruction of bone at the head of the talus.
2. Marked doughy swelling.
3. General demineralization.

4. The subperiosteal bone may be infected, but periosteal new bone rarely forms in tuberculosis.

5. Bone ends may be destroyed, the joint becomes involved, and ankylosis develops.

6. Destruction of bone may result in a cold abscess with a fistulous tract burrowing along muscles and fascia and opening through the skin.

7. Tuberculosis of the phalanges causes enlargement of the medullary canal by erosion from within. The shaft is dilated in a fusiform manner by deposition of new, light-density bone. This is called tuberculous dactylitis.

Leprosy (Hansen's Disease)

CLINICAL ORIENTATION

1. Multiple deformities are noted in the extremities due to soft-tissue contractures.

2. In advanced stages, the fingers and toes appear to have soft-tissue masses replacing the phalanges.

3. The characteristic anesthesia of digits subjects the ends of the toes to ulceration by trauma.

4. The mechanism of the destruction is unknown. It is thought that neural pathologic processes play an important part in this disorder.

5. Close examination of hands and feet is mandatory in patients presenting an anesthesia of the fingers and toes.

ROENTGENOLOGIC INTERPRETATION
(Fig. 64)

1. Active destruction with loss of bone substance is prominent.

2. Destruction and often complete absence of phalanges are noted.

3. There is usually an increase in soft-tissue density.

4. Sixty percent of patients without clinical signs of involvement present varying degrees of demineralization, atrophy, hypertrophy, or hyperostosis.

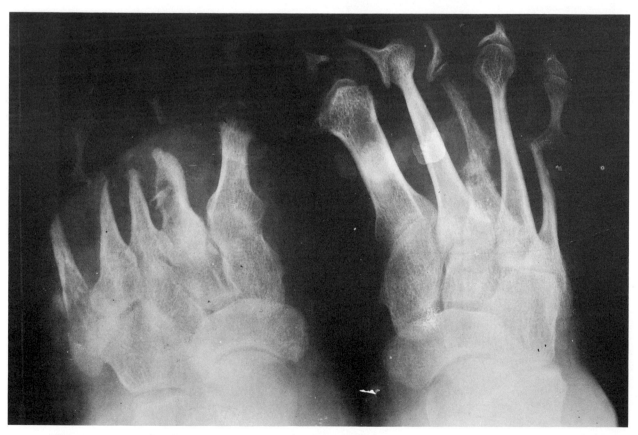

Fig. 64. Leprosy of the feet. (Courtesy Armed Forces Institute of Pathology, #48463.)

Garré's Nonsuppurative Osteitis

CLINICAL ORIENTATION

1. Garré's nonsuppurative osteitis commonly affects the tibia in persons under age 25.

2. The acute onset is accompanied by fever and leukocytosis.

3. Pain is aggravated by exercise, abuse, and fatigue.

4. Discomfort is noted in the legs, especially at night.

5. There may be a history of previous systemic infection, such as typhoid, pneumonia, influenza, or streptococcic septicemia.

6. This disease has a benign, slow, gradual, chronic course extending over a period of years.

7. It must be differentiated from Ewing's sarcoma or osteoid osteoma.

ROENTGENOLOGIC INTERPRETATION

1. The "onion peel" formation typical of Ewing's sarcoma is lacking.

2. Fusiform widening of the shaft is present in Garre's osteitis.

3. A thickened cortex of increased density should be looked upon with suspicion.

4. Medullary bone may be altered with condensation and sclerosis obliterating the normal trabecular patterns.

FUNGAL INFECTIONS OF BONE

Fungal infections of bone are rather uncommon but deserve mention. Osseous lesions may occur in actinomycosis, blastomycosis, mycetoma (maduromycosis), and coccidioidomycosis. These are slowly developing, destructive bone lesions. Granulomatous lesions of the skin, subcutaneous tissue, and lungs are suggestive of mycotic infections. A differential diagnosis is made by smear, culture, and tissue sections. The prognosis is poor if the disease is systemic with bone lesions but good if the origin of the bone lesion is adjacent to the infected site. We will briefly consider a few of these problems.

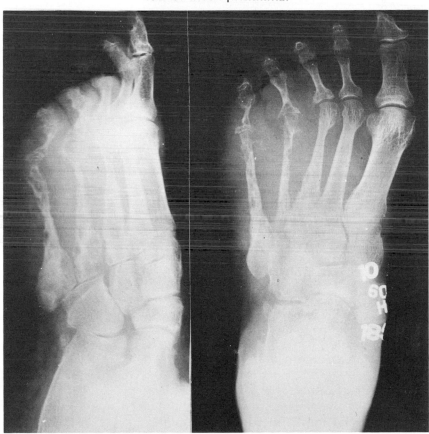

Fig. 65. Madura foot. (Courtesy Armed Forces Institute of Pathology, #61-8595.)

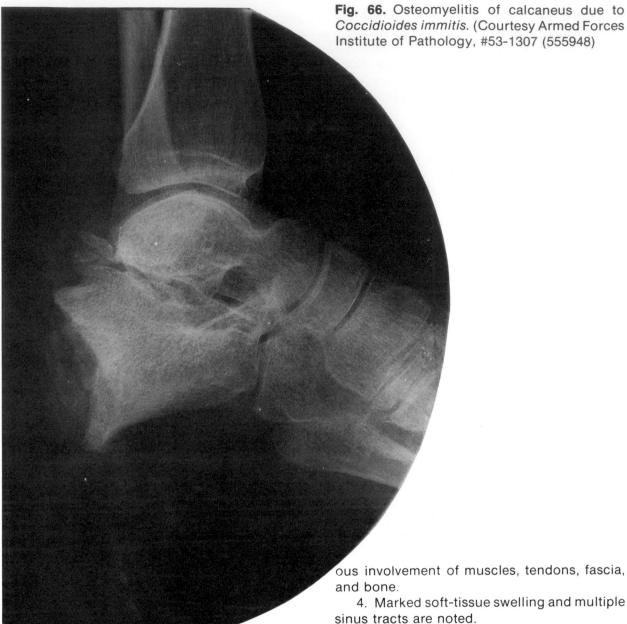

Fig. 66. Osteomyelitis of calcaneus due to *Coccidioides immitis.* (Courtesy Armed Forces Institute of Pathology, #53-1307 (555948)

Mycetoma (Maduromycosis, Madura Foot)

CLINICAL ORIENTATION

1. This disease occurs most frequently in tropical or subtropical regions and is known to occur in the southern states of the United States.

2. It usually affects the foot.

3. This is a painless, destructive fungus infection of the foot with chronic and insidi-ous involvement of muscles, tendons, fascia, and bone.

4. Marked soft-tissue swelling and multiple sinus tracts are noted.

5. Orange, yellow, and black-looking, ir-regularly shaped granules ooze from the soft-tissue sinuses.

6. The patient appears to have a markedly enlarged foot.

7. Comparative measurements of affected foot and ankle indicate swelling is about twice normal size (Marcus, 1963).

ROENTGENOLOGIC INTERPRETATION
(Fig. 65)

1. There is a marked increase in soft-tissue

density noted.

2. Sinus tracts may become visible in the roentgenogram in long-standing disease.

3. Secondary infection of the bones presents characteristic condensation, active destruction, cortical irregularity, and infectious subperiosteal transformations in bone.

4. Large spotted areas of decreased density are visualized.

5. Destruction of bone obliterates joint outlines (Marcus, 1963).

6. Bone structure appearing moth eaten is pathognomonic.

7. Khmelnitsky et al. (1971), following a histologic and roentgenologic study of madura mycetoma, considered it to be a specific osteomyelitis.

Coccidioidal Granuloma of Bone

CLINICAL ORIENTATION

1. Coccidioidomycosis is endemic to the Mohave, Sonora, and Chihuahua deserts of southwestern United States.

2. Dissemination with bone lesions is commonly seen in dark-skinned races in the third and fourth decades.

3. There is a history of pulmonary lesions with invasion to other organs.

4. Swelling, heat, and tenderness accompany the bone lesions.

5. Destructive bone lesions may cause soft-tissue involvement advancing to ulceration and abscess formation.

6. Cases have been reported involving the talus, navicular, cuboid, fifth metatarsal, patella, and lower end of the femur.

ROENTGENOLOGIC INTERPRETATION
(Fig. 66)

1. Reactive soft-tissue swelling is a usual finding.

2. Linear calcifications may be seen in the soft tissues.

3. A loss of substance, marked thinning of cortices, active destruction, and sclerosis may be noted.

Ainhum (Dactylolysis Spontanea)

CLINICAL ORIENTATION

1. This is an uncommon disorder usually found in Negroes and believed to be parasitic or viral in origin.

2. It usually is manifested as a firm, constrictive fibrous band on the undersurface of the fifth toe in the subcutaneous tissue.

3. The end of the toe becomes bulbous with a marked soft-tissue swelling.

4. The severity of the pain is in proportion to the extent of the constricting band and overlying hyperkeratosis.

5. The toe is cool to touch.

6. If a fibrous band envelops the entire toe, dry gangrene and loss of the toe are usual.

ROENTGENOLOGIC INTERPRETATION
(Fig. 67)

1. There is a bulbous soft-tissue swelling at the end of the toe.

2. A constrictive band is visualized if fibrous tissue is dense.

3. A narrowed transverse diameter of sclerosed bone is noted beneath the constrictive band.

4. Necrosis of bone may be recognized in the late stages.

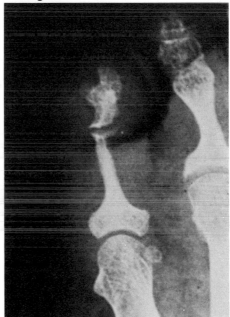

Fig. 67. Ainhum

1. Constricting fibrous bands about proximal interphalangeal joint, fifth toe.

2. Swelling of bulbous end of toe.

3. Atrophic changes and alteration of shape of proximal phalanx, fifth toe.

BIBLIOGRAPHY

Allen E., van N., Barker, N.W. and Hines, E.A.: *Peripheral Vascular Disease*. Philadelphia: W.B. Saunders Co., 1947.

Caffey, J.P.: *Pediatric X-ray Diagnosis*. Chicago: Year Book Publishers, 1946.

Davidson, J.C., and Palmer, P.E.S.: Osteomyelitis Variolosa, J. Bone Joint Surg. 45-B:687, 1963.

DeCarlo, R.: Sinuses, Chiropody Rec. 18:3, 1935.

Dell, J.M., Jr.: Demonstrations of Sinus Tracts, Fistulas and Infected Cavities by Lipiodol, Amer. J. Roentgen. 61:223, 1949.

Feigin, R.D., McAlister, W.H., San Joaquin, U.H., and Middlekamp, J.N.: Osteomyelitis of the calcaneus, Amer. J. Dis. Child., 119:61, 1970.

Ferguson, A.B.: *Roentgen Diagnosis of the Extremities and Spine*. New York: P.B. Hoeber, Inc., 1941 (Ann. Roentgenol. 17:10).

Gamble, F.O.: *Foot Roentgenology*, Lecture Notes, ed. 4. Philadelphia: Temple University, School of Chiropody, 1947.

Geschickter, C.F., and Copeland, M.M.: *Tumors of Bone*, ed. 3. Philadelphia: J.B. Lippincott Co., 1949.

Griffin, P.P.: Bone and Joint Infections in Children, Pediat. Clin. N. Amer. 14:533, 1967.

Gross, R.H.: *Modern Foot Therapy*. New York: Foot Therapy Publishing Co., 1948.

Hagler, D.J.: Pseudomonas Osteomyelitis Puncture Wounds of the Feet, Pediatrics 48:672, 1971.

Hauser, E.D.W.: *Diseases of the Foot*. Philadelphia: W.B. Saunders Co., 1939.

Hodges, F.J., Lampe, I., and Holt, J.F.: *Radiology for Medical Students*. Chicago: Year Book Publishers, 1947.

Homans, J.: *Circulatory Diseases of the Extremities*. New York: The Macmillan Co., 1939.

Johanson, P.H.: Pseudomonas Infections of the foot following puncture wounds, J.A.M.A. 204:170, 1968.

Khmelnitsky, O.K., Nekachalov, V.V., and Chistyakov, A.M.: A Comparative Histological and Roentgenological Study of Madura-mycosis (Mycetoma) of the Foot (Russian), Arkh. Pat. 33(6):55, 1971.

Kramer, D.W.: *Manual of Peripheral Vascular Disorders*. Philadelphia: Blakiston Co., 1940.

Lewin, P.: *The Foot and Ankle*. Philadelphia: Lea & Febiger Co., 1940.

Luck, J.V.: *Bone and Joint Diseases*. Springfield, Ill.: Charles C Thomas, 1950, pp. 43-141.

Madura Foot, J. Bone Joint Surg. 43-B:359, 1961.

Marcus, S.A.: Madura Foot (A Case Report, Civic Hospital, Detroit), The Michigan Podiatrist 1:9, 1963.

Miller, D., and Birsner, J.W.: Coccidioidal Granuloma of Bone, Amer. J. Roentgen. 62:229, 1949.

Minnifor, A.B.: Pseudomonas Osteomyelitis Following Puncture Wounds of the Foot, Pediatrics 47:598-601, 1971.

Newell, R.R.: Roentgenology: Contrast Media. In Glasser, O. (ed.), *Medical Physics*. Chicago: Year Book Publishers, 1944, vol. 1, pp. 1269-1271.

Rakow, R.B.: Obliterative Arterial Disease, J. Nat. Ass. Chiropodists 34:17, 1944.

Rigler, L.G.: *Outline of Roentgen Diagnosis*. Philadelphia: Lea & Febiger, 1955, pp. 307-354.

Sante, L.: *Principles of Roentgenological Interpretation*. Ann Arbor, Mich.: Edwards Bros., Inc., 1940.

Umansky, A.L., Schlesinger, P.T., and Greenberg, B.B.: Tuberculous Dactylitis in the Adult, Arch. Surg. 54:67, 1947.

Yale, I.: A Statistical Report on a Review of 1290 Foot Radiographs, J. Nat. Ass. Chiropodists 47:6, 1957.

Yater, W.M.: *Symptom Diagnosis*, ed. 4. New York: D. Appleton-Century Co., 1942.

4 ASEPTIC NECROSIS OF BONE

The process of aseptic necrosis of bone affects several bones of the foot. This type of lesion is essentially a noninflammatory, degenerative process, which may be termed an osteosis. The bone undergoes osteoclasis as intensive proliferation and formation of new blood vessels aid in the replacement by young connective tissue. Complete repair may be achieved. Permanent deformity may result if trauma or secondary infection interferes with this process of interplaying resorption and accretion.

If secondary infection occurs, the aseptic necrosis becomes septic and an osteitis develops in place of the noninflammatory osteosis.

Burns, frostbite, and trauma sufficient to cause gangrene of a distal part usually result in true necrosis of the skeletal part. Necrotic parts are separated from the healthy tissue by osteoclasis followed by invasions of granulation tissue. Due to the difference in blood supply, the epiphyseal cartilage may necrotize while articular cartilage remains viable.

Noninflammatory necrosis of bone may be caused by an overdosage of radiation.

Ischemia caused by arteriosclerosis or an embolic occlusion of a blood vessel may cause an aseptic necrosis. Trauma to a nutrient artery or one of its branches also may lead to necrosis of large areas of bone.

OSTEOCHONDRITIS— OSTEOCHONDROSIS— IDIOPATHIC OSTEOSIS (SPONTANEOUS OSTEOSIS OF UNKNOWN ETIOLOGY)

GENERAL CLINICAL ORIENTATION

Many of these disorders are known by their eponyms; e.g., Köhler's disease, Freiberg's disease, Legg-Calvé-Perthes disease, Kien-böck's disease, or Osgood-Schlatter disease. Such names fail to suggest the pathologic entity, and their use should be relegated to the history of the disorder. Their common usage should be discouraged.

1. The lesions are best described by the bone involved, the location in the bone, mode of onset, and the sequence of characteristic changes.

2. Idiopathic osteosis commonly affects children prior to maturation of bone.

3. It commonly affects the tarsal navicular, metatarsal heads, apophysis of the heel, apophysis at the base of the fifth metatarsal, the tibial tubercle, and the head of the femur. A rare case of the talus has been reported.

GENERAL ROENTGENOLOGIC AND HISTOPATHOLOGIC FEATURES (Fig. 68)

1. First stage.

a. Total necrosis occurs of bone tissue, marrow, epiphysis, part of epiphysis, or bone.

b. Damage to blood vessels cannot be noted microscopically.

c. There is no clinical evidence of the disorder noted at this time.

d. Changes are not visualized in the roentgenogram.

2. Second stage.

a. Resorption of the necrotic bone and invasion by young connective tissue occur.

b. There is substitution of new bone for the necrotic tissue.

c. The new bone is immature, coarse, and fibrillar.

d. The necrotic marrow is replaced by granulation tissue after the cell debris has been removed by macrophages.

3. Third stage — regenerative.

a. Complete healing is the exception

rather than the rule.

b. Abnormal stress on necrotic bone may cause a pathologic fracture. This fracture does not occur between healthy and diseased bone, and no signs of fracture are visualized in the roentgenogram at this time.

c. A pathologic or spontaneous fracture may weaken the support to the articular cartilage with alterations in bone visible in the roentgenogram.

d. It is obvious from studies that the necrosis precedes the fracture rather than the reverse (which has been the prevailing opinion).

e. Histologically, the fracture is bound by necrotic bone on both sides.

f. Friction at the opposing necrotic surfaces results in accumulated bone dust between the fragments walling off the distal from the proximal fragment.

g. Regeneration is slow in the distal portion as the bone dust barrier is replaced by young connective tissue.

h. Regeneration takes place.

i. A separation of new bone from necrotic bone is noted at this stage.

j. When the distal portion of necrotized bone is invaded by granulation tissue, regeneration may take place.

k. Necrotic and regenerated bone may unite, or only partial regeneration takes place.

l. A permanent separation has also been noted with loose bodies, chondromatosis, and degenerative calcifications.

m. From an early stage of osteoclasis and radiolucency the necrotic bone may progress to repair and greater radiopacity.

n. A summation of repeated trauma may cause ischemic necrosis of bone. Damage in the blood vessel morphology is not visible. It is believed that a neurovascular injury is probably a cause of the necrosis.

Osteochondritis of Metatarsals

(Syn.: Freiberg's disease; osteochondrosis of the second metatarsophalangeal joint; juvenile deforming metatarsophalangeal osteochondritis.)

CLINICAL ORIENTATION

1. This lesion occurs in young, active adults.

2. It usually is unilateral involving the second metatarsophalangeal joint but has been observed bilaterally and affecting multiple metatarsophalangeal joints.

3. Indurated edema with a sense of fullness over the dorsum of the affected joint is usually present.

4. There may be a limitation of active and passive flexion with crepitus.

5. Pain on palpation is common.

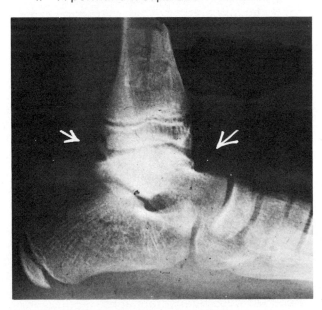 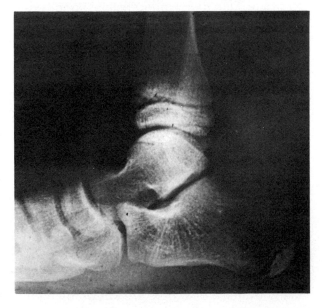

Fig. 68. Osteochondritis of the talus
  1. Flattening of the talus in its transverse diameter.   2. Marked sclerosis of the affected bone.

6.
ful jo

RC

1.
fected
norma
2.
tening
on its
diame
ficatio
fibrocy
3.
about
of the
boncs.
4.
itself u

(Syn.
chondr
osteoch

An ap
process
never be
which it
ter into
ered by
Calca
tlon of th
The calc
ing from
the body
berosity.
appears
for the a
eighth ye
union be
years to
sis ossifi
years ear

1. Ap
weight bo

Fig. 69. Osteochondrosis of second metatarsal head. (*1*) First evidence, flattened head, increased joint space. (*2*) Two months later, fibrocystic degeneration of head. (*3*) Two months later, repara- tive mineralization. (*4*) Three months later, more dense mineralization, normal epiphysis elimi- nated, maturity acceler- ated. (*5*) Six months later,

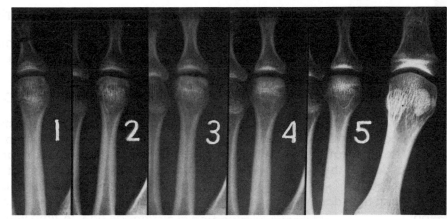

repair established, deformity at a minimum because of adequate protective care.

6. Poststatic dyskinesia may be present in acute or subacute stages.

7. Rarely is there heat or redness noted with this disorder.

ROENTGENOLOGIC INTERPRETATION
(Figs. 69-71)

1. This pathologic entity may affect any of the metatarsal heads but is most commonly seen in the second and third metatarsals.

2. Widening of joint spaces with effusion in the joint and slight soft-tissue swelling are seen early.

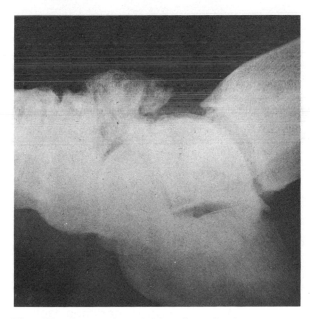

Fig. 70. Osteochondritis of navicular

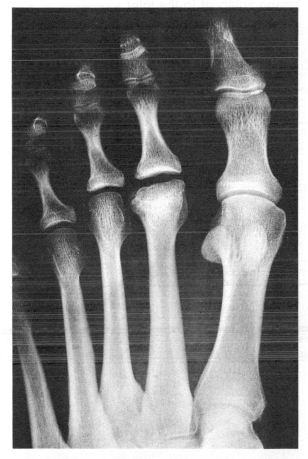

Fig. 71. Advanced osteochondritis, second metatarsophalangeal joint
1. Flattening and enlargement of the meta- tarsal head.
2. Thickening of the metatarsal neck.
3. Hypertrophy of the metatarsal shaft.

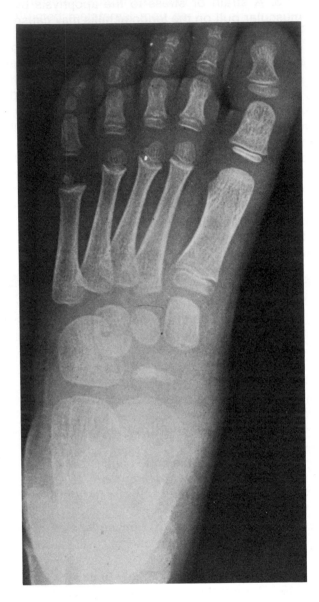

Fig. 73. Osteochondritis of the tarsal navicular

1. Marked flattening of the tarsal navicular in its long axis.

2. The navicular is narrowed anteroposteriorly and it is transversely broadened.

3. Irregular plaques of ossification are noted within the center of ossification.

4. A diffuse swelling is evident about the faulty developing bone.

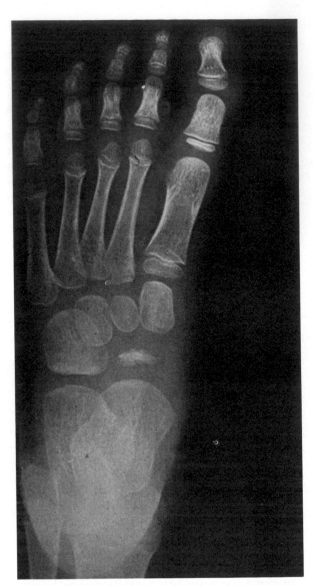

Fig. 74. Osteochondritis of the tarsal navicular

1. Examination 6 weeks after the onset reveals evidence of reparative calcification.

2. The disklike bone is broader in its long axis and the center of ossification is larger presenting a more uniform ossific pattern.

Fig.
1

56/

58/ASEPTIC NECROSIS OF BONE

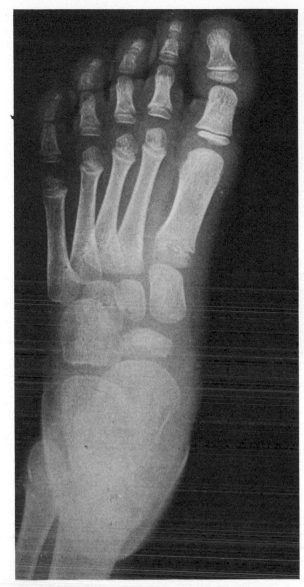

Fig. 75. Osteochondritis of the tarsal navicular. One year later shows evidence of an unusual development of the osteochondrosis to a normal tarsal navicular.

sifications, and early or late normal appearances of the apophysis. We do not believe that apophysitis can be diagnosed by roentgenologic findings alone.

1. In the lateral view of the heel, the apophysis appears moth eaten and somewhat flattened or fragmented, depending on the severity of the lesion.

2. Areas of decrease in density and eburnation or sclerosis are often seen on the opposing cartilaginous surfaces at the epiphyseal line.

3. The epiphyseal line has been seen to be cloudy and irregular.

4. Apparent fragmentation of the apophysis must not be interpreted without consideration that a normal apophysis may be bipartite, tripartite, or even further divided.

5. Several ossification centers in the posterior apophysis of the calcaneus have been seen.

6. It is questionable whether the apophysitis is visible and can be diagnosed roentgenologically.

7. It has been theorized that the alteration in local blood supply that produces the pathologic process is possibly the result of undue trauma to the peripheral nerves.

8. The hypothesis of Leriche and Policard's stated that the injury was in the nature of an "axon reflex" trauma to nerves causing vasodilation, hyperemia, and subsequent deossification of bone and local tenderness.

9. Afterward there occurs local edema, which stimulates increased calcification as seen on the roentgenogram.

10. When the osteochondrotic changes become severe, an osteitis and destructive lesions may occur. In some patients, a periostitis may be evident.

Epiphysitis of the Metatarsals

CLINICAL ORIENTATION

1. In examining youngsters prior to complete union and ossification of the epiphyses, interpretation of forefoot symptoms must be made cautiously.

2. A history of injury to the forefoot from a misstep, jump from a height and landing on the ball of the foot, or direct trauma should lead one to suspect epiphysitis of the metatarsals.

3. This condition is characterized by swelling on the dorsum of the foot over the affected epiphysis.

4. The second, third, and fifth metatarsal epiphyses are usually involved.

5. Often the inconstant styloid epiphysis of the fifth base may be displaced.

6. Pain on palpation is noted at the head of the affected metatarsal.

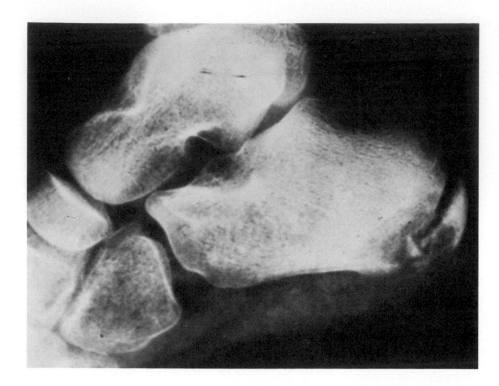

Fig. 76. Apophysitis — fractured apophysis

1. Fracture of posterior apophysis of calcaneus with triangular bone fragment transversing epiphyseal line.

2. Differentiate from aseptic necrosis (Fig. 68).

7. Slight heat and bluish-red discoloration are present about the affected parts, involving the toes.

8. The extensor tendons are usually contracted and very often inflamed with limitation of function accompanied by pain.

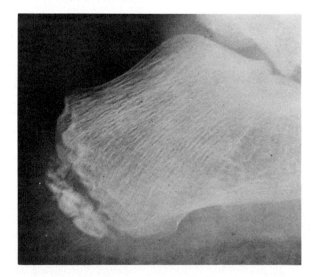

Fig. 77. Idiopathic osteosis of calcaneal apophysis. Irregular ossification of apophysis of the heel.

9. Osteochondritis of the medial sesamoid of the hallux has been reported in three cases (Atterborough, 1956).

ROENTGENOLOGIC INTERPRETATION

1. A soft-tissue swelling follows the fascial planes.

2. The joint may have an effusion that presents a symmetrical, fusiform outline.

3. The epiphysis may be subluxated at the metaphysis.

4. In long-standing disease, a local decrease in density may be evident anterior to the epiphyseal line.

5. Very often a fracture may involve the metaphyseal end of the bone.

6. Fibrocartilaginous tears at the epiphyseal line may be suggested but not visible.

7. If the injury occurs in early childhood and is of sufficient severity, it is possible to note a failure in future normal longitudinal development of the bone.

8. Early signs of osteochondritis of the metatarsophalangeal joint may develop following trauma to the metatarsal epiphysis.

BIBLIOGRAPHY

Archer, V.W.: *The Osseous System, Handbook of Roentgen Diagnosis.* Chicago: Year Book Publishers, 1947.

Atterborough, C.G.: Osteochondritis of the Medial Sesamoid of the Great Toe, Proc. Roy. Soc. Med. 49:809, 1956.

Axhausen, G.: Köhler's Disease and Perthes' Disease, Z. Chir. 50:553, 1923.

Bernstein, M.A.: Osteochondritis Dissecans, J. Bone Joint Surg. 7:319, 1925.

Brachman, P.: *Mechanical Foot Therapy.* Ann Arbor, Mich.: Edwards Bros., 1940.

Cinzio, J.R.: Freiberg's Infraction as an Initiating Factor of Secondary Arthritis in the Foot, J. Nat. Ass. Chiropodists, 1957.

Comroe, H.I.: *Arthritis and Allied Conditions.* Philadelphia: Lea & Febiger Co., 1940.

DeLorimer, A.A.: *The Arthropathies, A Handbook of Roentgen Diagnosis.* Chicago: Year Book Publishers, 1946.

Ferguson, A.B.: *Roentgen Diagnosis of the Extremities and Spine.* New York: P.B. Hoeber, Inc., 1941.

Freiberg, A.H.: Infraction of the Second Metatarsal Bone, Surg. Gynec. Obstet. 19:191, 1914

Gross, R.H.: *Modern Foot Therapy.* New York: Foot Therapy Publishing Co., 1948.

Harbin, M., and Zollinger, R.: Osteochondritis of Growth Centers, Surg. Gynec. Obstet. 51:145, 1930.

Hauser, E.D.W.: *Diseases of the Foot.* Philadelphia: W.B. Saunders Co., 1939.

Hodges, F.J., Lampe, I., and Holt, J.F.: *Radiology for Medical Students.* Chicago: Year Book Publishers, 1947.

Holmes, G.W., and Ruggles, H.E.: *Roentgen Interpretation,* ed. 5. Philadelphia: Lea & Febiger Co., 1936.

Lerner, L.H.: Radiographic Evaluation of Calcaneal Apophysitis, J. Nat. Ass. Chiropodists 1957.

Luck, J.V.: *Bone and Joint Diseases.* Springfield, Ill.: Charles C Thomas, 1950.

Meryerding, H.W., and Stuck, W.G.: Painful Heels among Children (Apophysitis), J.A.M.A. 102:1658, 1934.

Overton, L.M.: Osteochondritis of Growth Centers, Ann. Surg. 101:1062, 1935.

Rigler, L.G.: *Outline of Roentgen Diagnosis.* Atlas ed. Philadelphia: J.B. Lippincott Co., 1938.

Ritvo, M.: *Bone and Joint X-ray Diagnosis.* Philadelphia: Lea & Febiger Co., 1955.

Sante, L.: *Principles of Roentgenological Interpretation.* Ann Arbor, Mich.: Edwards Bros., Inc., 1940.

Sever, J.W.: Apophysitis of the Os Calcis, New York J. Med. 95:1025, 1912.

Urban, L.C.: Roentgenological Interpretation of Diseases of the Foot, Chiropody Rec. 21:60, 1938.

Weinmann, J.P., and Sicher, H.: *Bone and Bones.* St. Louis: C.V. Mosby Co., 1947.

Yale, I.: *Clinical and Roentgenological Interpretations in Lower Extremities.* Chiropody Literature, Ansonia, Conn., 1952.

Yale, I.: A Statistical Report on 1290 Foot Radiographs, J. Nat. Ass. Chiropodists, 47:6, 1957.

5 JOINT DISEASES

Feet are frequently afflicted by arthritic changes. Many arthritic persons seek their first medical attention because of painful feet. Early diagnosis is essential to help the patient maintain maximal usefulness. The chronicity of arthritis has caused the number of days lost from work by persons afflicted by rheumatic diseases to be second only to nervous and mental disease.

A comprehensive physical, laboratory, and roentgenologic examination is necessary to differentiate the type of arthritis or to recognize another disease causing the symptoms.

The American Rheumatism Association has proposed a tentative nomenclature and classification of arthritis and rheumatism. It will be obvious that many of the disease entities classified are not easily incorporated nor properly considered in a manual of foot roentgenology. This is the American Rheumatism Association (ARA) classification:

1. Polyarthritis of unknown etiology.
2. "Connective tissue" disorders.
3. Rheumatic fever.
4. Degenerative joint disease (osteoarthritis, osteoarthrosis).
5. Nonarticular rheumatism.
6. Diseases with which arthritis is frequently associated.
7. Associated with known infectious agents.
8. Traumatic and/or neurogenic disorders.
9. Associated with known biochemical or endocrine abnormalities.
10. Tumor and tumor-like conditions.
11. Allergy and drug reactions.
12. Inherited and congenital disorders.
13. Miscellaneous disorders.

GENERAL CLINICAL ORIENTATION

1. A comprehensive history of the patient is absolutely necessary because, when embarking upon a differential diagnosis of these 13 classifications, we may find many contributing diseases that are significant.

2. The physical examination supplements the history in its detail.

3. Adhesions in a joint may follow injury, infection, chronic strain, prolonged immobilization, arthritis, or a failure to rehabilitate an involved joint.

4. An infection of the joint may abolish all movement but usually, in less serious conditions, produces a periarticular fibrositis.

5. Chronic strain leads to inflammation with adhesions and stiffness in the small joints of the foot.

6. Injudicious and excessive immobilization of a joint leads to contractures of muscles and ligaments that produce considerable loss of function with pain on slight motion.

7. Arthritic changes may involve the articular ligaments, periarticular structures, articular cartilage, villi, and synovia.

GENERAL ROENTGENOLOGIC INTERPRETATION

1. The joints are made up by the articulating ends of bone. These ends are covered by hyaline cartilage which is not visible on the roentgenogram. A space of increased radiolucency is termed the joint space and is occupied by the articular cartilage. A cartilage line (joint space) is uniform in width, and the articular surfaces of the bones are smooth and have rounded margins.

2. If cartilage is destroyed, underdeveloped, overossified, or displaced, the joint space may be imbalanced or narrowed, roentgenographically speaking.

3. The joint space is widened when the articular cartilage is hypertrophied, overdevel-

oped, underossified, or if effusion exists.

4. Effusion is seen on the roentgenogram as an increase in soft-tissue density adjacent to the joint margin. This area of increase in density is smooth in outline and usually uniform. It lies within the confines of the joint capsule. The distention of the joint capsule may appear nodular or fusiform or be widespread about the joint. The effusion may contain hemorrhage, pus, synovia, hypertrophied villi, foreign bodies, tumor, and occasional chondromatosis. Tumors are nodular. Infections are spread throughout the joint with other physical signs of infection evident. Synovia usually appears fusiform within the articular capsule.

5. Loose bodies are usually calcareous deposits about the joints attached to strands of fibrous tissue. They are multiple and occur with degeneration of the periarticular connective tissue.

6. Osteochondromatosis results from degenerative changes in the cartilage with fibrosis, resorption, and calcification. These may be noted between the articulating margins of the joint.

7. Osteophytes, lipping, and spurs develop as degenerative changes. Arteriosclerosis, when present, is suggestive of the same degenerative changes in the vessel wall that occur at articular margins.

8. Lipping and spurs occur where the fibrous tissue meets the bone. Calcifications may develop and are confined within the contours of the fibrous ligaments and capsules.

9. Osteophytes are larger and develop from a broad base. They usually project at right angles to the bone axis.

10. Thermography is useful in the early diagnosis of neuropathic arthropathy in the feet of diabetics (Sardrow et al., 1972).

ARTHRITIS FREQUENTLY AFFECTING THE FEET

Degenerative Joint Disease

(Syn.: Hypertrophic arthritis; osteoarthritis; senescent arthritis.)

CLINICAL ORIENTATION

1. This degenerative joint disease is insidious, occurring most commonly after 40 years of age in overweight individuals. Patients complain of pain and stiffness with little obvious disability.

2. The painful effects of degeneration are seen most often in the fourth and fifth decades of life.

3. Numbness and stiffness with pain on arising after prolonged rest are common symptoms. The patient is generally well. The toes may be flexed and stiff at their proximal interphalangeal joints.

4. Passive or active motion in the extremes of range will cause pain.

5. Spasm and tenderness of the surrounding musculature are evident.

6. The articular margins of the affected joints are tender.

7. With progress of degenerative joint disease, there is a gradual, firm, irregular enlargement of the joint and on occasion the soft tissues are thickened.

8. Palpation may demonstrate crepitus of the joint during motion.

9. Trauma caused by faulty foot function and imbalanced weight distribution may cause an acute flareup of symptoms in a joint already degenerated but without changes demonstrable in the roentgenogram.

10. Heberden's nodes are found more frequently in women than in men. These small nodes develop as bony outgrowths from the lateral margins of the terminal phalanges of the fingers, less often the toes. They develop during middle life, persist throughout later life, and lead to stiffness and pain on slight flexion of the terminal phalanx. Rarely do individuals with Heberden's nodes develop any unusually severe generalized arthritis.

11. Ankylosis is uncommon in osteoarthritis even though the joint space is narrowed.

12. In osteoarthritis, the disability is usually not as great as that of rheumatoid arthritis. However, pain and swelling in the tarsus are the result of degenerative changes at the bony margins. Spurs may develop at the points of muscular, fascial, and ligamentous attachment.

13. Postmortem examination demonstrates that the primary changes are the result of degeneration in advancing age and functional stress of weight bearing. The feet are readily

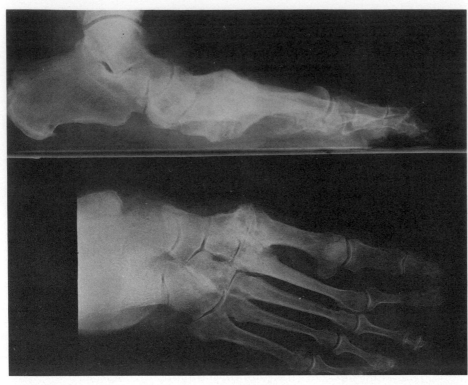

involved in patients suffering increased wear and tear through excessive or abnormal use of a joint. Mechanical defects will cause degenerative changes to develop sooner. Female patients are more commonly affected by clinical manifestations.

ROENTGENOLOGIC INTERPRETATION
(Fig. 78)

1. Degenerative changes in the form of metaplasia of fibrous tissues, such as lipping, osteophytes, spurs, and loose bodies, may develop early. The joint space is often imbalanced. With marked destruction of cartilage, the ends of the bones come into contact with each other, resulting in sclerosis or eburnation with fraying of the joint margins.

2. Loose bodies are visible only when calcified. Chondrifications and calcification of portions of synovial villi or soft tissue may form loose bodies. Torn portions of cartilage or osteophytes calcify and become loose bodies attached to bone by fibrous strands of villi.

3. A chondromatosis may occur outside the joint proper with no indication of degenerative changes in the joint.

4. The following joints of the foot are most commonly affected by osteoarthritis: the talocrural, subtalar, talonavicular, naviculocuneiform, and the first metatarsophalangeal articulations. The second metatarsophalangeal joint is affected through abnormal weight distribution, whereas all other joints mentioned may develop osteoarthritic changes with only ordinary function in everyday stress under normal environmental conditions.

Traumatic Arthritis

CLINICAL ORIENTATION

1. This form of arthritis is of greatest interest to the podiatrist because of its affect on the pedal extremities.

2. Traumatic arthritis is a frequent cause of disability following sudden or multiple minimal injuries or a single heavy blow.

3. The foot is subject to trauma from malfunction, occupational stress, and postural imbalance. It is an excellent example of a site that receives multiple minimal traumata. Ninety percent of a group of linemen on a football team with an average age of 23 years have shown pathologic changes in the ankle joint and feet on roentgenologic examination. Linemen who were usually heavy and had played

football 9 years or more had the highest incidence and most severe types of joint problems (Vincelette, 1972).

4. The use of a foot press, sewing machine, or automobile brake has a traumatizing effect on feet.

5. Pressure on a part of the foot from ill-fitting shoes, braces, or arch supports may cause traumatic arthritis in one or more joints of the foot.

6. The pressure of narrow, pointed shoes on the first and fifth metatarsophalangeal joints, as well as the back pressure on the metatarsal heads from short shoes, may produce arthritic changes in the articular cartilage of the metatarsophalangeal joints. Hallux abductus valgus or hallux rigidus may result from trauma. The fifth metatarsophalangeal joint may develop a typical tailor's bunion of digiti quinti varus with subsequent arthritic changes.

7. Ill-fitting hose may result in mild traumata to the interphalangeal and metatarso phalangeal joints.

8. Traumatic arthritic changes may develop in the interphalangeal joints causing the typical hammer toe or digiti flexus.

9. The metatarsal heads are commonly traumatized by short shoes and hose which cause an improper ratio of weight distribution on the metatarsus with associated traumatic arthritis.

10. Pressure over the dorsum of the foot from heavy eyelets may produce degenerative arthritis in the cuneo-first metatarsal joint.

11. Calcaneal spurs develop as a result of a periosteal tear, sudden strain, or repeated trauma. Degenerative calcification at the attachment of the plantar fascia is not uncommon. This may be occupational, functional, or accidental and may produce arthritic changes in the heel.

12. A misstep, sudden twist, or severe sprain can cause arthritic phenomena and changes in the calcaneocuboid and talocrural

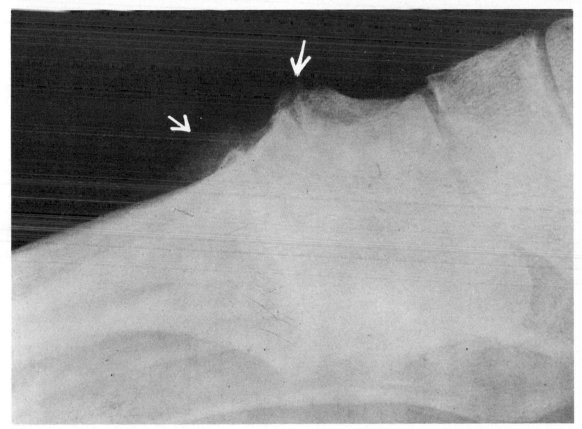

Fig. 79. Traumatic arthritis
1. Degenerative calcification at first metatarsocuneiform joint.
2. An osteochondroma is seen developing just distal to the traumatic arthritis.

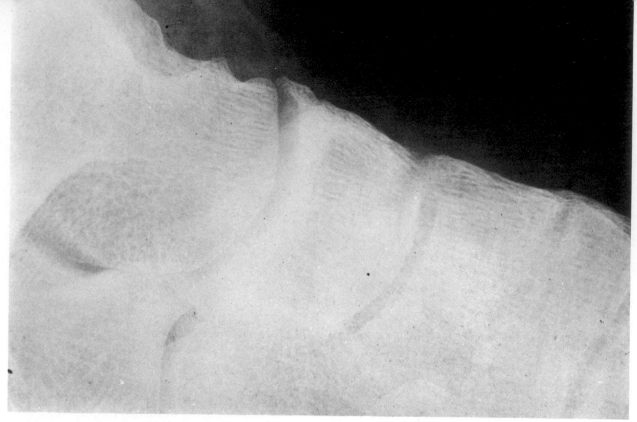

Fig. 80. Traumatic arthritis
1. Spur projecting back from the concave posterior articular surface of the navicular.
2. Subarticular sclerosis, posterior concave surface of navicular.

articulations. The concave posterior surface of the navicular shows evidence of a subarticular sclerosis from the stress of the pressure exerted through its articulation with the head of the talus.

13. Abnormal function in a joint because of bony deformity may cause arthritic changes.

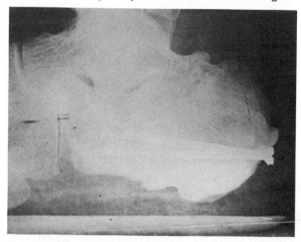

Fig. 81. Traumatic arthritis
1. Note narrowed subtalar joint and irregular destruction of bone.
2. Metallic density is evidenced by screws of greater density than cortex.

14. Obesity, flat feet, and poor posture will damage the weight-bearing joints. Articular cartilage when damaged will not regenerate and therefore may produce traumatic arthritis when injured. Synovial tissue does regenerate.

15. As a result of faulty biomechanics of the foot, the metatarsus and tarsus are put through abnormal ranges of motion causing injury to the joints.

16. Muscle spasm and limitation of motion are common symptoms of traumatic arthritis, although many times trauma may produce pain on motion and muscle spasm without obvious joint changes.

17. Traumatic arthritis is usually monarticular. The patient complains of pain in the affected joint on passive or active function. Motion is limited by contractures. Edema and muscle spasm are present. Joint effusion may or may not be present, depending on the stage of the lesion.

18. The onset of the articular changes may develop within a short time following trauma. The first symptoms may result from reaction in the periarticular structures followed by pathologic changes in the joint and bone.

19. Pathologically, there are degeneration

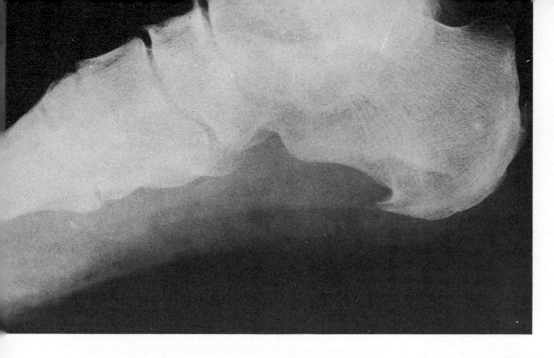

Fig. 82. Calcaneal spurs. Also note squaring off of articular margins of navicular with lipping and osteophytes.

of the articular cartilage and fibrosis of the joint capsule. Thickening of the synovial membrane occurs with production of new bone around the articular margins.

20. Many times repeated minor traumata may have gone by unnoticed, and a careful history will be required to differentiate between traumatic and degenerative joint disease.

21. To establish a diagnosis of traumatic arthritis, a knowledge of the previous condition of the affected joint is necessary. An examination of the opposite foot will give a fairly accurate picture of what is normal in this particular patient.

22. When the joint functions normally without pain, one can rule out a traumatic joint disease. Periarticular structures may be involved.

23. The first change following trauma to a joint is synovitis.

24. The formation of periarticular fibrous connective tissue may cause stiffness in the joints of the feet after an injury.

25. Limitation of motion with pain is evident; muscular spasm and contractures occur later. Tears of the joint capsule may result in adhesions and cause a stiffness of the joint. Calcareous degeneration may result in formation of lipping and osteophytes.

26. Third-degree burns may result in scars and disabling contractures. No growth discrepancies in bone and joints have been noted following pinning to avoid the deforming states of contractures that follow burns.

ROENTGENOLOGIC INTERPRETATION
(Figs. 79-86)

1. Significant changes are not recognized on the roentgenogram in the early stages of traumatic arthritis.

2. A synovitis may result in profuse swelling and effusion, while a sprain may cause pain and limitation of motion for years.

3. An intra-articular injection of a contrast medium will often disclose damage to the joint structures.

4. Hypertrophic changes, such as lipping and osteophytes that develop after weeks or months, may be demonstrated.

5. Injuries to a joint may present the appearance of hypertrophic arthritis, and existing arthritides are many times aggravated by injuries to the involved joint.

Polyarthritis of Unknown Etiology

(Syn.: rheumatoid arthritis; proliferative arthritis; chronic rheumatic arthritis; primary progressive polyarthritis; nonspecific infectious polyarthritis.)

CLINICAL ORIENTATION

1. This chronic systemic disease of unknown etiology is manifested by a chronic progressive polyarthritis with systemic and local symptoms.

2. Migrating symptoms of pain, stiffness, and swelling in the early stages are followed by deformities, contractures with fibrous and

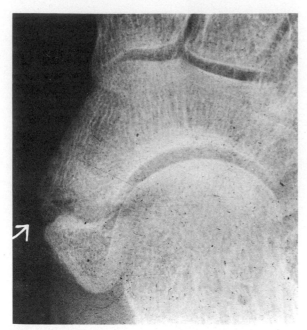

Fig. 83. Os tibiale externum. Traumatic arthritis at the fibrocartilaginous attachment of the accessory bone to the tuberosity of the navicular.

bony ankylosis, and subcutaneous nodules in the later stages.

3. The etiologic factors are so variable and unrelated that a search for the cause usually results in confusion. Infectious disease, bacterial allergy, peripheral circulatory involvements, an endocrinologic base, virus infection, trauma, and avitaminosis have all been suggested as etiologic.

4. The rheumatoid arthritic is generally ill and must be handled accordingly.

5. This disease commonly occurs in thin, asthenic persons between 20 and 40 years of age. In the early stages, the patient may be well nourished. Loss of weight is moderate, and the hands and feet perspire profusely. Often, the initial complaints are fatigue, exhaustion, vasomotor disturbances, muscular stiffness, loss of weight, and general debility. A low-grade temperature which persists for many months may be an early symptom.

6. The feet may be the first joints involved with characteristic changes in the hands occurring later. This early onset must be differentiated from biomechanical dysfunction of the feet. Biomechanical problems are usually relieved with rest. The foot pain of rheumatoid arthritis is severe after inactivity.

7. The proximal interphalangeal joints of the fingers are affected early. In severe disease, however, practically every joint in the body may be involved.

8. The onset is usually insidious, affecting joints by swelling, stiffness, and pain bilaterally and symmetrically. Commonly, the patient presents a fusiform swelling at the proximal interphalangeal joints. The synovial and periarticular tissues thicken, and atrophy of the muscles, proximal and distal to the involved joints, gives them this spindle-shaped appearance. Contractures may result from shrinkage of the noncontractile connective tissues. The toes have a fibular deviation. The skin on the foot in advanced stages becomes atrophic, smooth, shiny, discolored, cold, and clammy. Synovitis with pain of the metatarsophalangeal joints is an indication for synovectomy.

9. Muscular weakness and atrophy are

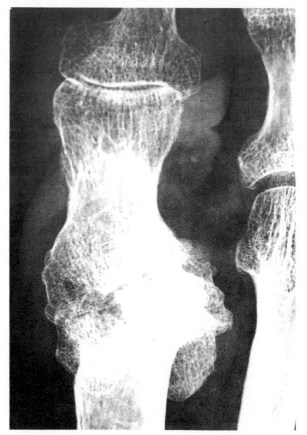

Fig. 84. Postoperative arthritis. Complete ankylosis of first metatarsophalangeal joint, right foot.

prominent objective findings.

10. Subcutaneous nodules may develop at sites of trauma.

11. The peripheral circulation may be decreased, and moderate tachycardia is often present. The surface temperature of the skin is diminished.

12. While rheumatoid arthritis may become quiescent, the persistent compensatory splinting of the painful joints by muscular contractions results in an undue function of the antagonists. The flexors, usually the stronger muscles, exert a great pull on the toes and cause a marked flexion with fibular deviation of the toes. The hallux is usually everted, and an overlying bursal sac, reddish-blue in color, is prominent.

13. A high blood sedimentation rate helps

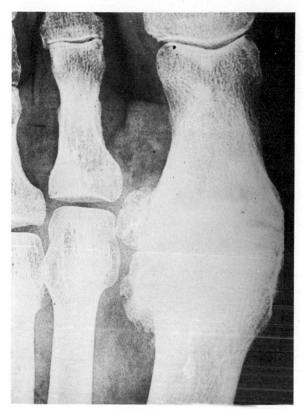

Fig. 86. Traumatic arthritis. Note narrowed joint space, sclorosis, and extraskeletal calcification.

differentiate rheumatoid arthritis from osteoarthritis.

14. A secondary anemia is common and responds very little to the usual therapy. There is a diminution in the number of erythrocytes with a corresponding drop in hemoglobin. The red cell count may drop to 2.5-3 million and the hemoglobin about 50% in the severe process. The white cell count is normal except in acute disease where a leukocytosis may be present.

15. Patients with ulcerative colitis may show joint changes similar to rheumatoid arthritis, and a careful history and consultation is always advisable.

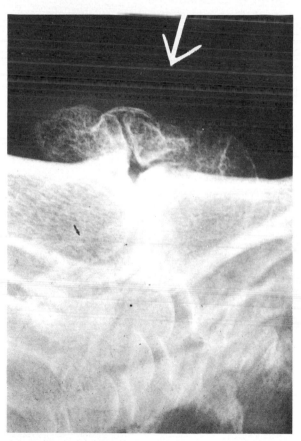

Fig. 85. Osteochondromatosis secondary to trauma

1. Note the loose body.
2. Osteophytes and irregular ossification with scalloped margin growing out from the articular surfaces.

ROENTGENOLOGIC INTERPRETATION
(Figs. 87-93)

1. A decrease in density of the ends of the long bones is demonstrated early.

2. Fusiform effusion within the capsule at the proximal interphalangeal joints of the fin-

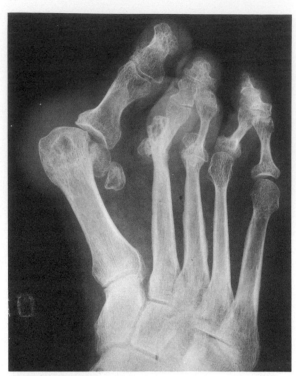

Fig. 87. Polyarthritis of unknown cause — rheumatoid arthritis

1. Systemic deossification of bone.

2. Dislocation and subluxation of metatarsophalangeal joints.

3. Pathognomonic fibular deviation of all toes.

gers is also an early finding. When the effusion is great, the patient complains of stiffness and pain.

3. The fusiform increase in density within the articular capsule is not to be confused with soft-tissue swelling. *Effusion* is confined within the joint capsule. Its density is increased and uniform with a smooth outline. *Swellings* are diffuse with infiltrated markings of increased soft-tissue density external to the joint capsule.

4. Cortical destruction or atrophic loss of substance of the metatarsal heads appears early.

5. Later findings present narrowed joint spaces, general demineralization and punched-out areas of atrophic loss of substance, subluxations, deformity, ankylosis, or possibly reparative calcifications.

6. Atrophic loss of substance occurs at the chondro-osseous margins of the joints. In gout, the areas of loss of substance are larger than those seen in rheumatoid arthritis.

7. The systemic demineralizations occur later due to limited mobility and loss of function in severely affected joints. Degenerative joint changes secondary to rheumatoid arthritis may occur late in the disease. Osteophytes and lippings may be present to becloud the diagnosis.

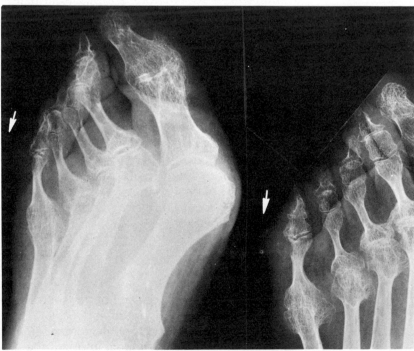

Fig. 88. Polyarthritis — infected bursa

1. Atrophic loss of bone substance at chondro-osseus margins.

2. Note fusion of interphalangeal joint of hallux and fifth metatarsophalangeal joints with narrowed joint spaces.

3. Systemic demineralization.

4. Marked increase in density of soft tissue, clearly outlined fifth toe.

8. With correlation of clinical and laboratory findings, the typical rheumatoid arthritis offers little difficulty in diagnosis.

Acute Rheumatic Fever

CLINICAL ORIENTATION

1. Acute rheumatic fever is thought to be an infectious but noncontagious disease characterized by irregular fever, polyarthritis, subcutaneous nodules, inflammation of cardiac tissue, pleuritis, and with a dramatic response to antirheumatic drugs.

2. It occurs in youth and early adult life. In childhood, girls are more commonly affected, and in adult life, men are more prone to the disease.

3. There are many predisposing factors to this disease. There is a hereditary history of rheumatism in one third of the cases.

4. Acute rheumatic fever is aggravated by damp and changeable weather. Occupational stress is a common cause in persons exposed to the elements.

5. The prodromal symptoms last for a few days or hours and consist of general malaise, shooting pains in the limbs, and a sense of fatigue.

6. The onset is sudden with chills, eleva-

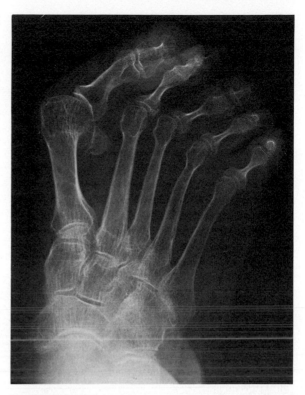

Fig. 89. Polyarthritis — rheumatoid arthritis
1. Dislocated metatarsophalangeal joints.
2. Lateral deflection of toes.
3. Systemic demineralization.

Fig. 90. Polyarthritis of unknown cause
1. The first metatarsophalangeal joint is ankylosed in the left foot
2. Loss of interarticular spaces in the tarsus of the right foot.
3. Systemic deossification of bone.
4. Thinning of the cortices.
5. Lateral deflection of toes is pathognomonic.

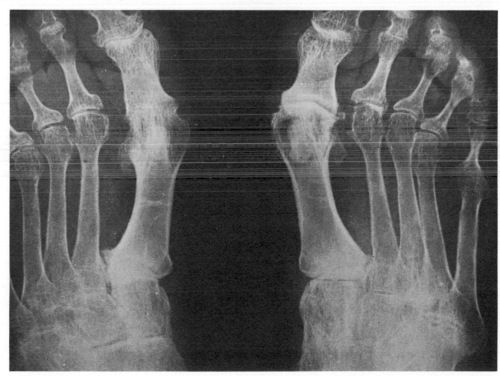

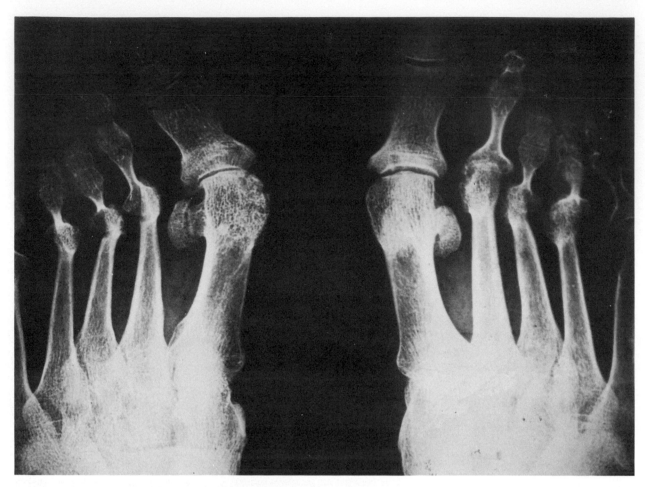

Fig. 91. Polyarthritis of unknown cause — rheumatoid arthritis
1. Systemic demineralization of bones.
2. Destruction of metatarsophalangeal joints.
3. Atrophic loss of substance, margin of joints.
4. Lateral luxation of toes.

tion of temperature, and pain in one or more joints.

7. Arthritis affects the lower extremities first. This involves the larger joints, usually in the following order: knees, ankles, shoulders, and wrists. No joint is immune, however, and several joints are affected simultaneously or successively. The infection shifts from joint to joint, and one joint may be affected several times. The joints are painful, tender to touch, and reddened. The patient lies motionless to avoid pain, which is worse at night. The pain is greatest in superficial joints.

8. The temperature ranges between 101°F to 104°F. It is irregular, remittent, and declines by lysis.

9. The skin is covered by copious perspiration, and the tongue is thickly coated and whitish. The patient is constipated.

10. Blood findings usually show a decreased red blood count and hemoglobin with a leukocytosis present. The erythrocytic sedimentation is rapid.

11. The urine is scant, dark, loaded with uric acid and urates, and the specific gravity is increased.

12. Heart involvement results in 40% of all cases. Myocarditis usually accompanies endocarditis and pericarditis as secondary sequelae to rheumatic fever.

13. The disease may terminate in 10-14 days; commonly it lasts 4-5 weeks. It may last several months.

ROENTGENOLOGIC INTERPRETATION

1. Soft-tissue swelling is visualized with increase in density and thickness of the soft tissues.

2. Effusion is noted with an increase in density of the joint soft tissues within the capsule.

3. Joint spaces are widened where acute inflammation exists.

Gout (Podagra)

CLINICAL ORIENTATION

1. Fifty percent of the cases give a history of heredity and practically no racial group is free of this disease.

2. Gout occurs in middle life (30-45) and more commonly in men. About 6% of the gouty cases reported are women.

3. Predisposing factors are heavy wines, beers, or ales, sedentary habits, and excessive eating, especially of meat.

4. The first attack usually occurs in winter and is precipitated by overindulgence, emotional upset, change in environment, fatigue, and local injury. It is conceivable that gout is an allergic manifestation.

5. Acute inflammation of a small joint, the first metatarsophalangeal joint, occurs in 60%-78% of the cases and is indicative of gout. The attack begins late at night or in the early morning. The patient is aroused by an excruciating pain, burning, throbbing, or aching. The painful joint is swollen, red, violaceous, and tender. Slight motion or pressure causes great distress. The toe is shiny, often slightly cyanotic, and the superficial veins are distended. The attack resumes at night with pain, usually subsiding somewhat during the day. Swelling and tenderness disappear in about 2 weeks after the initial onset. Itching and desquamation of the part may ensue following acute symptoms.

6. There may be a temperature of 100°F-101°F, restlessness, chilliness, and the digestion may be disturbed.

7. Attacks may occur at long intervals of years or may develop every few months. The attacks become less severe, last longer, involve a greater number of joints, and may result in residual stiffness and deformity in the chronic state. Attacks may last 2-8 days, become more frequent, and overlap.

8. The normal level of uric acid in the blood is 2.5-5.5 mg/100 ml of blood. A level

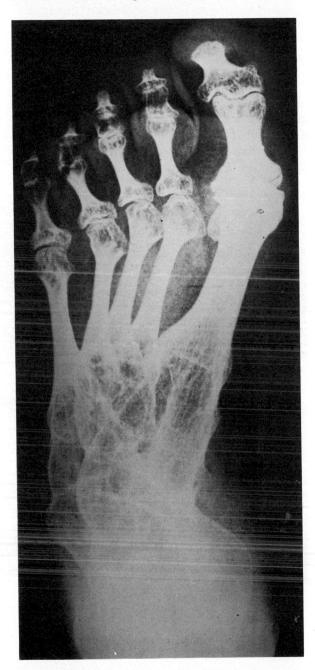

Fig. 92. Polyarthritis juvenilis of unknown cause — Still's disease — juvenile rheumatoid arthritis

1. Spotty deossification, ends of long bones.
2. Complete bony ankylosis of tarsal and tarsometatarsal articulations.

over 6.0 is indicative of gout. This rise is also seen in leukemia, starvation, lead poisoning, and kidney disease.

9. The blood uric acid level may be decreased before an attack, increased during an attack, and normal between attacks.

10. The urine is acid, dark, and of a high specific gravity. It contains an overabundance of uric acid crystals.

11. Variable-sized urate concretions can be palpated in the margins of the ears and in and about joints with permanent thickening of periarticular tissues with deformity.

12. The diagnosis may be confirmed by examination of the tophaceous deposits. The characteristic needle-shaped crystals of monosodium urates are visible.

13. This disease must be differentiated from acute rheumatic fever, atypical rheumatoid arthritis, gonorrheal arthritis, periarticular fibrositis, psoriatic arthritis, and hemophilic arthritis.

14. Recently, the author has observed a significant number of acutely inflamed joints in the foot simulating the clinical findings in gout. The patients have been taking thiazide diuretics for a prolonged period of time resulting in an induced hyperuricemia. The excretion of fluids had obviously increased the solid urates.

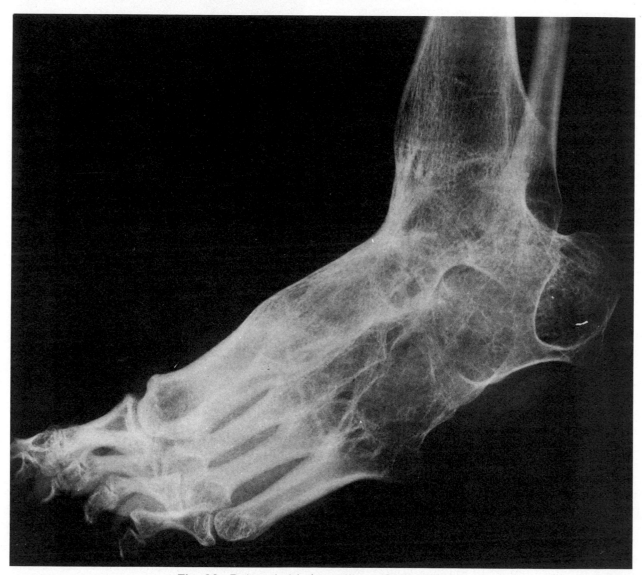

Fig. 93. Polyarthritis juvenilis — Still's disease

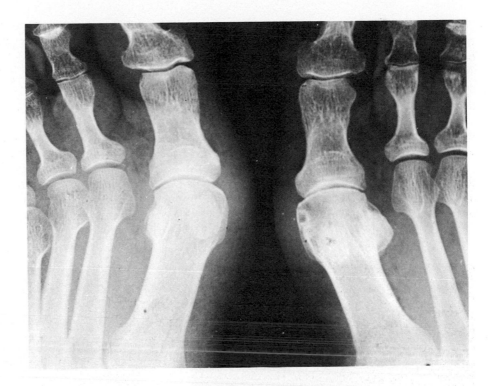

Fig. 94. Early acute gout

1. Note the swelling of the soft tissues as evidenced by a thickening of the soft tissues about the left hallucal joint.

2. A small, punched-out area of atrophic loss of substance is present at the medial aspect of the first metatarsal head, right foot, due to a previous attack.

ROENTGENOLOGIC INTERPRETATIONS
(Figs. 94-96)

1. The marked increase in thickness and density of soft tissues that develops adjacent to a painful joint may be visualized in the roentgenogram.

2. Changes in the bones and joints are observed only after repeated attacks. The diagnosis is made early through clinical and laboratory findings.

3. The characteristic roentgenologic findings are marked soft-tissue swelling, atrophic loss of substance, and eroded cystlike areas at or near the chondro-osseous margins of the afflicted joint. These areas of increased translucency resemble somewhat the changes that take place in rheumatoid arthritis and may also be confused with small bone cysts or fibrocystic degeneration.

4. Tophaceous deposits in the ends of bones expand greatly.

5. Entire joints may disappear leaving a shapeless tophaceous mass.

6. Subchondral lesions may simulate certain bone tumors or cysts.

7. The punched-out areas of atrophic loss of substance are usually larger in gout than those found in rheumatoid arthritis. In the ad-

vanced stages, there may be hypertrophic and destructive changes secondary to the gouty lesions.

8. Areas of loss of bone substance must be differentiated from those that occur in rheumatoid and degenerative joint disease, tuberculosis, syphilitic destruction of bone, certain of the mycotic bone disorders, reticuloendothelial disease, cysts, and tumors.

Differential Diagnosis of Rheumatic Fever from Biomechanical Dysfunction ("Growing Pains")

1. The term "growing pains" is confusing and doubtful. We believe that all such pains, when rheumatic disease has been excluded, are the result of biomechanical dysfunctions of the extremities.

2. In the so-called "growing pains" there is no swelling, redness or effusion, but the pains are noted in the muscles, ligaments, joints, and tendons of the feet and legs.

3. There is no tenderness, but the pain is more nagging and nonspecific.

4. In "growing pains," the patient is sullen, usually tired, and often affected by faulty foot balance.

5. Nodules occur in the rheumatic patient but are not found as the result of biomechanical defect.

6. In "growing pains" there are no cardiac symptoms, such as tachycardia, and the temperature is normal.

7. There is no anemia in "growing pains" and no history of focal infection, such as a sore throat.

8. The so-called "pavor nocturnas," a night terror or shrill cry uttered by a child in his sleep, may usher in an acute joint condition and is not related to faulty foot function.

ARTHRITIS DUE TO KNOWN INFECTIOUS AGENTS

GENERAL CLINICAL ORIENTATION

Joint diseases caused by staphylococcus, streptococcus, pneumococcus, gonococcus, meningococcus, tubercle bacillus, *Treponema pallidum,* and other bacteria or their toxins are found in this group.

About 50% of these arthritic involvements are due to infection by staphylococcus and the hemolytic streptococcus. Joints in the foot are

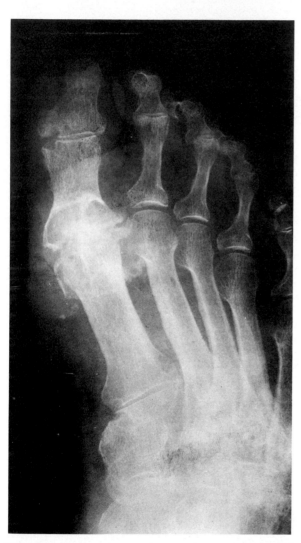

Fig. 95. Gout. Large defects of atrophic loss of substance, first metatarsophalangeal and interphalangeal joints at chondro-osseous margins.

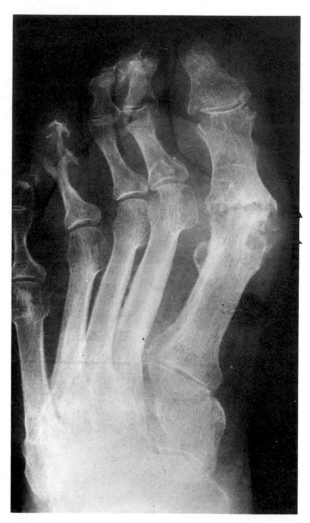

Fig. 96. Chronic gout
1. Note the large areas of atrophic loss of substance at the first metatarsophalangeal and interphalangeal joints.
2. Tophaceous deposits adjacent to joints.

reached through the circulatory system from a distant focus of infection. The bacteria may invade the joint by extension from a suppurative process in adjacent bone or soft tissue or infection may develop by direct entrance from a deep wound or sinus tract.

Pathologic Features

1. The articular structures present a histologic appearance of an acute suppurative inflammation.

2. Synovial tissue is hyperemic, swollen, thickened, and infiltrated with an abundance of polymorphonuclear leukocytes.

3. With prolonged infection, the leukocytic enzymes resorb the articular cartilage causing active destruction and loss of substance.

4. The periarticular connective tissues become inflamed, and when the infection is long standing, severe damage of the cartilage and ankylosis may occur.

5. Abscesses may develop in the epiphyseal tissue or the bone marrow.

Clinical Considerations

1. The joint infection is not as severe as the systemic symptoms, and very often the joint disease is overlooked.

2. The arthritis may be obscure at times without systemic symptoms.

3. There may be a sudden onset with fever, chills, hyperidrosis, fatigue, and anorexia.

4. The joint has all the cardinal signs of inflammation accompanied by exquisite pain.

5. The joint capsule is distended with effusion. Muscles inserting about the joint are in spasm.

6. The joints of the feet are infrequently affected.

7. Only one or two joints are involved in the average process.

8. When the infection is without treatment for a few weeks, the prognosis is poor.

Laboratory Findings

1. A leukocytosis with a rise in the polymorphonuclear cells is common, and a finding of 90% polymorphonuclear cells is not uncommon.

2. Sedimentation of erythrocytes is rapid. A smear or blood culture may isolate the of-

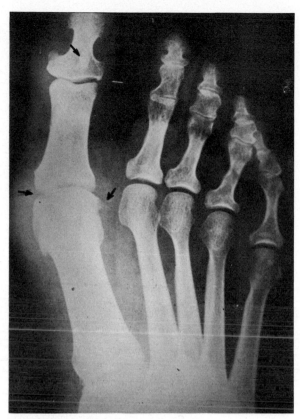

Fig. 97. Tuberculous arthritis
1. Monarticular involvement of marked doughy soft-tissue swelling.
2. Narrowing of joint space and early destruction of bone.
3. Hallux is pulled away from second toe because of spasm of the musculature.
4. Base of distal phalanx presents a compact island of academic interest.

---

fending organism.
3. The synovial fluid is cloudy or purulent, and leukocytes may number 100,000 per ml.

Diagnosis

1. The diagnosis is based on the acute onset of monarticular arthritis characterized by redness, exquisite pain associated with a fever, leukocytosis, elevated sedimentation rate, bacteremia, and the presence of a causative organism on smear or culture of the blood and synovial fluid.

Tuberculosis of Joints

CLINICAL ORIENTATION
1. Tuberculous joints usually occur in chil-

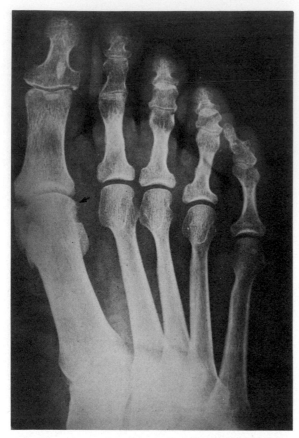

Fig. 98. Tuberculous arthritis. Several months later, spasm has subsided; active destruction at chondro-osseous margins of first metatarsophalangeal joint.

dren and are common in adults after trivial injury when there is a tuberculous history.

2. Nodular thickening of the synovial membrane with serous effusion is common with an extensive monarticular, palpable periarticular swelling.

3. Infection in the joints is usually by invasion from the cancellous ends of bone.

4. Joints are cool to mildly warm to touch, doughy, and swollen.

5. There is occasional pain with overuse, especially at rest after periods of activity.

6. A slight limp with poor function of the joint is followed by a gradual development of swelling and muscular atrophy.

7. If the ankle is involved, it becomes sensitive to sudden movements; stiffness and valgus deformity may develop.

8. Skin pallor, spasms, and tissue sensitivity become evident along with systemic symptoms of fever, loss of weight, and excessive perspiration.

9. Disease affecting the spine may cause neurologic symptoms referable to the extremities.

10. Following destruction and cavitation, joint function is lost.

ROENTGENOLOGIC INTERPRETATION
(Figs. 97-99)

1. Tuberculous arthritis is a slow, chronically progressive, usually monarticular disease.

2. The first roentgenologic signs consist of a haziness or cloudiness of the joint due to periarticular swelling, massive synovial effusion, and thickening.

3. Decreased density of the infected bone with abscess formation is a common sequel.

4. The gradual development of soft-tissue spasms may cause joint deformity.

5. After many months, the joint space is narrowed, and this is followed by erosion and destruction of cartilage and adjacent bone.

6. A dry tuberculous infection and destruction with irregular light sequestration may occur without first undergoing massive effusion.

7. Effusion generally subsides when an arthrodesis develops.

Gonorrheal Arthritis

CLINICAL ORIENTATION

1. This arthritis may develop suddenly in both sexes.

2. The causative organism spreads from a primary focus in the genitourinary tract through the lymphatics and blood stream to the synovial tissues.

3. Massive effusion develops quickly and subsides as rapidly in 3-6 weeks.

4. Joint lesions may develop 10-30 days after the initial infection.

5. The arthritis often develops several years after the onset of a prostatitis or urethritis.

6. The sudden onset, at first, may involve several joints, finally affecting a single joint in a few days.

7. Tenosynovitis and other forms of arthritis are common inflammatory diseases in the

foot to be considered in the differential diagnosis.

LABORATORY FINDINGS.

1. Aspiration of the joint fluid in the infected joint and its examination by smear, culture, or inoculation into guinea pigs are necessary to corroborate clinical and roentgenologic findings.

2. The reaction to a complement-fixation test becomes positive within 10-20 days of the onset of the arthritis in 90% of the cases.

ROENTGENOLOGIC INTERPRETATION

1. Effusion is extreme but subsides early.

2. The affected small bones and joints become decreased in density and the deossification lasts longer than the effusion.

3. The severe deossification appears as a destructive process, but destruction of bone itself does not occur.

Bacterial Arthritis

CLINICAL ORIENTATION

1. This type of arthritis is the result of infectious invasion of the joint by pyogenic organisms, such as staphylococcus, streptococcus, meningococcus, brucella, and pneumococcus.

2. Pyogenic arthritis may be acute or chronic.

3. In the acute phase, there are swelling, redness, heat, and pain with effusion.

4. Suppuration may follow with destruction of the joint tissue.

5. Early pyogenic infectious arthritis must be differentiated from the following:
   a. Sprain or contusion.
   b. Rheumatoid arthritis.
   c. Early gonorrheal arthritis.

ROENTGENOLOGIC INTERPRETATION
(Fig. 100)

1. A flat, hazy, indistinct articular bone is noted 1 or 2 days after onset and effusion and swelling may be evident.

2. A loss of substance *en masse* may be

visible in 2 or 3 weeks.

3. As the infection subsides, the soft-tissue changes clear.

4. Recurrences of the arthritis may present reactive swelling in a reaction area.

5. The infected joint space may appear widened due to cartilaginous destruction and effusion.

6. The joint space is narrowed when infec-

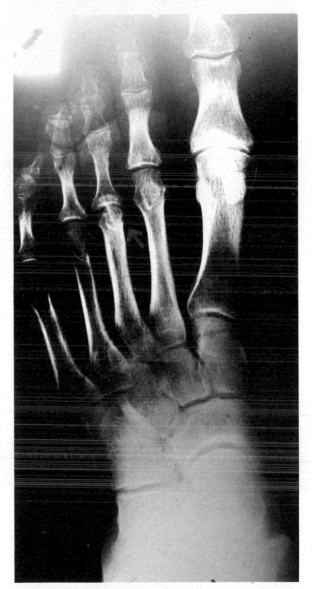

Fig. 99. Tuberculous arthritis

1. Note destruction of articular cartilage and narrowing of third metatarsophalangeal joint.

2. This is a slow, chronic, and insidious development.

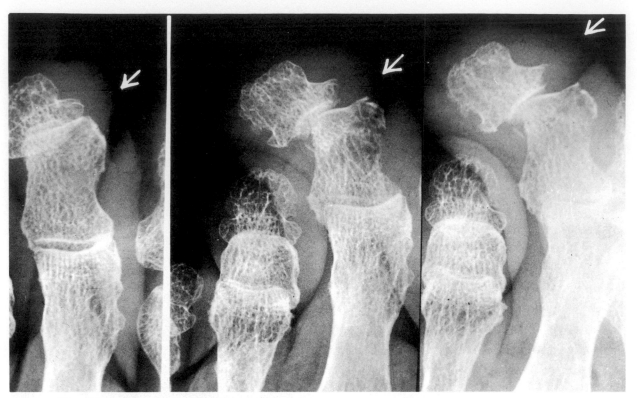

Fig. 100. Pyogenic arthritis
1. Progressive dislocation of distal phalanx with invasion of destructive infection.
2. Active destruction, middle phalanx.

tion of the joint has been severe.

7. Infectious subperiosteal changes may take place in the moderately advanced disease.

8. Ankylosis may occur late in pyogenic arthritis.

Syphilitic Arthritis

CLINICAL ORIENTATION

1. Syphilitic arthritis occurs in both the congenital and acquired types of syphilis in infancy, childhood, or early adult life.

2. Direct spirochetal invasion of the joint or a neurogenic factor causing a Charcot joint secondary to tabes is the causative factor.

3. Marked objective findings of swelling, discoloration, and deformity of a joint manifesting few or no subjective complaints are suspicious of a luetic arthritis. The feet are rarely affected.

4. This arthritis has an insidious onset without fever, and there is no evidence of muscular spasm, atrophy, or loss of function as seen in a tuberculous arthritis.

5. The joints are more painful at rest than after motion, a differentiation from the chronic arthritides.

6. The diagnosis of joint syphilis can rest on serology, guinea pig inoculation of infected joint fluid, or a therapeutic test.

CLINICAL TYPES OF SYPHILITIC ARTHRITIS.

1. Arthralgia due to syphilis.

a. There may be vague muscle and joint pains.

b. There are no joint changes in early acquired syphilis.

2. Osteochondritis, periostitis, and synovitis.

a. Syphilitic infants may present osteochondritis, periostitis, and epiphysitis as early manifestations of the disease.

b. Motion is limited and the joints are swollen but painless on manipulation.

c. A painless, symmetric synovitis is seen in older children, 8-10 years of age. It usually affects knee joints.

d. No bony changes or ankylosis are noted at this time.

e. This condition must be differentiated from knee disturbances caused by faulty foot biomechanics.

3. Gummatous arthritis.

a. Gummatous lesions are seen in the tertiary stage of syphilis.

b. They are frequently monarticular.

c. A gumma may start in the bone or periarticular structures and invade or extend into an adjacent joint.

d. Swelling is noted without heat, and there is little or no pain, stiffness, or local muscle spasm.

e. Bone destruction is noted on the roentgenogram.

4. Charcot joint secondary to syphilis.

a. This type of lesion may develop in peripheral neuropathies due to syringomyelia, diabetes, as well as syphilis.

b. Loss of the sensation of pain and position results in trophic and degenerative changes in the joints.

c. The joint is used in an awkward and disorganized manner.

d. Monarticular and occasionally symmetrical development in joints is characteristic.

e. The affected joint becomes large and deformed, flail-like in motion, and painless. It may be flexed, extended, and rotated to a marked degree.

f. There is no redness, tenderness, or warmth.

g. Neurologic signs, such as loss of deep muscle reflexes, positive Romberg's sign, and Argyll Robertson pupils, may be present.

h. Response to antiluetic treatment may prove the diagnosis.

ROENTGENOLOGIC INTERPRETATION
(Figs. 101-104)

1. Evidences for bone destruction are recognized in the roentgenogram in gummatous arthritis.

2. The Charcot joint presents a characteristic "bag of bones" appearance with destructive and productive bone disturbance associated with pathologic fractures, disorganiza-

tion, and disintegration of the joint. The destruction is transverse to the long axis of the bone.

3. Irregular detritus is seen at the margins of the massive effusion.

OTHER JOINT-RELATED DISEASES

The differential diagnosis of the arthritides and other joint-related diseases requires a broad knowledge of many systems and the roentgenogram is but one diagnostic tool. Within the scope of this text, however, it is necessary to limit the discussion to the clinical and roentgenologic features.

Periarticular Fibrositis

CLINICAL ORIENTATION

1. Fibrositis commonly affects the feet following injury and is characterized by soreness, stiffness, and pain on arising after periods of rest.

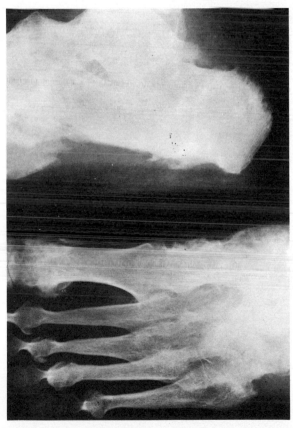

Fig. 101. Syphilitic arthritis and periostitis. Destruction of joints with a lacework periosteal reaction.

2. On arising in the morning, the first few steps are made with a limp. This gradually disappears only to come back after prolonged weight bearing.

3. The disease involves the periarticular fibrous connective tissue.

4. The most commonly affected joints are the talocrural, first metatarsophalangeal, talonavicular, and first and second metatarsocuneiform joints.

ROENTGENOLOGIC INTERPRETATION

1. In the early stages, there is no evidence of bony changes.

2. Following the acute episodes of pain, swelling of soft tissues may be visualized.

3. In the subacute and chronic state, lack of use of the part results in a disuse atrophy and deossification of adjacent bone.

Neuroarthropathy

CLINICAL ORIENTATION

1. Articular and periarticular changes may develop in the lower extremities of paraplegics and hemiplegics. Neuroarthropathy may be seen in patients with spina bifida or neurologic disorders of the vertebral column or spinal cord and in those who have sustained injury to the posterior nerve roots or a peripheral nerve injury.

2. Ataxic joints that are completely anesthetized are most commonly involved. This is believed to be secondary to trauma.

3. Brawny swelling is noted with deformity of the joint.

4. Crepitus is common on passive motion.

5. Neuropathic arthropathy is common in the diabetic.

6. Dinkel (1969) noted that changes found in diabetic arthropathy can also be observed

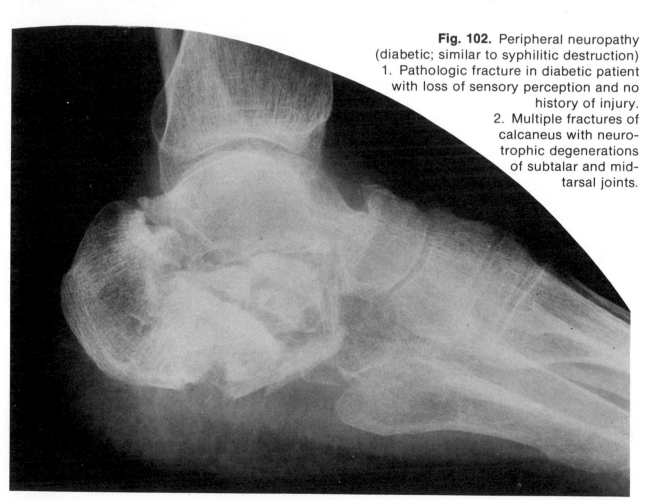

Fig. 102. Peripheral neuropathy (diabetic; similar to syphilitic destruction)
1. Pathologic fracture in diabetic patient with loss of sensory perception and no history of injury.
2. Multiple fractures of calcaneus with neurotrophic degenerations of subtalar and midtarsal joints.

in neuropathies due to nerve injuries, anesthetic leprosy, arthritis, inflammatory diseases and other forms of tissue damage.

ROENTGENOLOGIC INTERPRETATION

1. Roentgenologic evidence of periarticular swelling and marked intraarticular massive effusion is noted.

2. The joint changes may be hypertrophic, atrophic, or both.

3. Irregular detritus and destruction of bone transverse to the long axis of the bones are seen and the joint appears as a "bag of bones." Calcifications in the periarticular tissues and massive effusion are characteristic joint changes.

Chronic Idiopathic Hypertrophic Osteoarthropathy

CLINICAL ORIENTATION

1. This rare osteoarthropathy develops slowly and is found in boys at puberty or adolescence.

2. The digits are clubbed, bones and joints enlarged, and the skin of the face thickened in the absence of demonstrable primary disease.

3. There is swelling, pain, and limitation of motion in the affected joints.

4. These symptoms may also occur in early association with a primary pulmonary neoplasm.

5. Hypertrophic bone changes appear late in patients having chronic suppurative disease.

6. An acute onset, rapid development, and associated primary disease differentiate the secondary from the chronic idiopathic type.

ROENTGENOLOGIC INTERPRETATION

1. Symmetrically distributed subperiosteal calcification is associated with an exaggerated lateral growth in the long bones.

2. The medullary cavity is not narrowed.

3. The bone proliferation is greatest over the diaphysis and becomes narrower at the epiphysis.

4. The ungual tufts undergo absorption or atrophy while the bone length remains normal.

Peripheral Neuritis

CLINICAL ORIENTATION

1. Tingling and numbness with a muscular atrophy may develop early followed by a peroneal paralysis.

2. Nausea, chills, fever, general fatigue, and exaggerated tendon reflexes may precede

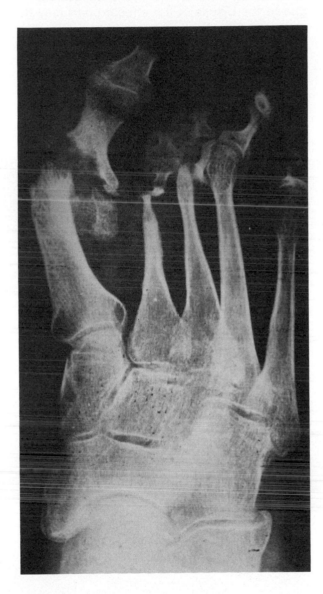

Fig. 103. Charcot joint — neurotrophic
1. Destruction of first metatarsophalangeal joint transverse to long axis of bone.
2. Irregular detritus.
3. Destruction and pencil pointing of second and third metatarsals.

a deformity, such as drop foot.

3. Later, the deep reflexes decrease, and the condition may be easily differentiated from arthritis or fibrositis.

ROENTGENOLOGIC INTERPRETATION

1. There are no early changes visualized.
2. Later, bone atrophy and deossification due to the disuse of the affected part may be recognized.

Psoriatic Arthritis

CLINICAL ORIENTATION

1. Lesions of the skin and nails are usually associated with psoriatic arthritis.
2. The extensor surfaces of the body may present silvery white, imbricated scales on a red base.
3. Secondary infections of the nail bed are common.
4. Swelling and tenderness of the joints simulate rheumatoid arthritis.

ROENTGENOLOGIC INTERPRETATION
(Fig. 105)

1. The toes and metatarsophalangeal joints are commonly affected.
2. The shafts appear ragged and irregular in outline.
3. Proliferative and destructive changes are present in the joints.
4. The chondro-osseous margins of the joints appear "moth eaten."

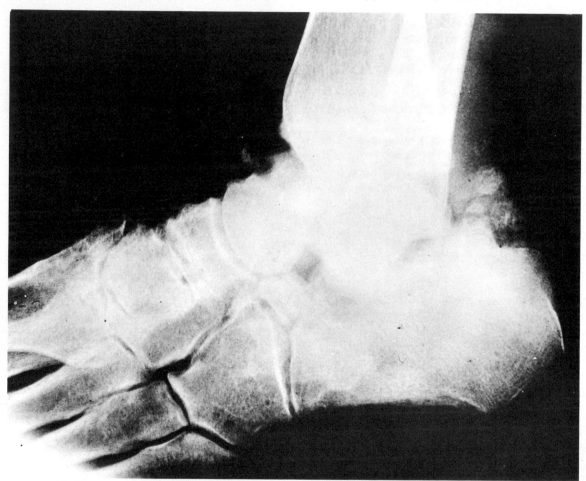

Fig. 104. Charcot joint
1. Massive swelling.
2. Destruction of bone transverse to long axis.
3. Irregular detritus at periphery.

Syringomyelia

CLINICAL ORIENTATION

1. Muscular atrophy, contractures, and spasticity occur in this disease of cavitation within the spinal cord.

2. Pain and temperature sensations are disturbed while the touch sensation remains normal.

3. Reflexes are hyperactive and the Babinski's sign is positive.

4. Painless ulcerations are seen early.

ROENTGENOLOGIC INTERPRETATION (Fig. 106)

1. Neurotrophic loss of substance and bone destruction at the chondro-osseous margins are common.

2. Metatarsals and phalanges may show resorption resulting in an appearance of pencil pointing of the distal parts.

3. Destruction of the articular cartilage is present, and the hands and feet become deformed.

Myxedema

(see also under "hypothyroidism," Chapter 6.)

CLINICAL ORIENTATION

1. This is a chronic disease of gradual onset in middle-aged women with atrophy of the thyroid gland and hypothyroidism.

2. The patient is often obese with an appearance of being mentally and physically lazy.

3. The face is bloated, expressionless, coarse, and pallid yellow; hair scant; skin and nails atrophic.

4. There are vague aches and pains with a sensitivity to cold.

5. A nonpitting, firm edema is characteristic.

6. Parasthesias are noted in feet and legs.

7. Diminished deep tendon reflexes accompany hypothyroidism.

Hyperthyroidism

CLINICAL ORIENTATION

1. The skin and nails are thick and dry.

2. The nails are often a gray yellow, appear powdery, hypertrophied, and sometimes loose from the nail bed.

3. Exophthalmos, fullness of the neck, and a high metabolic rate are often associated with hyperactivity of the thyroid gland.

4. The patient complains of generalized aches and pains.

ROENTGENOLOGIC INTERPRETATION

A mixed arthritis may be present.

Hemophilia

A hemoarthrosis may be present in male pa-

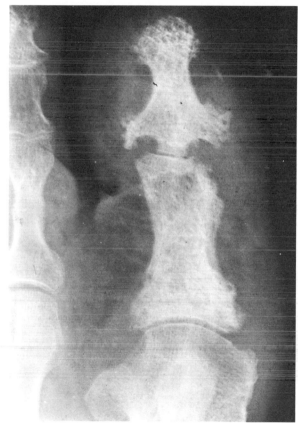

Fig. 105. Psoriatic arthritis

1. Psoriatic nails.

2. Soft-tissue markedly thickened.

3. Shaft of proximal phalanx presents a highly irregular cortex with inert subperiosteal calcification.

4. Chondro-osseous margin of interphalangeal joint presents atrophic loss of substance with widening of joint space.

tients who have tendencies for an abnormal clotting time. Massive hemorrhagic extravasations are evident within the articular capsule which is stretched. Scurvy may simulate these objective findings. Active destruction may be present at sites of joint hemorrhage.

Arthritic Purpura

Pain, edema, and tenderness of multiple joints with no evidence of bone pathologic changes are seen in asthenic individuals presenting a high temperature and purpuric hemorrhages.

Scleroderma

Scleroderma is often preceded by vasomotor symptoms or may begin with an arthralgia,

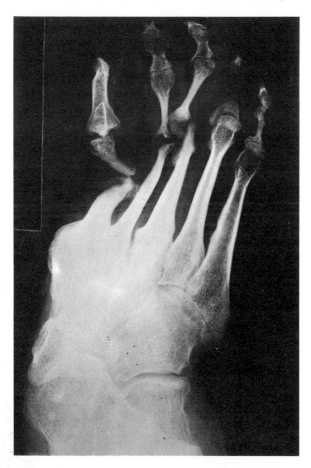

Fig. 106. Syringomyelia
  1. Fusion deformity of the tarsal and tarso-metatarsal articulations.
  2. Absorption and pencil pointing of the metatarsal heads and proximal phalanges.

malaise, sensory disturbances, and loss of weight. The skin and subcutaneous tissues become fibrosed with resultant stiffness and deformity. Later the skin on the extremities becomes parchment-like. Nails may be atrophied or completely absent. Trophic ulcers result from faulty weight distribution brought on by inadequate adipose tissue and contractures of the fibrosed tissues.

Intermittent Claudication

Arthritic changes are not a prominent feature in claudication. The dorsalis pedis and posterior tibial pulsations may be palpable but weak. When the cramp affects the ankle joint, intermittent claudication must be differentiated from muscular spasm or periarticular fibrositis.

Scurvy

A lack of adequate vitamin C may produce massive hemorrhage in the joints and subperiosteum. Superficial subcutaneous bleeding is common. The joints may become painfully swollen with the greatest pain elicited on palpations along shafts of long bones. Bleeding of gums is common. This deficiency disease is usually found in young people.

Vitamin B Deficiency

A multiple neuritis that is relieved by large doses of vitamin B must be differentiated from arthritic symptoms.

Rickets

In rickets, there is a generalized muscular atrophy and systemic demineralization of bone accompanied by flaring at the ends of the long bones in children. It is due to a lack of vitamin D. The roentgenologic features are bowing of the long bones, irregular metaphyses with saucerization, systemic decalcification, and rachitic lipping.

Hyperparathyroidism

The faulty calcium metabolism very often causes a cystic and fibrous degeneration with systemic demineralization of the long bones.

Osteitis Deformans (Paget's Disease)

In Paget's disease, the patient may complain of cramps and pain in the extremities which simulate arthritis. The long bones are bowed, and the head is enlarged. Roentgenographic findings are pathognomonic with thickening and increased radiolucency of the cortex, narrowing of the medullary bone, and a heavy crisscross trabecular pattern. The calvarium is widened.

Trichinosis

A history of ingestion of poorly cooked pork followed by muscle inflammation, nausea, and abdominal pain suggests trichinosis. The larvae may be recognized in tissue obtained from the inflamed musculature by biopsy. The pain may simulate arthritis.

Epidemic Arthritic Erythema (Haverhill Fever)

A multiple arthritis may be the sequel of this syndrome characterized by chills, fever, malaise, vomiting, and headache. This is soon followed by morbilliform eruptions of the extremities which become hemorrhagic. This disease has been described as an epidemic erythematous arthritis.

Boeck's Sarcoid

The bone lesions are usually part of a general disturbance in adults and are thought to be related to pulmonary disease. Symmetrical subcutaneous nodules occur about the interphalangeal joints of the hands and feet. Lymphadenopathy is common.

The roentgenologic features are thickening of the trabeculae with small cystic changes separated by a dense sclerosis.

Reiter's Syndrome

CLINICAL ORIENTATION

1. This symptom complex was first described by Reiter in 1916. It consists of a classic triad of urethritis, conjunctivitis, and arthritis following an episode of diarrhea or a venereal contact.

2. The causative agent has not been determined.

3. The postvenereal form occurs almost exclusively in men, the post-dysenteric form may affect entire families.

4. The arthritis tends to remain after the other manifestations have vanished and recurrence may produce chronic joint deformity.

5. Effects vary from extreme incapacitation to mild illness.

6. The arthritis is abrupt in onset, usually severe, and may involve many joints, including those of the ankle and feet.

7. Pain, swelling, stiffness, and effusion are present, and tenderness about the heels at the insertion of the tendo achillis is common.

8. Although recovery without permanent bony changes is common, there may be permanent residuals in the feet, such as painful talipes cavus, flat feet, hammer toes, lateral deviation of toes, calcaneal spurs, and metatarsophalangeal subluxation.

9. In recurrent Reiter's syndrome, ankylosing spondylitis occurs in 20% of the patients (Rosen, 1964).

ROENTGENOLOGIC INTERPRETATION

1. Roentgenologic changes are not apparent except in a chronic disease.

2. In chronic Reiter's syndrome, destructive changes with narrowing and fusion of the joint may be observed.

BIBLIOGRAPHY

American Rheumatism Association: Primer on the Rheumatic Diseases, J.A.M.A. 139:1068, 1949.

Amtrup, F.: Diabetic Arthropathy, Nord. Med. 83:627, 1970.

Anderson, W.A.D.: *Synopsis of Pathology*, ed. 2. St. Louis: C.V. Mosby Co., 1946.

Archer, W.W.: *The Osseous System, a Handbook of Roentgen Diagnosis.* Chicago: Year Book Publishers, 1947.

Arnott, G., Petit, H., Benoit, M., and Fourlinnie, J.C.: Syndrome of the Tarsal Scaphoid Revealing Latent Diabetes, Rev. Neurol. (Paris) 124:233, 1971.

Belser, F.: The Lower Extremity as the Organ of Predilection for Late Diabetic Syndromes, Schweiz. Med. Wschr. 100:1737, 1970.

Billig, H.E., and Brennan, R.I.: Foot Pains, J. Nat. Ass. Chiropodists 33:34, 1943.

Budin, H.: Pain in the Great Toe Joint. J. Exp. Podiat. 1(2), 1940.

Caffey, J.P.: *Pediatric X-ray Diagnosis.* Chicago: Year

Book Publishers, 1946.

Collis, W.J., and Jayson, M.I.: Measurement of Pedal Pressures, Ann. Rheum. Dis. 31:215, 1972.

Comroe, B.I.: *Arthritis and Allied Conditions.* Philadelphia: Lea & Febiger Co., 1940.

Copeman, W., and Sydney, C.: *History of Gout.* Berkeley: University of California Press, 1964.

Degenhardt, D.P., and Goodwin, M.A.: Neuropathic Joints in Diabetes, J. Bone Joint Surg. 42-B:769, 1960.

DeLorimer, A.A.: *The Arthropathies, A Handbook of Roentgen Diagnosis.* Chicago: Year Book Publishers, 1946.

Dinkel, L.: Changes of the Foot Bones in Diabetes Mellitus: Fortschr. Roentgenstr. 110:223, 1969.

Dixon, A. St. J.: Medical Aspects of the Rheumatoid Foot, Proc. Roy. Soc. Med. 63:677, 1970.

Evans, E.B., and Smith, J.: Bone and Joint Changes Following Burns, J. Bone Joint Surg. 41- :785, 1959.

Evans, E.B., Larson, D.L., Abston, S., and Willia, B.: Prevention and Correction of Deformity after Severe Burns, Surg. Clin. N. Amer. 50:1361, 1970.

Evans, E.B., Larson, D.L., and Yates, S.: Preservation and Restoration of Joint Function in Patients with Severe Burns, J.A.M.A. 204:843, 1968.

Ferguson, A.B.: *Roentgen Diagnosis of the Extremities and Spine.* New York: P.B. Hoeber, Inc., 1941.

Gicker, L.W.: Differential Diagnosis of Diseases of the Foot, Chiropody Rec. 22:151, 1939.

Godfrey, C.M., Lawson, G.A., and Stewart, W.A.: A Method for Determination of Pedal Pressure Changes during Weight Bearing: Preliminary Observations in Normal and Arthritic Feet, Arthritis Rheum. 10:135, 1967.

Grokoest, A.W.: *Juvenile Rheumatoid Arthritis.* Boston: Little, Brown and Co., 1961.

Gross, R.H.: *Modern Foot Therapy.* New York: Foot Therapy Publishing Co., 1948.

Harford, E.G.: Charcot's Disease, J. Amer. Podiat. Ass. 49:458, 1959.

Heimburger, R.A.: Burned Feet, Amer. J. Surg. 125:575, 1973.

Hodges, F.J., Lampe, I., and Holt, J.F.: *Radiology for Medical Students.* Chicago: Year Book Publishers, 1947.

Holmes, G.W., and Ruggles, H.E.: *Roentgen Interpretation,* ed. 5. Philadelphia: Lea & Febiger Co., 1936.

Kahone, S.B.: Seropositive Cases and Detected by the R-A Latex Tests, unpublished M.P.H. thesis, Yale University, New Haven, Conn., 1962.

Kersley, G.D.: *The Rheumatic Diseases,* ed. 4. London: Heinemann, 1962.

Kuhns, J.: The Foot in Chronic Arthritis, Clin. Orthop. 16:141, 1960.

Levinson, S.A., and McFate, R.P.: *Clinical Laboratory Diagnosis.* Philadelphia: Lea & Febiger Co., 1939.

Levitus, I.M., and Scheimer, O.M.: Gout as a Complication, J. Nat. Ass. Chiropodists 28:34, 1938.

Lewin, Philip: *The Foot and Ankle.* Philadelphia: Lea & Febiger Co., 1940.

Lievre, J.A. et al.: Prediabetic Nervous Osteoarthropathy, Rev. Rhum. 36:609, 1969.

Luck, J.V.: *Bone and Joint Disease.* Springfield, Ill.: Charles C Thomas, 1950.

Lichwitz, L.: Gout, Bull. N.Y. Acad. Med. 10:306, 1934.

Nutt, J.J.: *Diseases and Deformities of the Foot,* ed. 2. New York: E.B. Treat and Co., 1925.

Ondrouch, A.S.: Cyst Formation in Osteoarthritis, J. Bone Joint Surg. 45-B:755, 1963.

Partsch, H.: Ulcero-mutilating Neuropathies of the Lower Extremities: Clinical Aspects of Ulcero-mutilating Acropathy, Hautarzt 122:283, 1971.

Raunia, P., and Laire, H.: Synovectomy of the Metatarsophalangeal Joints in Rheumatoid Arthritis, Acta Rheum. Scand. 16:12, 1970.

Rigler, L.G.: *Outline of Roentgen Diagnosis.* Atlas ed. Philadelphia: J.B. Lippincott Co., 1938.

Ritvo, M.: *Bone and Joint X-ray Diagnosis.* Philadelphia: Lea & Febiger Co., 1955.

Rosen, P.: Reiter's Syndrome, Mod. Med.

Sante, L.: *Principles of Roentgenological Interpretation.* Ann Arbor, Mich.: Edwards Bros., Inc., 1940.

Sardrow, R.E., Torg, J.S. et al.: Use of Thermography in the Early Diagnosis of Neuropathic Arthropathy in the Feet of Diabetics, Clin. Orthop. 88:31, 1972.

Schuster, O.N.: A Case of Hallux Rigidus, J. Nat. Ass. Chiropodists 27:8, 1937.

Schuster, O.N.: *Foot Orthopedics,* ed. 2. Albany, N.Y.: J. Lyon Co., 1939.

Simpson, J.R.: Hypertrophic Osteoarthropathy, An Early Sign of Pulmonary Neoplasm, Harper Hosp. Bull.

Solovay, J., and Solovay, H.W.: Paraplegic Neuroarthropathy, Amer. J. Roentgen. 61:475, 1949.

Stroescu, I., Stoicescu, M., and Stoia, I.: Recherches concernant la statique et la dynamique de pied rhumatismal et le diagnostic fonctionnel des troubles de la marche, Rev. Rhum. 38:173, 1971.

Talbot, J.H.: *Gout.* New York: Greene and Stratton, 1957.

Ulmansky, A.L., Schlesinger, P.T., and Greenberg, B.B.: Tuberculous Dactylitis in the Adult, Arch. Surg. 54:67, 1947.

Urban, L.D.: Roentgenological Interpretation of Diseases of the Feet, Chiropody Rec. 21:60, 1938.

U.S. National Institute of Arthritis and Metabolic Diseases, "Current Clinical Studies," Bethesda, Md.: National Institutes of Health, 1960.

Vincelette, P.: The Footballer's Ankle and Foot, Canad. Med. Ass. J. 107:872, 1972.

Weinmann, J.P., and Sicher, H.: *Bone and Bones.* St. Louis: C.V. Mosby Co., 1947.

Wilson, M.G.: *Advances in Rheumatic Fever (1940-1961).* New York: Hoeber Medical Division, Harper & Row, 1962.

Yale, I.: A Statistical Report on Roentgen Findings in a Review of 1290 Foot Radiographs, J. Nat. Ass. Chiropodists 47:6, 1957.

6 ENDOCRINOPATHIES
AND ASSOCIATED DISORDERS

Diseases caused by dysfunction of the endocrine glands are very complicated. The effects of endocrinopathies upon the skeletal system are profound and varied. The broad aspect of roentgenologic diagnosis will be given to enable the reader to appreciate the pathogenesis involved. Specific endocrine disturbances that have manifest roentgenologic features in the feet will be identified.

Roentgenograms are a valuable aid in evaluating endocrine activity when a comparison is made to established normal patterns of bone growth.

The interrelationship between the endocrine glands should be recognized. A dysfunction of one gland may become manifest in bone by its influence upon the function of another.

Normal bone growth and development in youth prior to union of the epiphysis is controlled by the pituitary gland. Marked endocrine dysfunction affects the development and time of appearance of the centers of ossification of the epiphysis, the extent of the ossification of bone, and the development of cortical and cancellous bone. There are many endocrine gland interrelationships creating clinical symptoms that are not fully understood.

HYPERENDOCRINISM
Hyperpituitarism

CLINICAL ORIENTATION

1. Overactivity of the pituitary gland may be stimulated by hypogonadism.

2. With overactivity, the bone is increased accompanied by systemic demineralization in the advanced stages.

3. Diminished bone metabolism in basophilic lesions of the pituitary cause a decrease in density of bone.

Eosinophilic lesions in the pituitary present acromegaly in the adult and giantism in children.

Clinical findings may be secondary to an adenoma of the pituitary cells.

Acromegaly

CLINICAL ORIENTATION

1. There is a hyperfunction or adenoma involving the acidophils in the anterior lobe of the pituitary gland.

2. This syndrome occurs postadolescence, in the third and fourth decades, due to secretion of growth-promoting hormone reactivating endochondral bone growth at epiphyseal cartilage plates.

3. In the adult stage, feet elongate and shoes become too short.

4. Hands and feet are unusually large, the fingers and toes broadened, and the nails are convex.

5. The head and face are enlarged, and the expression is "lionlike." The lower lip and ears are thick, forehead furrowed, and the nose broad. A progthnatic lower jaw is pathognomonic.

6. Splanchnomegaly is a common anatomicopathologic finding.

ROENTGENOLOGIC INTERPRETATION
(Fig. 107)

1. There is usually a thickening of the bones.

2. Tufting of the terminal phalanges is pathognomonic.

3. The cancellous tufts and adjacent soft tissues are overdeveloped and the phalanges are elongated.

Pituitary Giantism

CLINICAL ORIENTATION

1. Hyperfunction of cells of the pituitary prior to union of the epiphysis stimulates development of objective symptoms.

2. Rapid growth and unusual development of height occur in childhood and youth.

ROENTGENOLOGIC INTERPRETATION

1. The bone cortex is thickened and sometimes irregular due to periosteal new bone.

2. Bones develop unusually long. They are giant size prior to union of the epiphysis in hyperpituitarism. Tubercles on bones are often larger than normal.

3. The distal phalanges may show tufting at their terminal ends. Osteophytic changes are often noted at the articular margins simulating osteoarthritis.

Cushing's Syndrome

CLINICAL ORIENTATION

1. A tumor or basophilic adenoma of the pituitary gland with hyperplasia of the adrenals may be a significant factor.

2. Pathology of the basophilic cells may

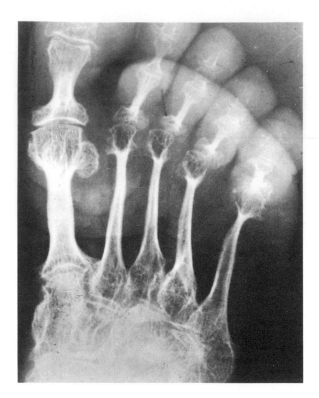

Fig. 107. Hyperpituitarism
1. Systemic deossification.
2. Hour-glass shaped metatarsals and phalanges.
3. Hypertrophy of ungual tufts.

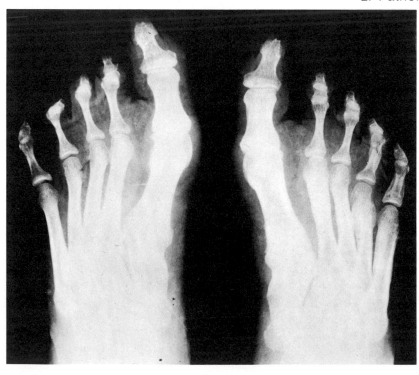

Fig. 108. Cushing's syndrome (pituitary basophilism)
1. Thickening and clublike shape of metatarsals.
2. Subperiosteal calcifications of inert type are present.

result in hyperplasia of the adrenals.

3. Hyalinization of the cells may or may not be present when the adrenals are affected by adenoma or carcinoma.

4. Hydrocortisone and cortisone are put out in excessive amounts by the adrenals. Protein is improperly synthesized, resulting in loss of nitrogen in the feces and urine.

ROENTGENOLOGIC INTERPRETATION
(Fig. 108)

1. Osteoporosis and bone atrophy are due to a diminished osteoblastic function.

2. Cortex is narrowed.

3. Joints may be affected and collapse from the excess of cortisone.

4. Faulty remodeling of bone may produce clublike metatarsals with inert subperiosteal calcifications along the shafts.

Chondrodystrophy

Chondrodystrophy is characterized by an al-tered rate in growth of bone from cartilage. It manifests itself as an acceleration of growth as in giantism or delayed growth of bone from cartilage as in cretinism (Fig. 109).

Chondrodysplasia

Chondrodysplasia is a failure in development of bone from cartilage.

CLINICAL ORIENTATION

1. Although not strictly of endocrine origin, chondrodysplasia may occur in pituitary, parathyroid, and thyroid disturbances.

2. It results in defective development in bone and may affect a single bone or all bones.

3. The limbs may be short in a general chondrodysplasic involvement.

4. If it affects only a single growth center, the bone is normal in length.

5. Trauma in growing bones may result in chondrodysplasia.

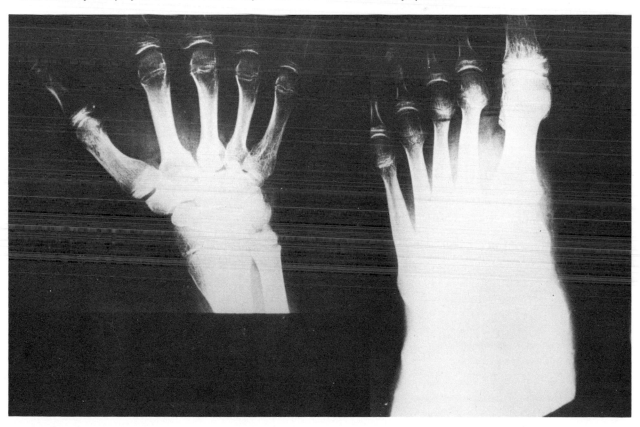

Fig. 109. Chondrodystrophy — Hypogonadism
1. Delayed union of epiphysis. 2. Note opened epiphyseal plates. 3. Man, age 26, appears younger than stated age. Secondary sex characteristics are poorly developed. No axillary or pubic hair.

ROENTGENOLOGIC INTERPRETATION
(Fig. 110)

1. Permanent bone tissue is not normally structured.

2. The bone may present marginal, sub-marginal, or central defects.

3. A defect may be cartilaginous, fibrous, cystic, or merely nontrabeculated osteoid which has failed to develop a reticular pattern.

4. There may be a lack of structure in bone. Nonosseous efects may be present.

5. Abnormal shape and faulty remodeling of bone occur.

6. The bones fail to develop and the growth length is deficient.

7. These bone changes may be localized or diffuse and a single bone or all the bones may be affected.

Hyperparathyroidism

Extensive osteoclastic activity on the walls of the Haversian canals takes place soon after injections of parathyroid hormone and the blood calcium level rises. Marked osteoclasis with limitation of osteoblastic activity occurs in hyperparathyroidism. The osteoclasis sites are replaced by extensive fibrosis. Later this becomes the basis for bone blending and deformity. Mobilization of calcium is increased with hyperfunction of the parathyroid. Newly formed bone fails to calcify after injection of parathyroid hormone. More commonly seen in women and is rare under 10 years of age. A familial tendency is noted. Hyperparathyroidism may be primary or secondary. A parathyroid adenoma may be etiologic.

CLINICAL ORIENTATION

1. Skeletal, renal, and gastrointestinal symptoms are common in hyperparathyroidism. Renal calculi and pyelonephritis are pathognomonic.

2. In long-standing disorder, the patient experiences pain, pathologic fractures, bone tumors, cysts, and deformities with faulty development of bone. The bones of the jaw and vertebral column may show changes earlier than the hands or feet.

3. The calcium and phosphorus metabolism is disturbed. There is a negative mineral

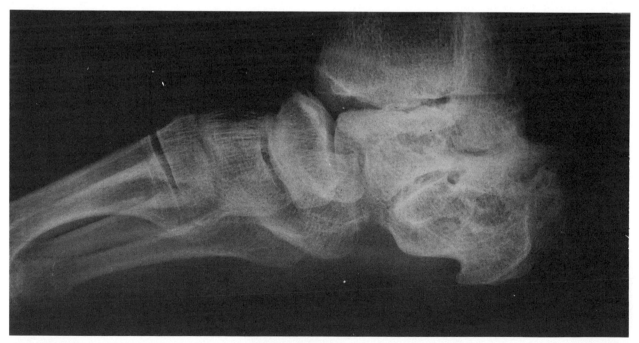

Fig. 110. Chondrodysplasia
1. Note destruction subtalar and talocrural articulations secondary to trauma during a period of growth and development.
2. Faulty development from cartilage of talus, navicular, and calcaneus.

balance.

a. An evaluation requires a serum analysis after several hours of fasting which may show an increased production of parathyroid hormone and a serum calcium level over 11.0 mg/100 ml. A low serum phosphorus below 2.0 mg/100 ml with a high serum calcium is almost always pathognomonic of hyperparathyroidism. Serum calcium levels may range between 12.0 and 15 mg/100 ml.

b. Hypercalcemia, diminished blood phosphorus levels, and an increase in serum alkaline phosphatase accompany hyperparathyroidism.

c. Values for urine calcium and phosphates are increased.

4. If left untreated, focal hyperplasia, adenoma, or neoplasia of one or more of the parathyroid glands is fatal.

5. The presence of renal calculi should heighten suspicion of hyperparathyroidism and lead to early diagnosis before bone manifestations.

6. In the presence of skeletal changes the serum alkaline phosphatase may range from 8-35 Bodansky units depending on severity. (Normal is 1.5 to 3.5 Bodansky units per 100 ml.)

7. Renal (secondary) hyperparathyroidism may be accompanied by hyperplasia of the parathyroid glands.

ROENTGENOLOGIC INTERPRETATION

1. Systemic demineralization, expansion of multiple cyst formation, and weakening of the bone evidenced by bending deformities are indicative of hyperparathyroidism. Cortices are thinned. Trabeculae in the spongy ends of bone appear blurred.

2. The systemic decrease in density is due to osteoclasis in the bones with fibrous substitution.

3. The texture of bone is lost, and the lesions appear diffusely throughout the diaphysis of the tubular long bones.

4. The bone diameter is increased by irregular scalloping accretion. This is especially common in the middle phalanx of the fingers and possibly the toes.

5. The osteomalacia, softening, and bowing are pathognomonic. Pathologic fractures are common.

6. Multiple fibrotic lesions are found in the middle of the shafts.

7. "Brown tumor" consisting of hemorrhagic deposits with cystic degeneration may be present.

8. According to Jaffe (1972, p. 312), "these lesions represent 'giant cell reparative granuloma.'"

Hyperthyroidism

CLINICAL ORIENTATION

1. A high metabolic rate accompanies this disorder.

2. Exophthalmos and fullness in the neck are noted.

3. Generalized aches and pains in the limbs are a common complaint.

4. The skin and nails are hypertrophied and dry.

5. Heloma miliare is often noted on soles with fissures about the margins of the heels and distal ends of toes.

ROENTGENOLOGIC INTERPRETATION

1. Osteoporosis is an early bone change.

2. Occasional cysts in bone are common.

3. A mixed arthritis is common but not definitive.

Hypergonadism

CLINICAL ORIENTATION

1. Tumors of the adrenal cortex predispose to hypergonadism.

2. Growth is accelerated with overactivity of the gonads.

ROENTGENOLOGIC INTERPRETATION

1. Accelerated maturation of the skeleton is the rule.

2. The epiphyseal plates close early in contrast to hypothyroidism and hypopituitarism where epiphyseal cartilage persists into old age.

Albright's Syndrome

CLINICAL ORIENTATION

1. Usually develops in young girls with an

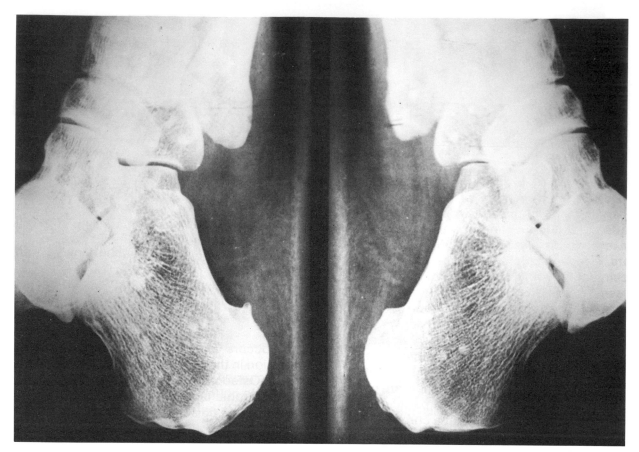

Fig. 116. Osteopoikilosis
1. Irregular, spotty areas of increase in density. 2. Generally systemic with familial predisposition.
3. Note the sclerosis at the posterior plantar aspect of the calcaneus.

mutant gene and is not endocrine in nature despite the failure of growth.

2. All the bones in the body are involved since this is a systemic defect in skeletal ossification.

3. The long bones fail to grow.

4. The hands and feet are stumpy.

5. The feet are small but strong.

6. True dwarfs have a large normal head and small face, and the cranial vault may be expanded.

7. The spine is often curved in scoliotic or kyphotic deformity.

ROENTGENOLOGIC INTERPRETATION

1. Achondroplasia is characterized by a faulty development of bone from cartilage and a failure of regular union of the epiphysis to the diaphysis.

2. The epiphyses appear slowly and are irregular and moth eaten in appearance.

3. There are narrow epiphyseal disks that ossify and unite to the diaphysis prematurely.

4. The bones are short but of normal thickness in achondroplasia.

5. Coxa vara is common.

Osteopoikilosis (Spotted Bone)

CLINICAL ORIENTATION

1. Being asymptomatic, osteopoikilosis is usually discovered when roentgenograms are performed in the study of other conditions.

2. It is generally systemic in nature and occurs commonly in the small bones of the hands and feet.

3. Familial predispositions have been reported.

ROENTGENOLOGIC INTERPRETATION
(Fig. 116)

1. Small, spotty islands of increase in density that range from 1 to 2 mm in diameter are seen in several bones.

2. A smooth outline and a central structureless condensation are characteristic.

3. A punctate or nodular spot may develop at ends of bones.

4. Linear shadows arranged longitudinally occur in another type of osteopoikilosis.

5. One must differentiate this condition from Sudeck's atrophy in which small, spotty islands of decrease in density are seen.

Familial Osseous Atrophy

CLINICAL ORIENTATION

1. This defect in ossification is of unknown origin, but a familial pattern on the male side is noted.

2. Pain in the feet is common.

3. There may be repeated recurrence of bullous lesions and large ulcerations on the foot with necrosis of bone that is of no other apparent cause.

4. A gradual loss of the distal ends of the feet has been reported.

ROENTGENOLOGIC INTERPRETATION

1. The destruction of bone is not unlike the neurotrophic changes in the metatarsals and toes seen in leprosy and must be differentiated.

2. Pencil pointing of the metatarsals and phalanges is a usual change.

3. Demineralization and atrophy of bone are common.

Osteitis Deformans (Paget's Disease).

CLINICAL ORIENTATION

1. Middle-aged men are affected more often than women.

2. Widening of the calvarium and bowing of long bones are pathognomonic.

3. The tibia and fibula may be bowed anteriorly and laterally.

4. Indurated swelling of the affected parts

is a usual finding.

5. Mild increase in skin temperature and a dull ache are noted.

6. Moderate limitation of functional capacity of the affected extremity is a symptom.

7. While the blood calcium level may be normal or slightly elevated, the serum phos-

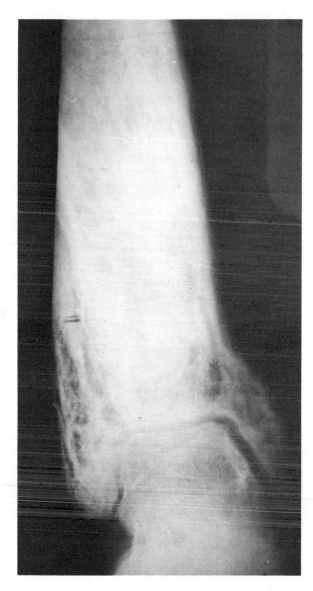

Fig. 117. Osteitis deformans (Paget's disease)

1. Thick calcareous trabeculations in bone crisscrossing at wide angles.

2. Bowing, thickening of the cortex and narrowing of the medulla.

3. Despite the thickening of the cortex, the peripheral bone is decreased in density.

4. Pseudocystic changes in bone at malleoli.

phatase is high and the phosphorus levels fluctuate above and sometimes below normal.

8. The severe bowing deformity may result in imbalanced, faulty functioning feet.

ROENTGENOLOGIC INTERPRETATION
(Figs. 117-118)

1. The thickened cortex is decreased in density and encroaches upon the medulla which is decreased in width.

2. The general pattern of bone is a crisscross of thickened, calcareous strands.

3. Heavy trabeculation with large spaces of soft-tissue density between strands is a typical finding.

4. Trabeculations cross each other at angles to assume a coarse appearance.

5. Woolly appearance of the skull is pathognomonic.

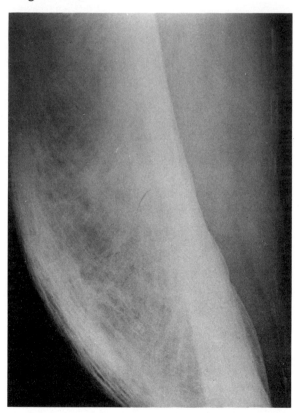

Fig. 118. Osteitis deformans (Paget's disease)

1. Thickened cortex with decrease in density.

2. Medullary bone is narrowed with crisscross pattern of thickened trabeculae.

3. Bowing of long bones is characteristic.

6. The roentgenologic findings must be differentiated from those in osteogenic sarcoma, which may be a late complication of this disorder.

BIBLIOGRAPHY

Albers-Schönberg, H.: Eine seltene bisher nicht bekannte Structuranomalie des Skelettes, Fortschr. Roentgenstr. 23:171, 1915.

Archer, V.W.: *The Osseous System, A Handbook of Roentgen Diagnosis.* Chicago: The Year Book Publishers, 1947.

Brailsford, J.F.: Osteogenesis Imperfecta. Brit. J. Radiol. 16:129, 1943.

Caffey, J.P.: *Pediatric X-ray Diagnosis.* Chicago: The Year Book Publishers, 1946.

Clifton, W.M., Frank, A., and Freeman, S.: Osteopetrosis (Marble Bones), Amer. J. Dis. Child. 56:1020, 1938.

Cooper, J.G., Adair, N., and Patterson, W.M.: Familial Osseous Atrophy, Radiology 48:509, 1947.

Davison, W.M., and Smith, D.R. (eds.): *Proceedings of the Conference on Human Chromosomal Abnormalities.* London: Staples Press, 1961.

Fairbanks, H.A.: Osteopetrosis, Osteopetrosis Generalista, Marble Bones, Albers-Schönberg's Disease, Osteosclerosis Fragilitas Generalisata, J. Bone Joint Surg. 30-B:339, 1948.

Ferguson, A.B.: *Roentgen Diagnosis of the Extremities and Spine.* New York: P.B. Hoeber, Inc., 1941.

First Inter-American Conference on Congenital Defects. compiled and edited for The International Medical Conference, Ltd. Philadelphia: J.B. Lippincott Co., 1963.

Fishbein, M. (ed.): *Birth Defects.* Philadelphia: J.B. Lippincott Co., 1963.

Jones, H.E.: Studies in Achondroplasia, J. Anat. 66:565, 1932.

Keefer, C.S.: Some Clinical Features of Deficiency Disorders. New York J. Med. 32:253, 1932.

Palma, A.F. (ed.): *Clinical Orthopaedics and Related Research.* Philadelphia: J.B. Lippincott Co., April, 1964, Vol. 33.

Weinmann, J.P., and Sicher, H.: *Bone and Bones.* St. Louis: C.V. Mosby Co., 1947.

9 BONE TUMORS OF THE FEET

Bone tumors may be either benign or malignant. For the instructional purposes of this manual, we shall first classify bone tumors and then proceed with a clinical and roentgenologic evaluation of those lesions found in the foot.

It is obvious that many specific classifications could be used in subdividing the benign or malignant lesions into categories for study. However, we have chosen to place tumors into special categories dependent on their sites of origin.

Bone tumors originating from bone and those from nonosseous tissues will form the basis of the classification. In addition, tumors of specialized skeletal structures will be considered, although these are difficult to diagnose roentgenologically.

CLASSIFICATION OF BONE TUMORS (AFTER GESCHICKTER AND COPELAND)

TUMORS OF OSSEOUS ORIGIN

Malignant Tumors

1. Osteogenic sarcomas.
   a. Primary chondrosarcoma.
   b. Secondary chondrosarcoma.
   c. Sclerosing form of osteogenic sarcoma.
   d. Osteolytic sarcoma.
2. Malignant variant of giant cell tumors.
   a. Giant cell tumors improperly treated may serve as a local site for the development of a metastatic lesion.

Benign Lesions

1. Osteochondromas.
2. Multiple exostoses.
   a. Hereditary deforming chondrodysplasia.
3. Chondromas.

   a. Chondromyxoma.
4. Bone cysts.
5. Variants of bone cysts.
   a. Acute bone cysts.
   b. Giant cell variants of bone cysts.
   c. Osteitis fibrosa cystica.
   d. Latent bone cysts.
6. Fibrous dysplasia.
   a. Polyostotic fibrous dysplasia.
   b. Monostotic fibrous dysplasia.
7. Giant cell tumors.

TUMORS OF NONOSSEOUS ORIGIN

Malignant Tumors

1. Ewing's sarcoma.
2. Metatases to the foot skeleton from carcinoma or sarcoma in other organs of the body.
3. Fibrosarcoma of bone by direct extension from adjacent soft tissue.

Benign Lesions

1. Invasion of bone from growths in adjacent soft-tissue elements.

TUMORS OF SPECIALIZED SKELETAL STRUCTURES

Tumors of Tendon Sheaths

1. Osseous and cartilaginous.
2. Ganglia.
3. Giant cell xanthoma or benign synovioma.
4. Lipoma, fibroma, and synovial sarcoma.
5. Angioma and lymphangioma.

Tumors of the Joints.

1. Cartilaginous tumors.
2. Cysts.
3. Giant cell tumor (xanthoma).
4. Lipoma, fibroma, and fibrosarcoma.

The clinical considerations and roentgenologic findings in those tumors of bone that are more commonly seen in the foot will be discussed. General characteristics of tumors are herein considered to differentiate and identify the growth according to its mode of development, potential danger, and roentgenologic criteria.

MALIGNANT TUMORS OF OSSEOUS ORIGIN

GENERAL CLINICAL CORRELATION

1. Malignant lesions are large growths that commonly grow in spherical fashion about a point of origin.

2. A malignant tumor is characterized as an invasively destructive cellular mass.

3. Destruction is too rapid for the bone to expand.

4. Tumor cells invade by way of least resistance; *e.g.,* through cellular and vascular tissues.

5. Coley and Sharp (1931) state that they have observed metastasis from the breast to the phalanges of the toes. Metastasis to the foot has been reported from hypernephroma.

6. A malignant mass is generally firm and indurated.

7. The veins may be distended.

8. The temperature of the part may vary from hot to cool depending on the activity of the lesion.

9. Active and passive motions are limited as the body makes an attempt to splint the painful part.

10. Consideration of clinical findings and roentgenologic changes is essential before subjecting the patient to a possibly unnecessary biopsy or amputation.

GENERAL ROENTGENOLOGIC INTERPRETATION

1. There may be active destruction of bone with no roentgenologic signs of infection.

2. There is no evidence of expansion of bone with the rapid destruction that takes place.

3. There are invasion and destruction of the surrounding tissue.

4. A slow-growing tumor may present dense condensation of bone.

5. Perpendicular lines in a "sunburst" ef-

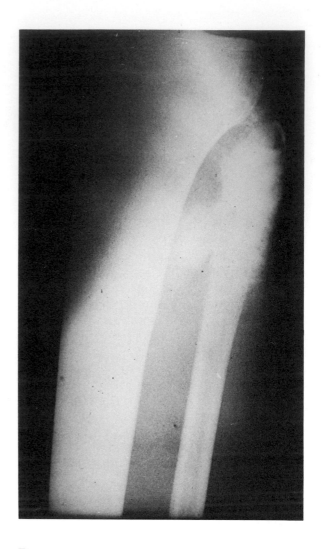

Fig. 119. Primary chondrosarcoma
1. Active destruction of the head and neck of the fibula with invasion of the surrounding bone and soft tissue.
2. Appears to spiral about point of origin with "sunburst-like" strands extending out into soft tissues.

fect are usually characteristic of a malignant growth.

6. When tumor bone is found in the medullary canal, it usually originates from periosteum at the surface of bone and grows in.

7. Cortex is generally swept away with malignancy.

8. Serial roentgenograms are necessary to follow the course in questionable lesions.

9. Early consultation is advised.

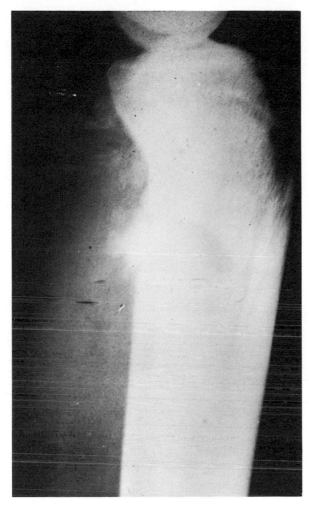

Fig. 120. Primary chondrosarcoma

OSTEOGENIC SARCOMA
Primary Chondrosarcoma

CLINICAL ORIENTATION

1. Primary chondrosarcoma usually occurs in adolescence through early twenties.

2. In the advanced stage, there is excruciating pain in the affected extremity.

3. An indurated, firm, nodular mass may be palpable.

4. Before a diagnosis can be made, laboratory criteria and biopsy results are necessarily established.

ROENTGENOLOGIC INTERPRETATION
(FIGS. 119-120)

1. The periosteum is elevated by subperiosteal extravasations.

2. A faint, translucent shadow is present in soft tissue adjacent to the bone.

3. Fine, radiating bone spicules may protrude at right angles to the cortex.

4. The cortex may be thickened or it may be perforated.

5. Late in its growth, there is an osteolytic destructive process in the cortex and medullary bone.

6. An area of destruction may contain scattered foci of calcification.

7. Subchondral bone may be destroyed.

Secondary Chondrosarcoma

CLINICAL ORIENTATION

1. This lesion may follow a benign osteochondroma or chondroma. An embryonic connective tissue may develop upon the above benign lesions.

2. Irritation of benign osteochondromata by incorrect treatment may be the cause of secondary chondrosarcoma.

3. Pain is severe, especially at night.

4. Early biopsy is indicated to establish a definitive diagnosis.

ROENTGENOLOGIC INTERPRETATION
(FIGS. 121-122)

1. The usual characteristics of a malignant tumor as previously given are to be evaluated.

2. A fuzzy, perpendicular, right-angle radiation into the soft tissues associated with an osteochondroma or chondroma may be diagnostic of a malignant process.

3. Active destruction with no evidence of infection in bone suggests malignancy of the lesion.

Sclerosing Osteogenic Sarcoma

CLINICAL ORIENTATION

1. Sclerosing osteogenic sarcoma is a malignant and fatal lesion in the 15-25-year age group.

2. Trauma is thought to be an exciting factor.

3. It usually affects the upper end of the tibia and the lower end of the femur, rarely the foot.

4. Severe pain is followed by an indurated massive swelling.

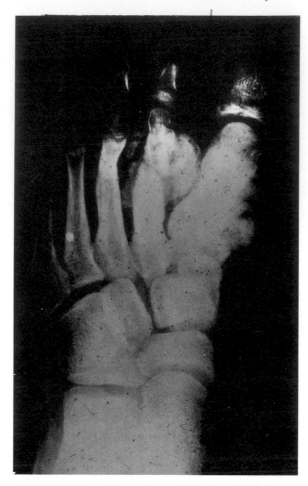

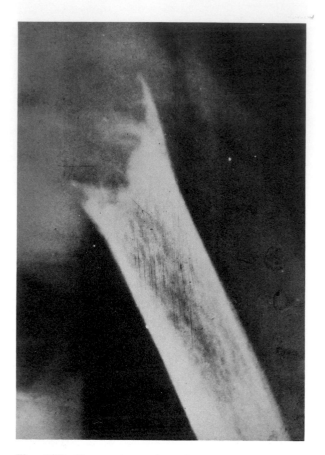

Fig. 121. Secondary chondrosarcoma
1. Severe destruction and invasion involving the first and second metatarsals in young patient.
2. Probably secondary to osteochondroma involving heads of metatarsals.

5. There may be swelling of the popliteal and inguinal lymph glands.
6. Serologic examination and blood chemistry are necessary to rule out simulating syphilitic and osteomyelitic infections.
7. A high serum alkaline phosphatase is found in osteogenic sarcoma.
8. Aspiration biopsy should be used to confirm the clinical and roentgenologic interpretations.

ROENTGENOLOGIC INTERPRETATION
(FIGS. 123-124)

1. The metaphyseal side of the epiphyseal line is the usual site of involvement.

Fig. 122. Secondary chondrosarcoma
1. Rapid, active destruction of bone with invasion.
2. No evidence of infection.
3. "Sweeping" away of bone.

2. Delicate, radiating lines from the periosteum are seen early. Later there is invasion of the medullary tissue.
3. There may be a destruction and condensation with invasion through the cortex and the development of a shelf-like mass on each side of the tumor.
4. Marked, irregular, active destruction with laying down of new bone in a sunburst fashion is a characteristic finding.

Myxochondrosarcoma

CLINICAL ORIENTATION

1. This has been reported in the literature

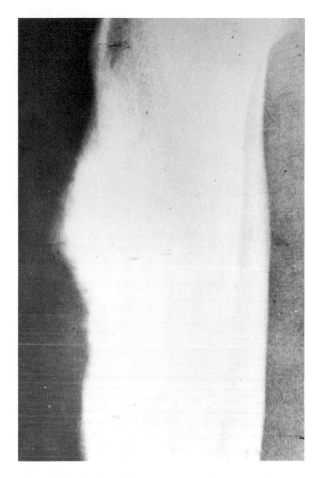

Fig. 123. Sclerosing osteogenic sarcoma

1. Active destruction, no evidence of infection.

2. Expansion of bone with invasion of irregular, perpendicular calcareous strands into soft tissue.

3. Condensation in bone is present with hypertrophy.

as a primary malignant tumor (the talus was involved in a 62-year-old patient).

2. A fluctuant, pseudocystic hemorrhagic mass is palpable.

3. A slow course with metastases via the veins to the lung has been observed.

ROENTGENOLOGIC INTERPRETATION

There is bone destruction visualized with no evidence of infection.

Malignant Variant of Giant Cell Tumor

1. A giant cell tumor that is abused by in-

judicious treatment or trauma may develop an active malignancy.

2. The roentgenologic features are the evidence of the original giant cell tumor plus the classical invasive destruction of a malignant lesion.

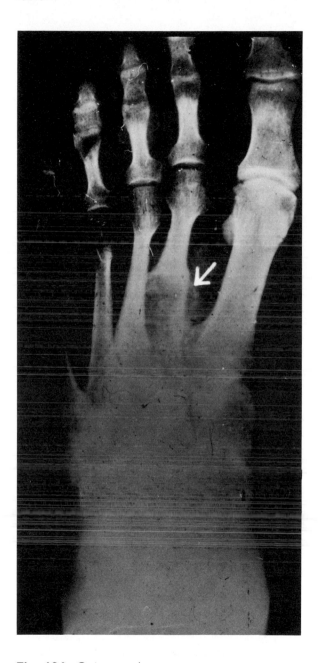

Fig. 124. Osteogenic sarcoma

1. Invasively destructive mass, proximal one-third second metatarsal.

2. Shelf-like projections at site of active destruction.

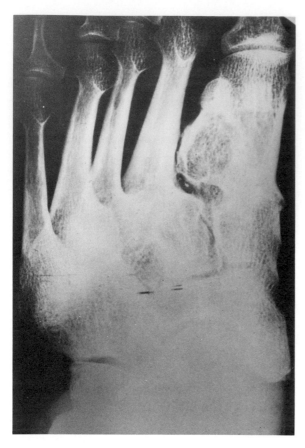

Fig. 125. Osteoma — bony ankylosis

1. Postoperative fusion of tarsometatarsal and intercuneiform cuboid articulations.

2. Lateral aspect shaft of first metatarsal presents an osteoma which appears to have originated from the metaphysis.

BENIGN TUMORS OF OSSEOUS ORIGIN

Osteoma

An osteoma is a benign tumor of bone characterized by development of an ossific pattern and cortex with a rounded smooth surface.

CLINICAL ORIENTATION

1. Osteoma may be found at any age.

2. It is a slow-growing bone tumor.

3. A sudden, rapid growth of a mass suggests malignancy.

4. Osteomata are often seen at sites of shoe pressure or about the joints in the foot that receive stress from malfunction or injury.

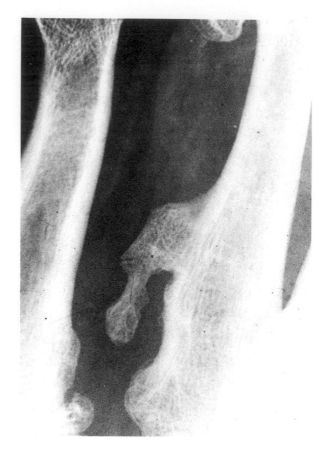

Fig. 126. Osteoma

1. Large, ossific mass extending from cortex perpendicular to shaft and then back toward base.

2. Soft-tissue thickening in the intermetatarsal space.

5. Palpation reveals a firm, rounded, hard mass extending from the bone into the soft tissues.

6. The margins are usually smooth and even to palpation.

7. Pain may be present due to a compression of the soft tissues from pressure of the bony growth.

8. There are occasional redness and soft-tissue swelling where pressure is great.

9. The lesion may limit function if it is large enough to interfere with muscle movement.

10. An *osteoid osteoma* has been seen at all ages but is most common in the young. Lesions have occurred in the phalanges of the feet, talus, and calcaneus.

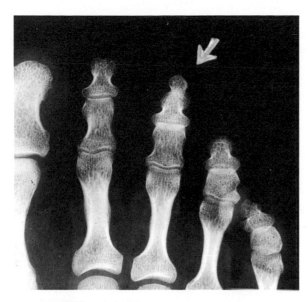

Fig. 127. Osteoma, distal end third toe

ROENTGENOLOGIC INTERPRETATION
(FIGS. 125-130)

1. These new growths originate from the cortex and extend out into the soft tissue.

2. The growth arises near the metaphyseal end of the diaphysis and grows back away from the joint. They are rarely seen at the center of a shaft.

3. As the bone grows, the osteoma gets farther away from the joint.

4. Osteomata may develop from a broad or narrow base.

5. The growth is continuous with the bone proper and presents a trabecular ossific pattern.

6. Osteomata are not to be confused with the rare osteoid osteoma.

7. An osteoma may develop cartilaginous elements at its tip with scalloped margins.

8. Osteoid osteomata are monocentric. They have occurred in both cancellous and cortical bone.

   a. This is a rounded, dense, pea-sized bone tumor with a surrounding zone of decrease in density.

   b. When located near the periosteum, a thick circumscribed periosteal bone develops with a blending at the margins with adjacent bone.

   c. Trabeculae are usually in an osteoid state.

   d. Often an osteoid osteoma is mistaken for osteomyelitis with sequestration.

Exostosis

Exostoses are benign overgrowths of bone. Chronic irritation may result in a proliferation

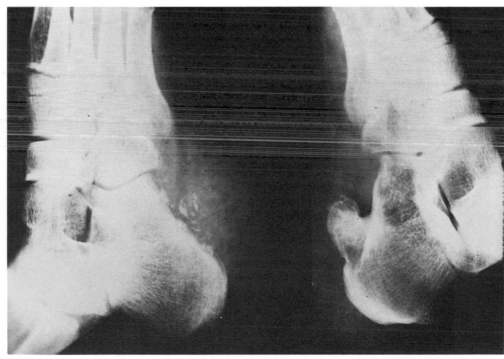

Fig. 128. Osteoma calcaneus. Preoperative and postoperative.

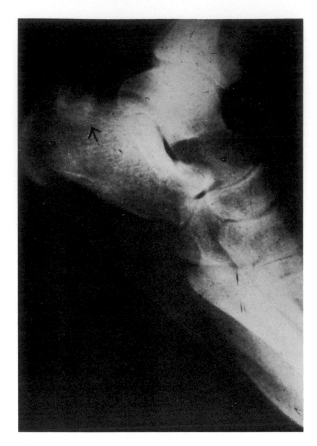

Fig. 129. Osteoid osteoma. Circumscribed, dense, irregular area of condensation, dorsal aspect posterior one third of calcaneus.

on the bone with development of an overlying protective bursa.

CLINICAL ORIENTATION

1. An *exostosis* and *spur* are one and the same as interpreted clinically and roentgenologically.

2. Exostoses occur at sites of chronic irritation, especially in those bones of the foot subject to trauma.

3. They may develop on those joints receiving undue strain and stress from faulty weight distribution.

4. Pressure from a strap or low-cut shoe, irritation from a metal eyelet, or a direct trauma may cause an exostosis to develop.

5. A plantar calcaneal spur develops from undue stress at the origin and attachment of the plantar flexor digitorum brevis muscle, plantar fascia, and plantar ligaments.

6. Pain may be present at the medial tubercle of the plantar surface of the calcaneus.

7. Calcaneal spurs are generally painful on arising after periods of rest.

8. A posterior calcaneal exostosis extending upward into the tendo achillis is common in obese persons, in those using foot pedals or brakes, or in any occupation or trauma pro-

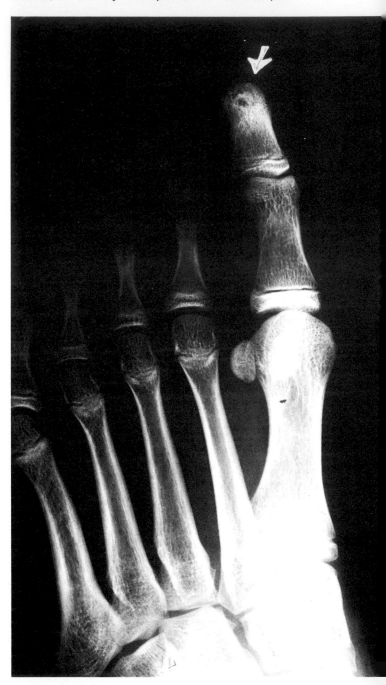

Fig. 130. Osteoid osteoma, distal end of hallux

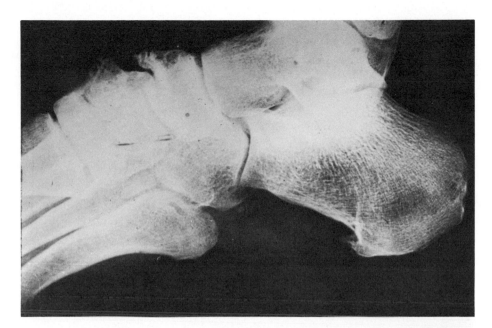

Fig. 131. Ecchondroma —exostosis

1. Bone in various stages of ossification extending into soft tissue on dorsum of navicular and cuneiform secondary to trauma.

2. Calcaneal spur.

ducing great strain on the tendo achillis.

9. These exostoses are rarely painful and are usually caused by imbalanced feet, abnormal weight distribution, and marked rotation of the calcaneus accompanied by pull and pressure from shoes on the tendo achillis.

10. A direct trauma or tear, friction, pressure, or traction on the attachments of articulating ligaments and capsules is often the exciting factor in the development of exostosis on the dorsomedial margin of the head of the talus.

11. A bursa may overlie an exostosis on the dorsum of the first metatarsocuneiform articulation.

12. A dorsal bunion over the first metatarsophalangeal joint is often secondary to an exostosis.

ROENTGENOLOGIC INTERPRETATION (FIGS. 131-133)

1. An exostosis may develop from the slightest periosteal proliferation to the size of a standard fountain pen point.

2. An exostosis usually projects in the direction of stress, pointing at varying angles. It may be continuous with the bone.

3. Occasionally, exostoses are found in two or more parts separated by radiolucent tissue.

4. In the absence of a fracture line through an exostosis, it is conceivable that calcareous

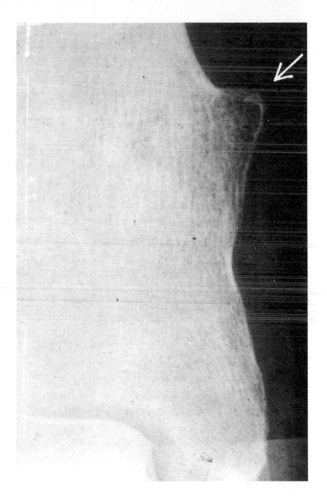

Fig. 132. Table-top exostosis

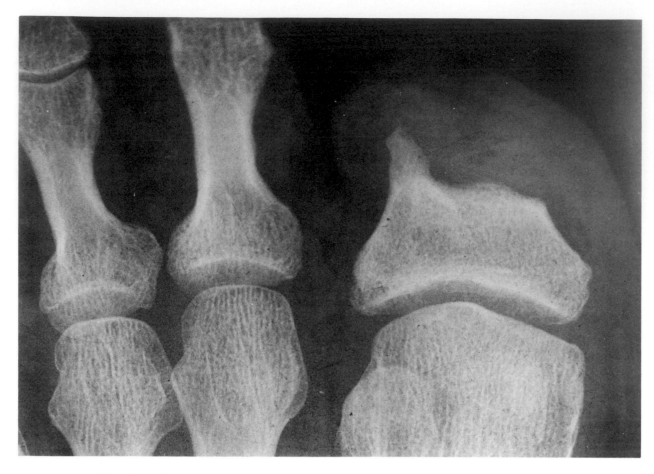

Fig. 133. Exostosis
   1. Distal end of amputated stump creating ulceration in the soft tissue.
   2. This may be the sequel to incomplete amputation.

changes have taken place in the fibrous expansions of the tendon or ligament at its attachments to bone.

5. Sometimes they develop from one or more sites on the bone with several points projecting into the soft tissues.

6. Exostoses may vary in size and shape and be pointed, smooth, or highly irregular.

7. The size of a spur or its sharpness does not indicate the severity of the symptoms.

8. A long-standing exostosis may become smooth, rounded, and develop a cortex with a central trabecular pattern.

9. A spur (exostosis) that has been asymptomatic is often found by chance on a roentgenogram.

10. The talus may present an exostosis projecting upward from its head with an abutting exostosis on the posterior articulating surface of the navicular.

11. An exostosis over the metatarsocuneiform joints must be differentiated from an accessory ossicle.

12. One on the lateral aspect of the base of the first metatarsal projecting into the intermetatarsal space must be differentiated from an os intermetatarseum or the sclerosed communicating artery.

13. Exostoses are commonly found on the dorsal aspects of the first metatarsal head projecting upward and backward from the joint.

14. Exostoses have been seen on the heads of metatarsals, bases and heads of phalanges, and throughout the tarsometatarsal and tarsal articulations, with or without other roentgenologic signs of disease.

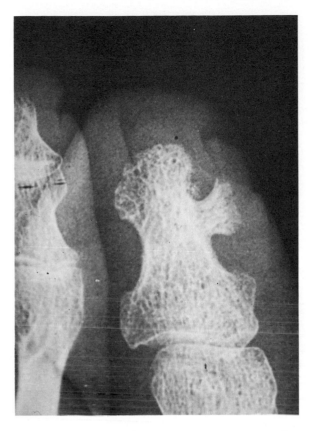

Fig. 134. Subungual exostosis — preoperative. Note site of origin from the cortex.

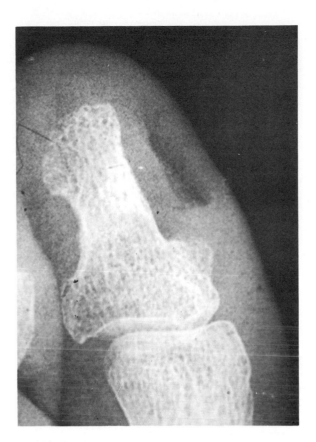

Fig. 135. Subungual exostosis — postoperative.

Subungual Exostosis

CLINICAL ORIENTATION

1. Subungual exostoses may be caused by direct trauma, unremitting irritation from ill-fitting footgear, or torn linings in the toe cap of a shoe.

2. Although more commonly seen under the hallux nail, they may occur under the nails of the lesser toes.

3. Painful, hypertrophied nails may present underlying bone pathology.

4. A low-grade inflammation, infection, and suppuration may be the first signs of a subungual exostosis, and the nail plate may be elevated.

5. Subungual ulcerations in the nail bed may develop from compression of the nail plate on an exostosis.

6. Removal of the nail plate overlying the subungual elevation discloses either a rough, calloused nail bed with tyloma or a subungual heloma dura.

7. Occasional breaks in the subungual tissue result in ulceration and the presence of profuse granulations in the ulcer bed.

8. The subungual tissue overlying an exostosis may be fibrous, thin, and shiny.

ROENTGENOLOGIC INTERPRETATION
(FIGS. 134–136)

1. The distal phalanx presents a small bone tumor extending upward beneath the middle and distal end of the nail plate.

2. Early, there may be an increase in soft-tissue density beneath the nail plate.

3. The proliferation of bone from the distal phalanx presents a cortex with a medullary reticulum and base originating from the phalangeal cortex.

4. The exostosis may be rounded, pointed, or table top in shape and may be from 1 mm to 1 cm in size.

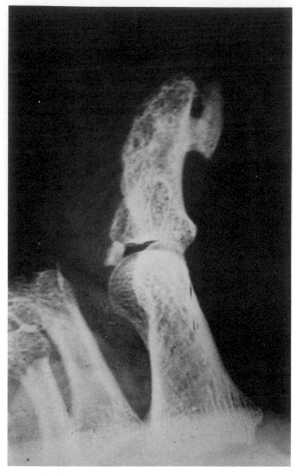

Fig. 136. Table-top subungual exostosis — calcification in joint space

1. Exostosis originates from the cortex and is flattened out in its development due to nail pressure above.

2. Calcareous deposit in joint space spreads the joint.

Enchondroma (Chondroma)

CLINICAL ORIENTATION

1. Enchondromata develop in the phalanges of the hands and feet and may occur at any age.

2. Preexisting cartilage cells of an embryonic origin commence developing in adult tissue resulting in these tumors in bone.

3. An indurated thickening of a toe may be a clinical sign of enchondroma.

4. Trivial trauma may cause symptoms of a toe fracture. Pathologic fracture may occur through an enchondroma. It is usually transverse.

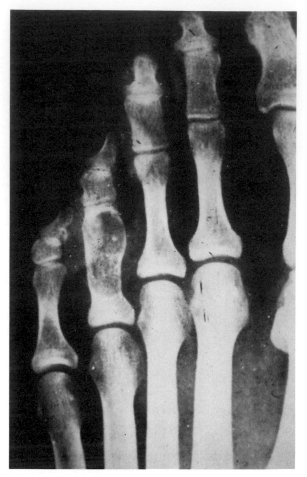

Fig. 137. Enchondroma. Proximal phalanx, fourth toe, presents expansion, thinning of cortex, and lack of structure involving the distal two thirds of bone.

5. An enchondroma does not affect function unless a pathologic fracture develops.

6. These tumors may have malignant tendencies but should only be diagnosed as malignant when mitotic figures are noted on histopathologic examination.

ROENTGENOLOGIC INTERPRETATION
(Figs. 137-139)

1. An enchondroma appears centrally as a localized area of decrease in density in the shafts of long bones. It has occurred in tendon sheaths.

2. There is a loss of the trabecular pattern of bone.

3. The growth of an enchondroma is from many centers expanding in all directions.

4. The outline is regular and rounded.

5. The cortex is expanded and thinned.

6. Enchondromata resemble bone cysts but are usually multilocular and often multiple.

7. A transverse pathologic fracture through an enchondroma may occur spontaneously or follow trivial trauma.

8. An enchondroma must be differentiated from an intramedullary lipoma of bone (Mueller and Robbins, 1960).

Osteochondroma (Ecchondroma, Cartilaginous Exostosis)

CLINICAL ORIENTATION

1. Ecchondromata commence growth before puberty.

2. These growths occur near the ends of the shaft growing away from their origin at the epiphysis or joint.

3. Pain is noted when pressure on soft tissues causes inflammatory changes.

4. Although these are benign growths, they can become malignant with trauma or injudicious treatment.

ROENTGENOLOGIC INTERPRETATION
(Figs. 140-141)

1. An osteochondroma is a small or large benign growth of bone originating from the epiphyseal or articular cartilage.

2. Bone and cartilaginous elements result in the appearance of a scalloped margin.

3. Prior to ossification, the hypertrophic overgrowth of cartilage is called an ecchondrosis.

4. A partially ossified chondroma or ecchondrosis is termed an osteochondroma.

Giant Cell Tumor

CLINICAL ORIENTATION

1. Cell origin is unknown. Large giant cells

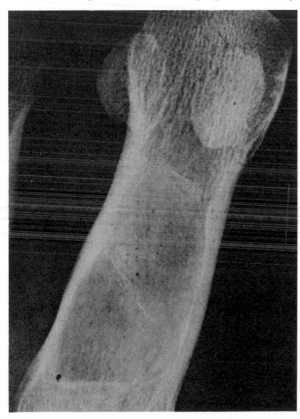

Fig. 138. Large enchondroma. Area of lack of structure in first metatarsal shaft.

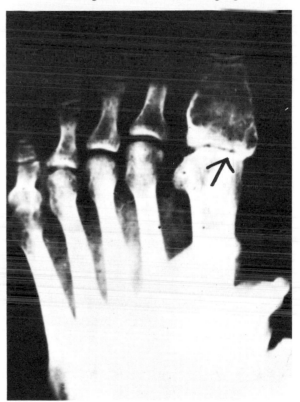

Fig. 139. Enchondroma

1. Expansion of the central area of the proximal phalanx of the hallux.

2. Thinning of the cortices.

3. Multilocular areas of nonreticulation of bone.

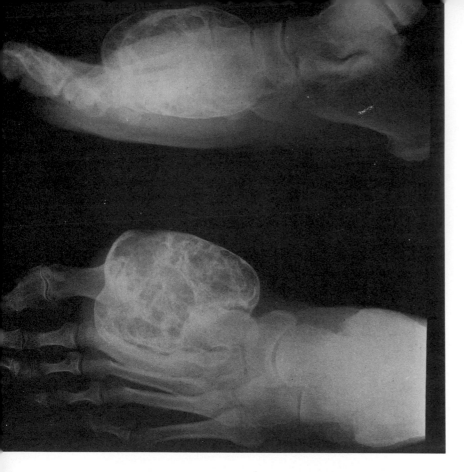

Fig. 140. Giant Cell Tumor. Large, multilocular, ovoid expansion of bone. Thinned cortex and muliple trabeculations. This lesion would have to be differentiated pathologically from an osteochondroma.
(Courtesy of Earl Zatz, D.P.M.)

are present, but it is questionable that they replace bone.

2. Giant cell tumor occurs near the end of a growth period for bone, *e.g.*, just prior to union of epiphysis to shaft.

3. It occasionally develops in metatarsal heads and the proximal phalanges near the joints.

4. Vague pains are usually an early symptom of giant cell tumor.

5. Not infrequently, slight swelling or pathologic fracture may be the first sign of the lesion.

6. Limitation of motion is common.

7. There is no evidence of infection.

8. The growth is slowly progressive in its development.

9. Induration at the site of tumor requires careful evaluation.

ROENTGENOLOGIC INTERPRETATION
(Figs. 143-145)

1. Giant cell tumors occur after the epiphyseal line is ossified. Cells at the former epiphyseal cartilage replace bone tissue to form a growth.

3. Benign, large, round, or ovoid, multilocular-appearing lesions are noted.

4. Loculation and decrease in density with expansion of bone are characteristic.

5. The reticular bone structure is absent in the epiphyseal and distal end of the diaphysis.

6. Periosteal new bone may result in trabeculations extending out into the soft tissues. This must be differentiated from a malignant process or periosteal hemangioma.

7. The cortex is thinned but intact. Accretion is noted on the cortical surface.

8. Many fine trabeculations are noted in the tumor, thus differentiating it from an enchondroma.

9. Loxley, Thiemeyer, and Ellsasser (1972) reported two cases of periosteal hemangioma as a painful mass over long bone without history of injury. Periosteal hemangioma was described as a shallow-shaped depression externally in the cortex, marked local sclerosis with thickening of the periosteum. The authors feel that this must be differentiated from periosteal giant cell tumor.

Solitary Bone Cysts (Unicameral Cysts)

CLINICAL ORIENTATION

1. These cysts may be seen at any age but usually occur about adolescence.

2. The lesion may follow old trauma with resorption of a hematoma.

3. A bone cyst can be innocuous and go unnoticed except by a chance roentgenogram.

4. Pain may be characterized by a dull ache or moderate swelling.

5. A pathologic fracture may initiate the pain.

6. Edema in the surrounding soft tissues may be slight.

7. In the systemic type of bone cysts, osteitis fibrosa cystica, the serum calcium levels are high, the serum phosphorus levels low, and phosphatase high.

8. In unicameral cysts, no changes take place in the blood.

9. The solitary bone cyst must be differentiated from enchondroma or infection in bone.

10. Eight cases involving the calcaneus, five of them in children, have been reported by Kingsbery (1957).

11. At surgery, the lesion may contain cystic or fibrocystic elements tinged brown.

ROENTGENOLOGIC INTERPRETATION
(Figs. 146-148)

I. Solitary cysts occur singly and are centrally located, oval-shaped, and sharply defined. They are localized to a single bone, such as the diaphysis or metaphysis of the tubular

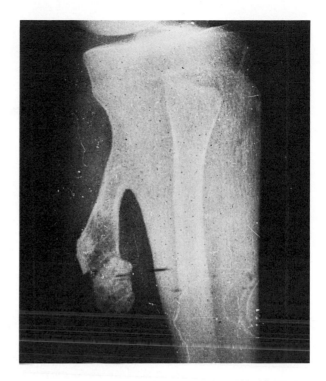

Fig. 141. Osteochondroma — fractured

1. Elongate ossific mass with cartilaginous tip which is fractured and slightly displaced.

2. Break in continuity of cortex and multiple fibrocartilaginous changes at tip.

3. Growth is continuous with the tibia at its base.

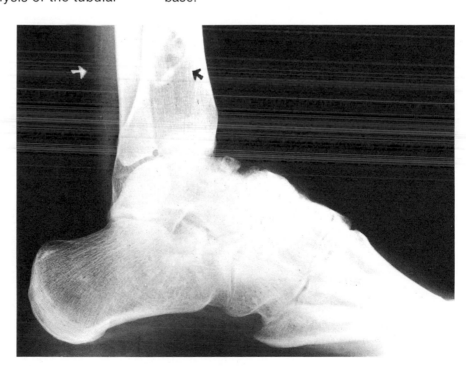

Fig. 142. Nonossifying fibroma and Charcot's joint — young diabetic

1. Note multilocular deossification of bone surrounded by definitive outline of dense bone, distal one third of tibia. Must be differentiated by biopsy from aneurysmal bone cyst.

2. Charcot's joint involving the tarsus.

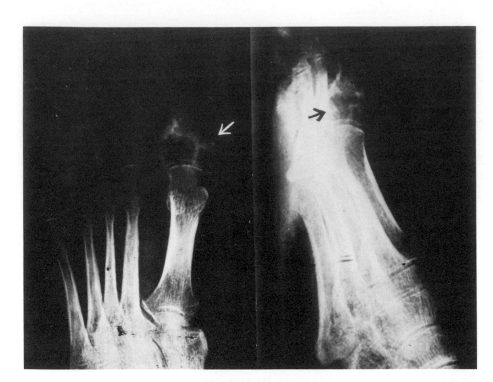

Fig. 143. Giant cell tumor. Multilocular areas of lack of structure with expansion by accretion.

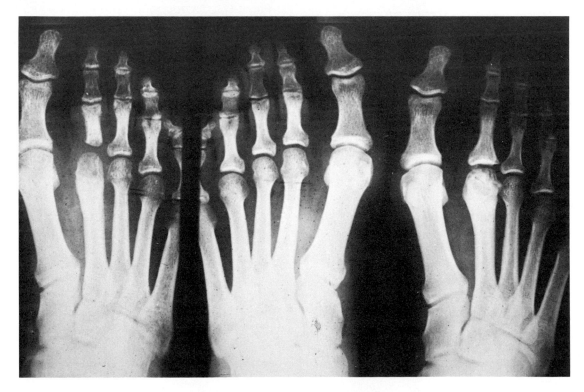

Fig. 144. Giant cell tumor — preoperative and postoperative
1. (*Right*) Second metatarsophalangeal joint presents a thickening of the metatarsal head.
2. Areas of increase and decrease in density with expansion.
3. Wide neck of metatarsal and thick cortices.
4. (*Far left*) Postoperative excision and remodeling of joint.

long bones.

2. A circumscribed area of lack of structure may be visualized on the roentgenogram.

3. The cortex is usually expanded, thinned from pressure, and the bone resorbed.

4. The cortex is sharply defined and thin except when pathologic fracture occurs. However, thickened inner cortical walls are common, and these must be differentiated from multilocular lesions.

5. Small cystic changes may be seen in bone adjacent to a hyperemic area, *e.g.,* first metatarsal head.

6. Pathologic fractures through a cyst are not uncommon. These occur spontaneously and vary in appearance from small cracks to that of a crushed egg shell.

Aneurysmal Bone Cyst

An aneurysmal bone cyst of a metatarsal was reported by Booher (1954, 1957).

ROENTGENOLOGIC INTERPRETATION

1. The aneurysmal bone cyst appears as a soft-tissue mass of increased density.

2. There is an early gradual development of a domelike calcified outline.

3. The cortex is thinned and expanded but intact without evidence of cortical destruction.

4. In young patients, the lesion occurs in the distal half of the diaphysis.

5. Booher described a lesion in the third metatarsal that measured 3.5 × 1.5 cm. This grew rapidly to 3.5 × 2.5 cm.

6. Late spontaneous healing may occur with ossification of the cyst.

Fibrous Dysplasia

Fibrous dysplasia may appear as a monostotic or polyostotic lesion.

CLINICAL ORIENTATION

1. There appears to be an endocrine or neurogenic course, but investigations have not been conclusive.

2. Fibrous dysplasia is commonly associated with precocious puberty in girls.

3. Fibrous dysplasia develops in preadolescents with the development of single or multiple lesions.

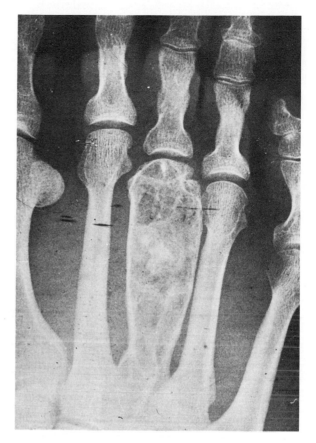

Fig. 145. Giant cell tumor. Note the clublike shape and expansion and lack of structure due to multilocular resorption.

4. There is a tendency for it to be unilateral, affecting the extremities, and it is more common in tubular long bones.

5. There is no evidence of pain unless a pathologic fracture occurs.

6. Areas of brown skin pigmentation may be present on the back and thigh.

7. Blood calcium and phosphorus levels are normal. With an increase in osteoblastic activity, the serum alkaline phosphatase may be increased.

ROENTGENOLOGIC INTERPRETATION
(Fig. 149)

1. A replacement of normal bone by fibrous tissue is visualized as a decrease in density in the cortex and medulla.

2. The cyst is considered to be a fibrous dysplasia if the density within it is greater than that of water.

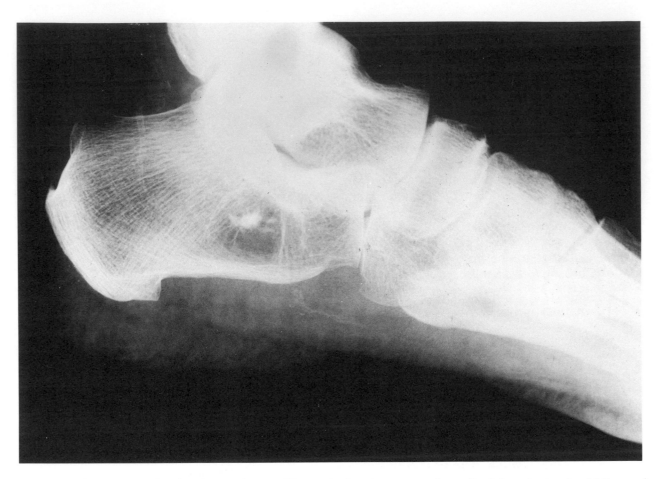

Fig. 146. Bone cyst. Lack of structure with central calcareous deposit at juncture of middle and distal one third of calcaneus.

3. Superimposed dense trabeculae produce a homogeneous increase in the density within the dysplasia.

4. The dysplasia appears as a smudge or as a ground-glass texture.

5. The bone may appear widened but is without alteration in size or shape in early stages.

6. A rather constant finding is the extension of the lesion into the adjacent bone with a shading off, "candle flame" appearance.

7. In monostotic fibrous dysplasia, the calcifications at the periphery of an apparent cyst may be dense and irregular. There is a sharp inner margin of increase in density.

8. Bending deformities occur as the bone weakens.

Osteitis Fibrosa Cystica

CLINICAL ORIENTATION

1. This disease occurs more commonly in young adults and in middle-aged women.

2. It is often associated with hyperparathyroidism due to a parathyroid adenoma.

3. The blood calcium levels may be high and phosphorus levels low, with a high serum alkaline phosphatase.

4. It must be differentiated from fibrous dysplasia, neurofibromatosis, and solitary bone cysts.

ROENTGENOLOGIC INTERPRETATION

1. The bone lesions are found systemically with a generalized deossification and bending.

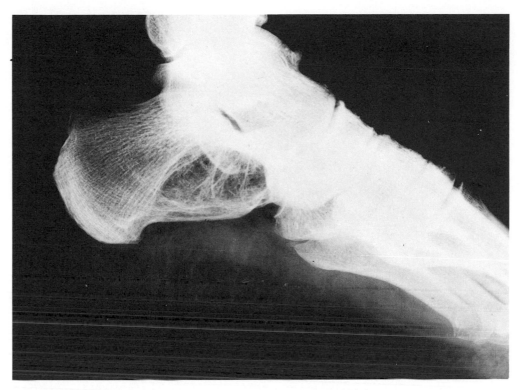

Fig. 147. Bone cyst (lack of structure). Lack of structure in preoperative area involving distal one third of calcaneus

Fig. 148. Surgical repair of cyst. Reparative calcification following curettage and implantation of bone chips from tibia.

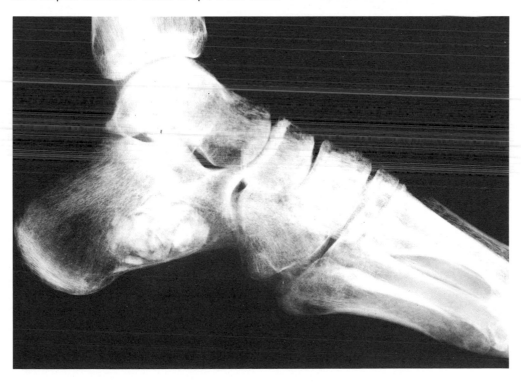

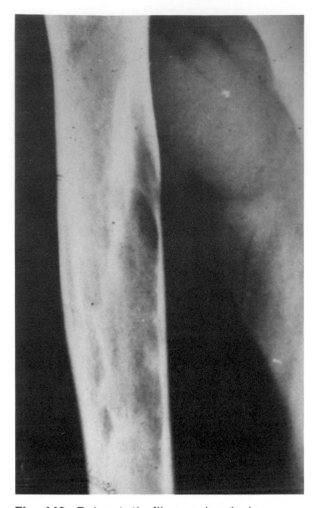

Fig. 149. Polyostotic fibrous dysplasia
1. Rounded and elongate areas of lack of structure in bone with some thinning of the cortices.
2. A smudging and shading off of the dysplasia is evident.

2. The changes are seen at the metaphyseal ends of long bones, but all bones are decreased in density.
3. The cortex is thinned and atrophic in osteitis fibrosa cystica.
4. Cystic degeneration in the shafts of the long bones results in a loss of the normal trabecular pattern.
5. There is a lack of bone structure, and expansion is seen about the elongate defect in the bone.
6. Pathologic fracture through the defect is not uncommon.

Chondroma — Soft Tissue
CLINICAL ORIENTATION

1. Chondroma may occur at any age.
2. A firm, movable subcutaneous mass is noted adjacent to bone.
3. Chondroma may recur following surgical excision.
4. Pathologic study may demonstrate calcareous degeneration intermingled with cartilaginous elements.

ROENTGENOLOGIC INTERPRETATION
(Fig. 150)

1. A calcareous deposit may be present in soft tissues adjacent to the cortex of bone.
2. The calcified deposit is irregular in outline with no evidence of a cortex or reticular pattern and must be differentiated from calcification by microscopic examination.
3. Pressure of the tumor on the cortex of bone may create slight deformation.

MALIGNANT TUMORS OF NONOSSEOUS ORIGIN
Ewing's Tumor (Endothelial Myeloma)
CLINICAL ORIENTATION

1. While Ewing's tumor rarely affects the foot, it must be ruled out in apophysitis of the calcaneus.
2. It has been recorded in the calcaneus and talus (Margo and Owens, 1960).
3. A Ewing's tumor was reported in a fourth metatarsal in an 11-year-old girl with metastasis to the calcaneus (Newman, 1961).
4. It is common in childhood and adolescence. Some cases have been recorded as early as age 4½.
5. Trauma may initiate symptoms, but the onset is usually indefinite.
6. There may be a tenderness and dull pain at the site of a small, palpable mass or swelling in the shaft of a long bone, usually the lower ends of the femur, tibia, fibula, and metatarsals.
7. Temperature may be increased with some redness of the overlying skin.
8. The extent of the leukocytosis is dependent on the severity of the lesion, and a moderate secondary anemia is noted.

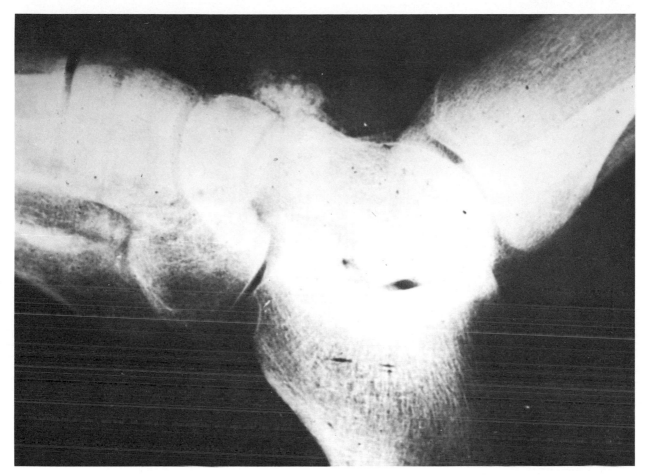

Fig. 150. Chondroma. 1. Irregular calcification.
2. This lesion must be differentiated from osteochondromatosis and calcification of the periarticular tissues.

9. The rapid growth is not too painful or disabling. The lesion grows by infiltrating adjacent tissues and by expansion of its extra-cortical mass.

10. Metastasis to regional lymph glands, to other bones, and to the lungs is the usual pathogenesis.

11. Ewing's tumor must be differentiated from infection by clinical findings and biopsy. Pyogenic, syphilitic, and tuberculous osteomyelitis, sarcoma, carcinoma, and reticuloendotheliosis must all be considered in the differential diagnosis.

12. Less than 10% recovery rate has been reported.

ROENTGENOLOGIC INTERPRETATION
(Fig. 151)

1. Parallel deposits of subperiosteal calci-

fications are visualized. These have an "onion-skin-like" appearance.

2. Some of the periosteal proliferations end freely in the soft tissues simulating the osteogenic sunburst.

3. Early, the cortex is mottled, and as the lesion progresses, the cortex shows active destruction with deposition of parallel calcifications.

4. It is believed that the lesion develops early in the cortex, then breaks through, infiltrating in several directions, thus stimulating the subperiosteal calcification.

5. A thin layer of fibrous bone is placed over the cortex breakthrough. Subsequent layers attach and become calcified in layers but do not keep the tumor from spreading.

6. The tumor spreads to the metaphysis of the bone and is slowed up at the epiphyseal

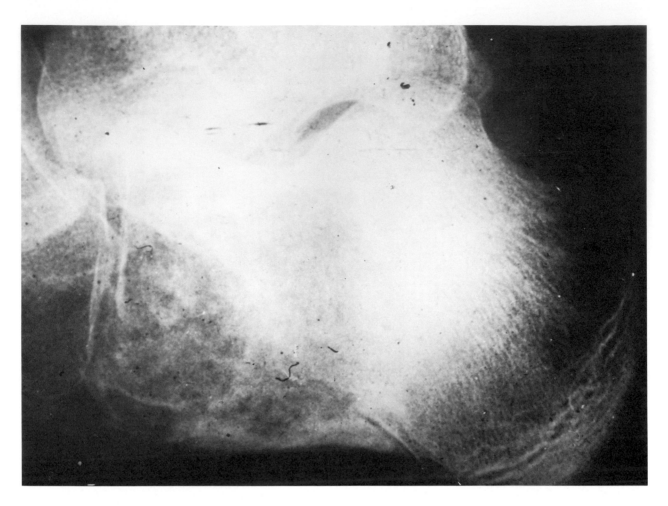

Fig. 151. Ewing's endothelioma
  1. Note parallel laying down of bone with mottling. Cortical outline is thinned.
  2. Anterior and plantar angle of calcaneus has been irradiated.

cartilage.

7. Ewing's tumor rarely invades joints.

8. The medullary portion of the bone reacts to the lesion and becomes osteosclerotic and widened.

9. Pathologic fracture and considerable activity in the bone are common in the calcaneus.

10. A mottled or "pock-marked" bone was described by Newman in 1961.

MALIGNANT TUMORS OF SPECIALIZED SKELETAL STRUCTURES

Synovioma (Synovial Fibrosarcoma)

CLINICAL ORIENTATION

1. Synovioma may occur from early in childhood through old age but usually develops about adolescence through the fourth decade.

2. The tumor is derived from the synovial lining of joints, bursae, and tendon sheaths.

3. Although derived from synovial tissue, the mass may develop beyond the capsular tissue.

4. It commonly affects the knee and is uncommon in the foot.

5. It has malignant characteristics.

6. Metastasis involving the lungs and lymph glands may be rapid or may take place over a period of years.

ROENTGENOLOGIC INTERPRETATION
(Fig. 152)

1. A synovioma presents as an ovoid or spherical increase in density of the soft tissues.

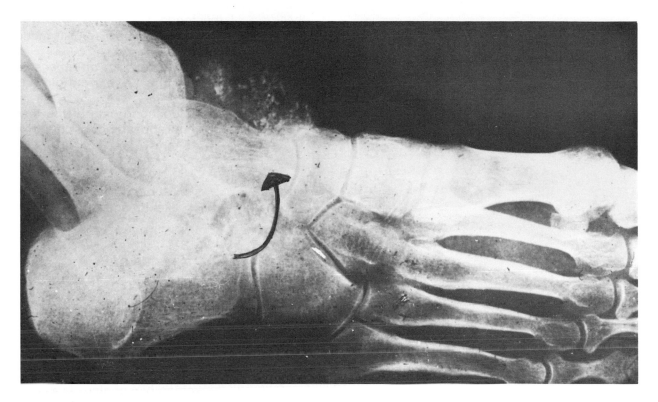

Fig. 152. Synovioma
1. Flaky, calcareous density within a circumscribed mass of increased soft-tissue density. A biopsy is necessary to differentiate.
2. Talonavicular joint presents active destruction due to invasion.

2. The mass appears of uniform density with a smooth, definitive outline.

3. Occasionally, calcific deposits are present in the mass.

4. Adjacent bone and soft-tissue reaction is uncommon.

5. Osteoporosis frequently accompanies synovioma.

6. If bone destruction does occur, it is not as massive as one might expect considering the size of the synovioma. The destruction appears hazy and indistinct.

Fibrosarcoma

Goldenberg (1960) describes a well-differentiated fibrosarcoma of the calcaneus as follows:

ROENTGENOLOGIC INTERPRETATION

1. There is enlargement of the tuberosity of the calcaneus.

2. Collapse of the articular surface occurs with a loss of the tuber angle.

3. The normal trabecular pattern is replaced by coarse multiloculation involving most of the bone.

4. The posterior superior aspect of the calcaneus is expanded and irregular, indicating a perforation of the cortex.

Phalangeal Metastasis

CLINICAL ORIENTATION

1. Colson and Willcox (1948) report two cases of metastasis from carcinoma of the bronchus to the terminal phalanges of the toes.

2. It is believed to be due to the easy access of bronchial lesions to the pulmonary veins and thence to the systemic arteries.

3. In one case, the first sign of a malignant disease was metastases to a phalanx and a metatarsal.

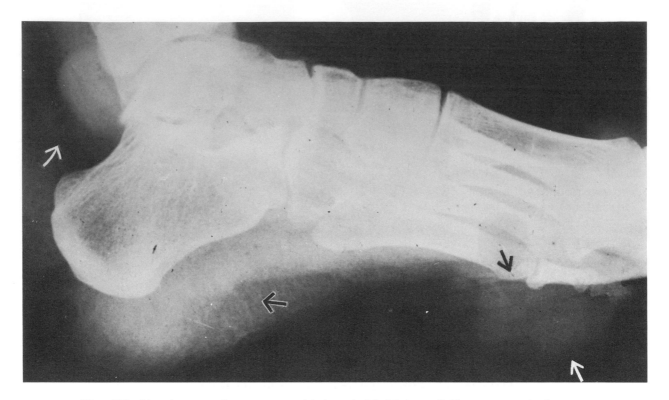

Fig. 156. Xanthoma tuberosum multiplex. 1. Multiple soft-tissue mass in foot. 2. Marked increase in density of soft tissues with definitive outline.

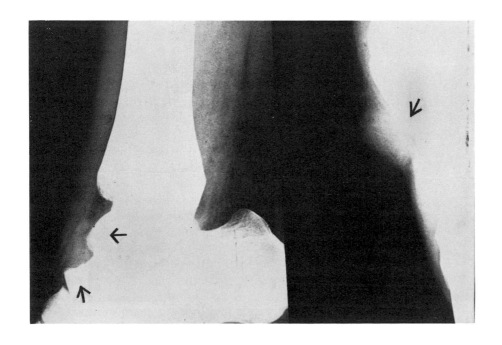

Fig. 157. Xanthoma. 1. Marked increase in density of soft tissues. 2. Appears rounded with definitive margins.

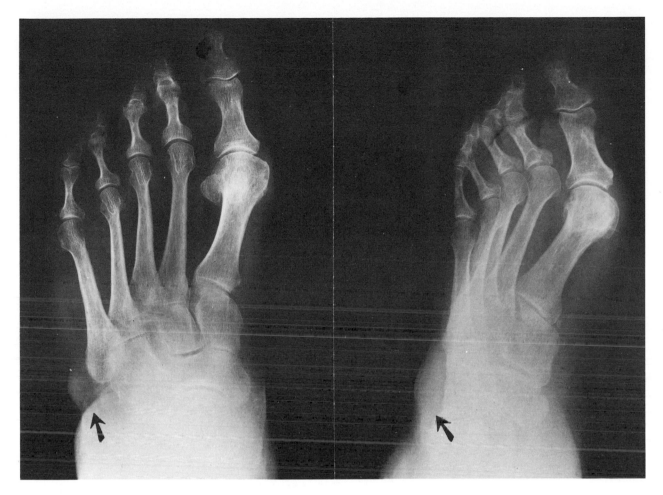

Fig. 158. Mass — ganglion
  1. Soft-tissue mass overlying cuboid.
  2. Note increase in soft-tissue density and definitive outline.

ROENTGENOLOGIC INTERPRETATION
(Figs. 156-157)

1. Multiple masses of soft tissue 1 mm to 2 cm in diameter are visible.

2. The increase in soft-tissue density is circumscribed and definitely delineated in outline.

3. Bone may be osteoporotic containing multiple areas of lack of structure which are possibly cystic, fibrous, or cartilaginous.

Nonosteogenic Fibroma (Fibrous Metaphyseal Defect)

CLINICAL ORIENTATION

1. This condition is rare after the age of 30.

2. It occurs at the ends of long bones.

3. It is suggested that the lesion is a localized disturbance in bone growth.

4. The lesion may disappear spontaneously.

ROENTGENOLOGIC INTERPRETATION
(Figs. 158-162)

1. A thin-walled area of lack of bone structure is visualized at the end of a long bone.

2. Occasional marked sclerosis about the defect is typical of this tumor.

3. There may be a gradual diminution of the size of the lesion with the passage of years.

4. The lesion may disappear entirely.

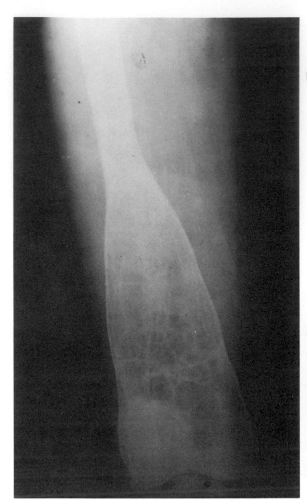

Fig. 159. Gaucher's disease

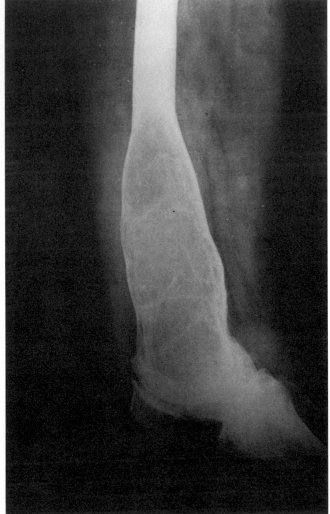

Fig. 160. Gaucher's disease

    1. Distal end of femur is expanded with thinning of cortex and multicentric areas of lack of structure.

    2. Bones are expanded and subject to pathologic fracture.

    3. Replacement of normal erythropoietic marrow results in anemia and enlargement of spleen.

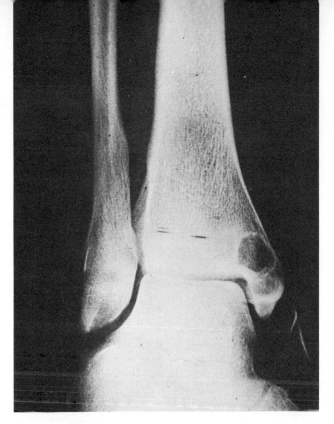

Fig. 161. Nonossifying fibroma

1. Occurs adjacent to the metaphysis and the cortex.

2. Note the surrounding dense sclerotic outline.

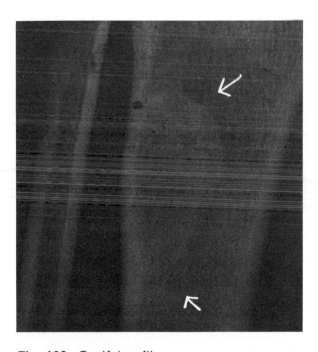

Fig. 162. Ossifying fibroma

1. Definitive increase in density adjacent to the cortex.

2. Clearly delineated.

BIBLIOGRAPHY

Ackerman, A.J., and Hart, M.S.: Multiple Primary Hemangioma of the Bones of the Extremity, Amer. J. Roentgen. 48:27, 1942.

Ackerman, L.V., and Spjut, H.T.: Tumors of Bone and Cartilage, Armed Forces Institute of Pathology, 1962.

Albright, F., Butler, A.M., Hampton, A.O., and Smith, P.: Syndrome Characterized by Osteitis Fibrosa Disseminata, Area of Pigmentation, and Endocrine Dysfunction with Precocious Puberty in Females, Report of 5 Cases, New Eng. J. Med. 216:727, 1937.

Badgley, C.E., and Battis, M.: Osteogenic Sarcoma, Arch. Surg. 43:4, 1941.

Bloodgood, J.C.: Benign Bone Cysts, Osteitis Fibrosa, Amer. J. Surg. 69:345, 1919.

Bloodgood, J.C.: Bone Tumors, Ann. Surg. 80:817, 1924.

Booher, R.J.: Aneurysmal Bone Cyst of a Metatarsal, J. Bone Joint Surg. 29-A:435, 1957.

Booher, R.J.: Tumors Arising from Blood Vessels in the Hands and the Feet, Clin. Orthop. 19:71, 1961.

Coley, B.L., and Sharp, G.S.: Paget's Disease: Predisposing Factor to Osteogenic Sarcoma, Arch. Surg. 23:918, 1931.

Colson, G.M., and Willcox, A.: Phalangeal Metastases in Bronchogenic Carcinoma, J.A.M.A. 137:995, 1948.

Dahlin, D.C.: *Bone Tumors: General Aspects and an Analysis of 2,276 Cases.* Springfield, Ill.: Charles C Thomas, 1957.

Durbin, F.C., and Smith, S.G.: A Chondromatous Tumor of the Calcaneum, J. Bone Joint Surg. 37-B:584, 1955.

DuVries, H.: Surgical Intervention for Calcaneal Spur, J. Amer. Podiat. Ass. (June), 1958.

Ewing, J.: *Neoplastic Diseases.* Philadelphia: W.B. Saunders Co., 1942.

Ferguson, A.B.: *Roentgen Diagnosis of the Extremities and Spine.* New York: P.B. Hoeber, Inc., 1941.

Geschickter, C.F., and Copeland, M.M.: Primary Tumors of the Cranial Bones, Amer. J. Cancer 26:155, 1936.

Geschickter, C.F., and Copeland, M.M.: *Tumors of Bone,* ed. 3. Philadelphia: J.B. Lippincott Co., 1949.

Geschickter, C.F., and Maseritz, I.H.: Ewing's Sarcoma, J. Bone Joint Surg. 21-B:26, 1939.

Goldenberg, R.R.: Well Differentiated Fibrosarcoma of the Calcaneus, J. Bone Joint Surg. 42-A:1151, 1960.

Gorham, L.W.: Albright's Syndrome, Clinics 1:358, 1942.

Haldemann, K.O.: Development of Bone in Relation to the Formation of Neoplasma, Radiology 40:247, 1942.

Huntington, R.W., Jr., Sheffel, D.J., Iger, M., and Honkolmann, C.: Malignant Bone Tumors in Siblings, J. Bone Joint Surg. 42-A:1065, 1960.

Jaffe, H.L., and Lichtenstein, L.: Solitary Unicameral Bone Cyst with Emphasis on Roentgen Picture, Pathologic Appearance and Pathogenesis, Arch Surg. 44:1004, 1942.

Janik, A.: Tumors of Tendon Sheaths, Ann. Surg. 85:897, 1927.

Kaump, D.G.: Laboratory Tests in General Practice, J.A.M.A. 132:253, 1946.

Kingland, H.D.: Recurrent Chondroma, J. Amer. Podiat. Ass. 52(11), 1962.

Kingsbery, L.B.: Solitary Cyst of the Os Calcis in Adults and Children,

Kolodny, A.: Bone Sarcoma, Surg. Gynec. Obstet. 44:126, 1927.

Lewin, P.: *The Foot and Ankle.* Philadelphia: Lea & Febiger Co., 1940.

Lichtenstein, L.: *Bone Tumors,* ed. 2. St. Louis: C.V. Mosby Co., 1959.

Lichtenstein, L., and Jaffe, H.L.: Fibrous Dysplasia of Bone, Arch. Path. 33:777, 1942.

Lichtenstein, L., and Jaffe, H.L.: Chondrosarcoma of Bone, Amer. J. Path. 19:533, 1943.

Loxley, S.S., Thiemeyer, J.L., Jr., and Ellsasser, J.E.: Periosteal Hemangioma, Clin. Orthopedics and Related Research, 85:151, 1972.

Margo, M.K., and Owens, J.N.: J. Okla. Med. Ass. 53:14, 1960.

Maudsley, R.H.: Non-ostogenic Fibroma of Bone (Fibrous Metaphyseal Defect), J. Bone Joint Surg. 38-B:714, 1956.

Miller, D., and Birsner, J.W.: Coccidioidal Granuloma of Bone, Amer. J. Roentgen. 62:229, 1949.

Mueller, M.C., and Robbins, J.L.: Intramedullary Lipoma of Bone, J. Bone Joint Surg. 42-A:517, 1960.

Newman, A.W.: Ewing's Sarcoma, J. Amer. Podiat Ass. 51(10):1961.

Oughterson, N.W., and Tennant, R.: Angiomatous Tumors of the Hands and Feet, Surgery 5:73, 1939.

Pachter, M.R., and Alper, M.: Chondrosarcoma of the Foot, J. Bone Joint Surg. 46-A:601, 1964.

Pack, G.T. (ed.): *Tumors of the Hands and Feet.* St. Louis: C.V. Mosby Co., 1939.

Pike, M.M.: Paget's Disease with Associated Osteogenic Sarcoma, Arch. Surg. 46:750, 1943.

Platt, H.: Cysts of the Long Bones of the Hand and Foot, Brit. J. Surg. 18:20, 1930.

Sossman, J.L.: X-ray Changes of Diagnostic Importance in the Commoner Types of Arthritis, Bull. Rheum. Dis. 7 (Suppl.): (April), 1957.

Unmansky, A.L., Schlesinger, P.T., and Greenberg, B.B.: Tuberculous Dactylitis in the Adult, Arch. Surg. 54:67, 1947.

Urban, L.D.: Roentgenological Interpretation of Diseases of the Feet, Chiropody Rec. 21:60, 1938.

Wyatt, G.M., and Randall, W.S.: Monostatic Fibrous Dysplasia, Amer. J. Roentgen. (March), 1949.

Yale, Irving: A Statistical Report on a Review of 1290 Foot Radiographs, J. Nat. Ass. Chiropodists 47:6, 1957.

10 TRAUMATIC EFFECTS

The foot is prone to trauma. A comprehensive discussion of traumatic effects will be given for the benefit of the student and as a demonstration of the specific problems that may occur in the foot. These effects may occur singly or in combination. Many roentgenologic features of traumatic tissue reactions are shown in Chapter 2.

INFLAMMATION

CLINICAL ORIENTATION

1. Following injury, effusion, subcutaneous hemorrhage, and synovitis may occur with a fluctuating edema over the inflamed parts.
2. Pain on palpation over the affected area is perhaps one of the most common complaints.
3. Bone, joint, muscle, tendon, or capsular injury must be clinically differentiated to provide proper perspective and definitive roentgenograms.

ROENTGENOLOGIC INTERPRETATION

Pathologic changes demonstrated roentgenologically are suggestive of the site, anatomic structure, extent, and course of the inflammatory disorder.

SYNOVITIS

Acute Synovitis with Effusion

CLINICAL AND PATHOLOGIC ORIENTATION

1. A trauma to a joint, usually the larger joints, may produce an intraarticular effusion composed of serous exudate or hemorrhagic extravasations.
2. The synovial membrane is congested; redness develops from the engorgement of the blood vessels, particularly about the attachments to the articular cartilage. The swelling lasts from 1 week to 10 days.

ROENTGENOLOGIC INTERPRETATION

1. Effusions are often accompanied by a superficial deossification of bone.
2. Effusion is identified by an increase in soft-tissue density within the confines of the joint capsule.

Purulent Synovitis

CLINICAL AND PATHOLOGIC ORIENTATION

1. In poorly handled cases or in complications of the acute synovitis, the joint may become enormous with increased synovial exudation.
2. The exudate may become turbid from cellular debris and accumulated wastes, finally becoming infected and purulent.

ROENTGENOLOGIC INTERPRETATION

1. Early, a widening of the joint from the increased pressure within it is demonstrated. An increase in soft-tissue density within the articular capsule suggests effusion.
2. Rapid destruction of the joint occurs when the abnormal fluid is not allowed an avenue of exit.
3. The roentgenogram presents a hazy, flat, indistinct bone structure.
4. When destruction occurs, a loss of substance is evident with reaction area and a reactive swelling
5. In the later stages, the joint space is narrowed with a decrease in articular cartilage.

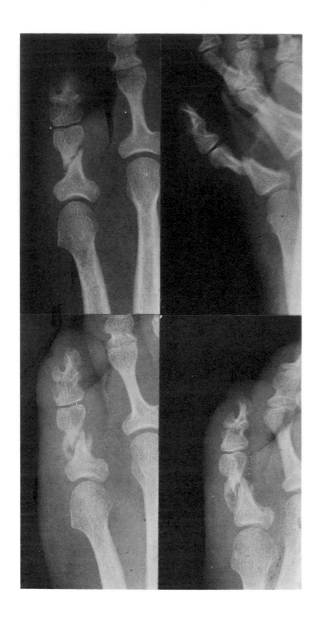

Nonunion of Fractures

1. Factors influencing fracture repair.

a. Repair of fractures may be affected adversely by old age, an abnormal edema, poor circulatory supply to the affected part, too early manipulation of the fractured fragments, the presence of a local disease process, faulty local calcium supply, unusually large hematoma, or by marked displacement.

b. The calcium supply to the fractured part is derived from the adjacent fractured margins of bone, walls of ruptured blood vessels, and nourishing fluids.

2. Causes of nonunion.

a. Nonunion of movable bone fragments may result from excessive mobility of the fragments, a decrease in the ability of the patient to regenerate bone, or from infection. Syphilis may cause dense callus with excessive calcification and condensation.

b. Failure of union may result from interposition of soft tissue in the fracture line.

c. A fibrocartilaginous disk or hyaline cartilage may develop between the movable bone fragments.

3. Failure of union may result in a pseudoarthrosis. The margins develop reparative calcifications but do not unite.

4. A fibrous union may unite after immobilization. The margins are spiculated and not rounded as in the already repaired pseudoarthrosis.

Epiphyseal Displacement

Epiphyseal displacement may result in fracture of the margins of the metaphysis. The apophysis when fractured must be differentiated from an accessory epiphyseal cartilage. Bipartite and tripartite apophyses are quite common.

Osteochondritis Dissecans (Fig. 181)

Osteochondritis dissecans results from injury by impaction to the epiphysis. A sclerotic bone plaque separates from the traumatized bone and forms in the joint space. The roentgenogram presents a fragment of bone, an in-

Fig. 179. Fracture and callus

1. Complete oblique fracture, proximal phalanx.

2. Calcareous strands (callus) unite fractured fragments.

b. After 3 or 4 weeks, demineralization and soft-tissue atrophy develop. This becomes severe in about 6 weeks.

c. Later calcareous density develops as evidence of repair.

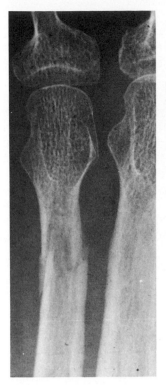
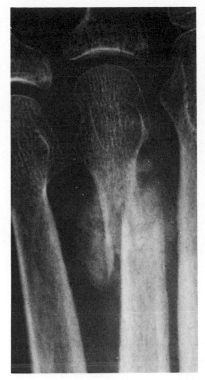
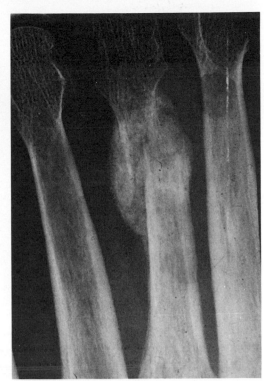

Fig. 180. Repair of fracture. 1. Complete transverse fracture.
2. Displacement of fragments with callus development.
3. Remodeling of bone with increased density of callus.

creased density, or local demineralization at the site of impaction, effusion, widening of the joint space, and irregular ossification

Tenosis

Tenosis, as seen in Osgood-Schlatter disease and at the posterior of the calcaneus, presents no evidence of fracture line. It does show edema, hemorrhage, and degenerative changes in a tendon at its attachment. Irregular ossification due to impared circulation occurs at the site of the tendon attachment and with decrease of the swelling, the tendon becomes thicker.

Sudeck's Atrophy (See Figs. 45-47)

1. Sudeck's atrophy may develop after fracture and repair or after trivial or severe trauma.

2. It commonly develops after prolonged immobilization and is associated with impairment of circulation by swelling, trivial injury, vascular disease, prolonged physiotherapy, infectious arthritis, and causalgic states.

3. The roentenologic feature is an irregu-

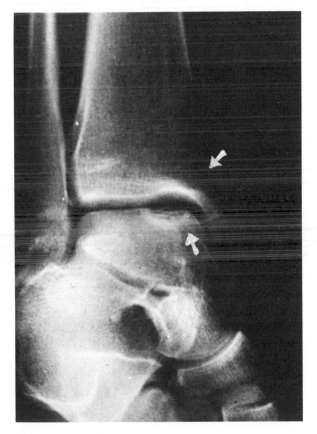

Fig. 181. Osteochondritis dissecans of talus

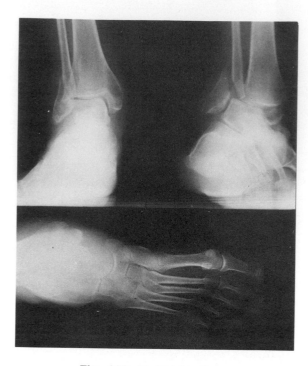

Fig. 182. Pott's fracture

lar, mottled resorption with minute, abundant, spotty areas of demineralization of bone distal to the site of injury.

4. Trophic osteitis or Sudeck's atrophy disappears when the physical cause of impaired circulation has subsided. Stiffness, pain, redness, and swelling are present with the bone changes.

Infection

Compound fractures often become infected and present the usual roentgenologic appearance of infection in bone, *e.g.,* reactive soft-tissue swelling, reactive area as evidenced by a hazy, flat, indistinct, and translucent bone of increased soft-tissue density, condensation, and irregular reactive calcifications.

SPECIAL FRACTURES

Pott's Fracture

CLINICAL ORIENTATION

Pott's fracture may follow a direct, forceful injury or twist of the foot. The usual signs of trauma exist, and the foot is held in eversion and abduction.

ROENTGENOLOGIC INTERPRETATION
(Fig. 182)

1. The fibula is fractured about 3 inches above the tip of the lateral malleolus; the internal malleolus is fractured; the tibiofibular ligament is ruptured; and the foot is displaced upward and backward.

2. When one or both of the malleoli are fractured, the backward and upward pressure of the talus produces a fragmentation of the posterior aspect of the articulating surface of the tibia.

3. The ankle mortise is widened and the foot is shorter from the tibia to the toes. It is assumed that the tibiofibular ligaments are torn.

4. Cortical tears are commonly seen at the tip of the lateral malleolus after a twist of the ankle.

5. The joint is distended with hemorrhagic extravasation and effusion.

Calcaneus

CLINICAL ORIENTATION

1. A history of a fall from a height with a direct blow on the heel, followed by the usual signs of fracture with inability to bear weight on the heel and excruciating pain is pathognomic.

2. A twist of the foot or a fall from a height may fracture the sustentaculum tali.

3. Sudden, severe dorsiflexion of the foot or inversion or extension may cause a fracture of the anterosuperior process of the calcaneus.

4. Occasionally, spontaneous fractures occur in the heel due to stress and multiple minimal trauma.

5. Stress fractures of the calcaneus may be transverse, oblique, stellate, or longitudinal.

6. Fractures may occur where a cyst, enchondroma, or giant cell tumor is present in the body of the calcaneus.

ROENTGENOLOGIC INTERPRETATION
(Figs. 183-185)

1. The fracture appears as a buckling with a fold of increased density at the site of fracture.

2. It may be transverse, comminuted, oblique, or longitudinal.

3. The upper anterior process of the calcaneus is a common site of a transverse fracture. Following a sprain of the ankle, special oblique views may be necessary to rule out fracture.

4. The posterior surface may be avulsed from severe contracture of the tendo achillis. A cortical tear may be noted.

5. The subtalar and calcaneocuboid joints may develop a degenerative joint disease following heel fractures.

Talus

CLINICAL ORIENTATION

1. Fracture of the talar neck results from extremely forceful dorsiflexion of the foot.

2. There may be a history of direct violence or of a fall on the sole of the foot.

3. These neck fractures are usually transverse and are often accompanied by forward and outward subluxation or dislocation.

4. If dislocations are not readily reduced, necrosis of the integument may result from pressure.

5. Pain and immobility are severe over the site of injury. The condition is often interpreted as a sprain with massive effusion.

6. Crepitus may be felt on rotating the foot while the heel is held firmly.

ROENTGENOLOGIC INTERPRETATION

1. These fractures may be transverse, longitudinal, or stellate.

2. The entire body of the bone may be crushed or comminuted with a resultant decrease in the distance between the ankle joint and the calcaneus.

3. Very often the lateral process of the posterior surface of the talus is fractured. This must be differentiated from the os trigonum, which may appear as this lesion on the roentgenogram.

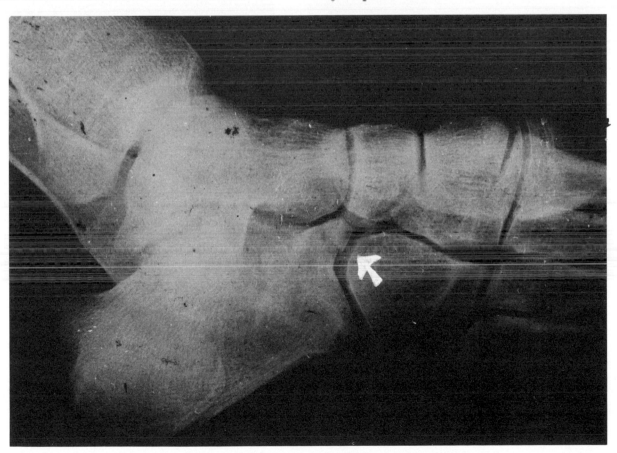

Fig. 183. Fracture, anterior superior process of calcaneus

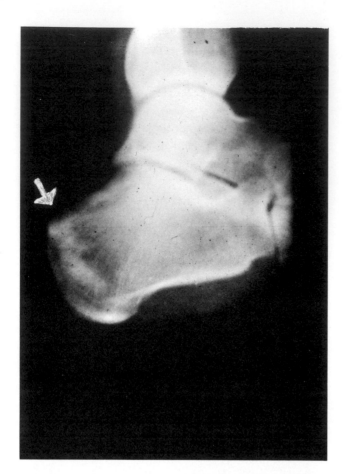 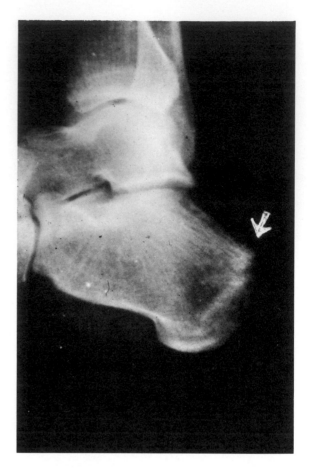

Fig. 184. Stress fracture, calcaneus. Observe irregular line of increase in density at site of fracture and impaction.

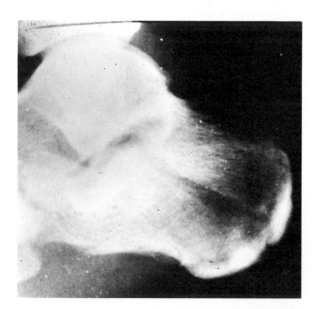

Fig. 185. Longitudinal and oblique stress fractures of calcaneus

Navicular

CLINICAL ORIENTATION

Usually, there is evidence of trauma and associated clinical signs of fracture with swelling, discoloration, pain on palpation, and limitation of function.

ROENTGENOLOGIC INTERPRETATION

1. Longitudinal or oblique, irregular lines of decreased density through the tuberosity of the navicular are common findings.

2. These fractures may be oblique, transverse, or longitudinal; crushing injuries may cause comminution or impaction.

3. The fractures may simulate tears of the fibrocartilaginous attachment of the os tibiale externum to the tuberosity of the navicular.

4. A cartilage line may exist between the os tibiale externum and the tuberosity of the navicular.

Metatarsal Fractures

CLINICAL ORIENTATION

1. These fractures must be differentiated from other pathologic processes in the static foot.

2. In stress fracture (march fracture), the second and third metatarsals are often fractured without history of sudden trauma.

3. It may occur without the usual clinical signs of fracture from the great stress of carrying heavy weights or following prolonged weight bearing.

4. The base of the fifth metatarsal is commonly fractured transversely or obliquely during severe ankle sprains.

5. Clinically, slight pain in the metatarsus may follow stress with resultant progressive disability.

6. The dorsum of the affected bone presents a firm, painful, indurated, nodular swelling, simulating tenosynovitis.

Stress Fracture (March Fracture)

CLINICAL ORIENTATION

1. In the early stage, there is soreness in the forepart of the foot, a feeling of weakness, and possibly some pain on walking which disappears when the foot is rested.

2. Excruciating pain may occur after 5-10 days.

3. The pain remains localized, and with continued weight bearing the color may progress from a marked rubor to a deep, cyanotic edema of congestion.

4. Pain is increased by pressure on the head of the affected metatarsal and at the site of fracture. When the head of the bone is grasped and gently manipulated, the pain is increased.

ROENTGENOLOGIC INTERPRETATION
(Figs. 186-188)

1. The roentgenographic examination disclosed edema, possibly inert subperiosteal cal-

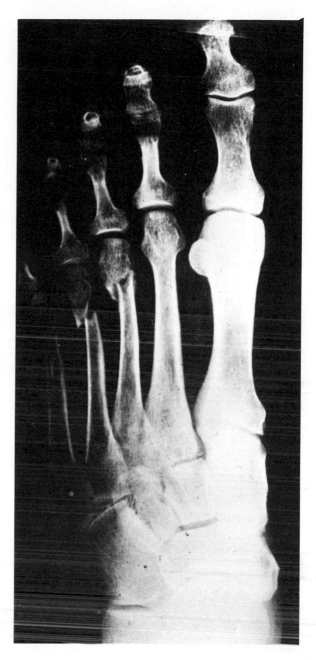

Fig. 186. Complete transverse fractures, third and fourth metatarsals

cification, and local demineralization.

2. Later, the fracture line appears as an irregular line of decreased density, uneven, and spiculated at the opposing surfaces.

3. The cortex is broken and the adjacent bone is deossified.

4. Callus becomes profuse as a result of failure of early immobilization.

5. Comparative bilateral roentgenograms will assist in differentiating fractures from dislocations, anomalous development of the navicular, and os tibiale externum.

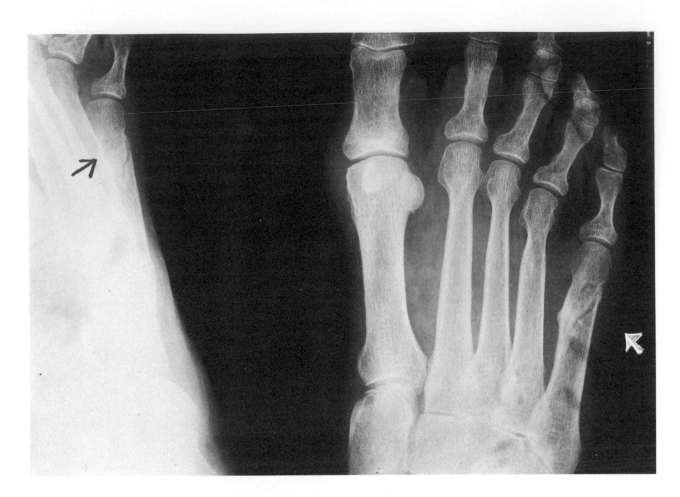

Fig. 187. Spiral fracture of fifth metatarsal

5. Union is usual and uneventful.

6. When the clinical findings are typical and the roentgenogram is negative, the lesion should be considered a fracture until proved otherwise. Serial roentgenograms are taken at 2-week intervals to verify a clinical diagnosis.

7. A complete, transverse pathologic fracture may occur through shaft tumors or cysts.

Fracture of Phalanges

CLINICAL ORIENTATION

1. The usual signs of trauma are evident with pain increased on motion. Sometimes a compound fracture occurs.

2. The swelling of the toe causes more discomfort in a well-fitted shoe than the extent of the injury would indicate.

3. The proximal phalanx of the second and fifth toes is commonly fractured by direct trauma to these toes.

4. "Bedroom fractures" are suggested when the history of injury indicates that the trauma was the result of bumping into a piece of furniture while not wearing protective foot covering after getting out of bed in the dark.

5. The distal phalanx of the great toe is commonly injured when a heavy object falls on the toe. This injury very often results in subungual hemorrhage with comminuted fracture of the distal phalanx, injury to the nail matrix, and subsequent development of onychogryposis.

ROENTGENOLOGIC INTERPRETATION
(Figs. 189-190)

1. Fractures of all proximal phalanges are usually oblique or comminuted.

2. Transverse pathologic fractures may occur in diseased bone or through a cyst.

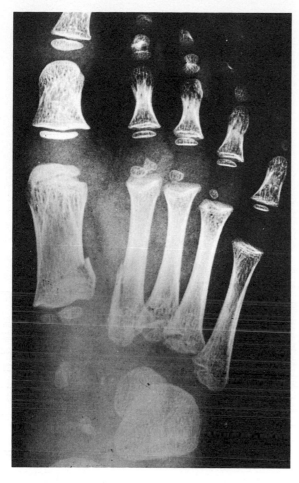

Fig. 188. Fracture, bases of first and second metatarsals

Fractured Sesamoids

CLINICAL ORIENTATION

1. These fractures are not very common.
2. The tibial or medial sesamoid is often bifurcate or bipartite.
3. A misstep into a hole or off a curb may result in a tear of the fibrocartilaginous attachment of the bipartite sesamoids.
4. A crushing blow may cause a comminution of the tibial sesamoid. The wearing of high-heeled shoes may predispose to this injury.

ROENTGENOLOGIC INTERPRETATION
(Fig. 191)

1. Roentgenograms taken in dorsoplantar, lateral, oblique, and special sesamoid views

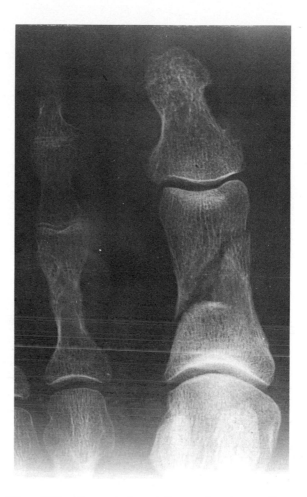

Fig. 189. Complete oblique fracture, first proximal phalanx
1. Break in continuity of cortex.
2. Irregular spiculated fracture line, which is wider at one end than the other.

are necessary to differentiate between a fracture and a cartilage line.
2. The sesamoids have been observed by the authors to be tripartite or even quadripartite.
3. The bones may present a spotty deossification in the presence of soft-tissue inflammation.

SUMMARY

1. Partially fused epiphyseal lines must be differentiated from fractures by comparative analyses and additional views if necessary.
2. Epiphyseal injuries are difficult to diag-

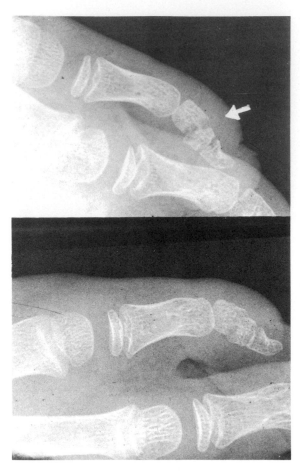

Fig. 190. Transverse fracture, middle phalanx of fifth toe

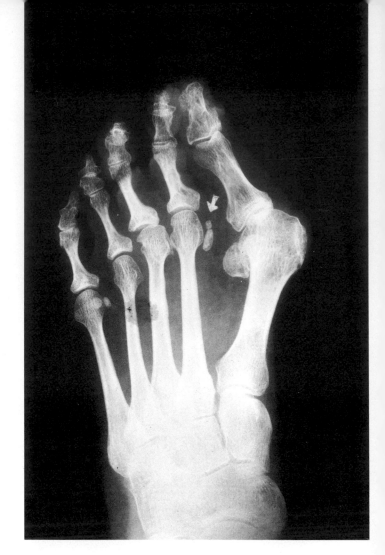

Fig. 191. Accessory ossicle provoking inter-metatarsal bursitis

nose roentgenologically.

3. Premature union and arrested growth are probable sequelae to damage of epiphyseal cartilage.

4. When the bones of a child's foot are painful after injury and no roentgenologic evidence of bone pathologic processes is demonstrable, discuss the possible damage to centers of ossification and epiphyseal cartilage with the parents to avoid legal problems in the future.

5. Calcifications are amorphous calcareous deposits which under certain circumstances may appear as a chip fracture or accessory ossicle.

6. Accessory bones at the distal ends of the malleoli are not uncommon. Calcifications of previously traumatized soft tissues adjacent to the joint may be mistaken as chip fractures.

7. One must look for the defect in bone from which the supposed fracture had arisen before rendering an opinion.

8. An aseptic necrosis or idiopathic osteochondrosis of the second metatarsal head, often with a development of calcification in the articular ligaments, must not be mistaken for fracture.

9. Sesamoids occurring under the first metatarsal head are usually no great problem because of their size, but accessory bones under the other metatarsals may be mistaken for chip fractures.

10. Evaluation of the smoothness in outline of these bones is necessary; they have a cortex and a normal medullary pattern when present as accessory ossicles.

11. Very often the os trigonum is confused as a fracture of the talus on its posterior aspect. This is differentiated by clinical findings and roentgenologic examination.

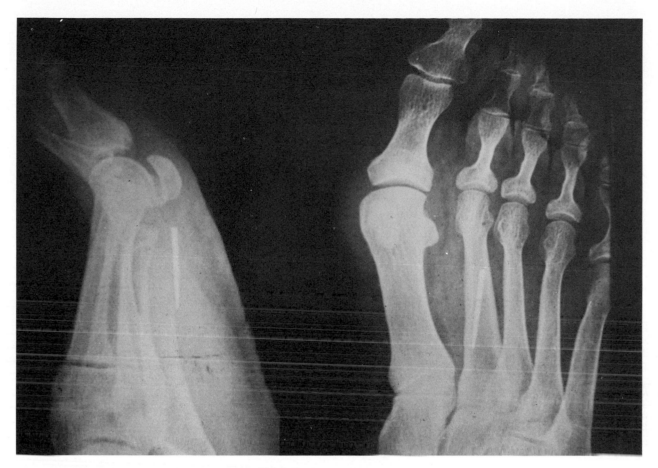

Fig. 192. Metallic density (foreign body). 1. Metallic density is of greater density than cortex. 2. Soft tissues about hallux joint are thickened and increased in density (swelling).

12. If hemorrhage fills the triangle bound posteriorly by the tendo achillis, anteriorly by the tibia, and at its base by the body of the os calcis, a fracture must be ruled out roentgenographically.

13. The proximal end or base of the fifth metatarsal may present an ununited separate center of ossification which may simulate a fracture. This is the os Vesalii. Lack of pain on clinical examination is confirmatory.

14. Overlapping of metatarsal bases may be confused as fracture lines. Other views will identify this phenomenon.

15. Overlapping shadows of soft tissue may be misinterpreted as linear fractures of bone.

16. Adhesive folds and heavy bandages may cause lines that simulate fractures.

17. Fractures involving joints have a questionable prognosis for return of normal joint function.

18. Often a local demineralization of bone will be the only early roentgenographic sign of fracture.

19. Serial roentgenograms may demonstrate the lesion in 2 or 3 weeks after the injury.

FOREIGN BODIES

CLINICAL ORIENTATION

1. There is a history of trauma and evidence of penetration of a foreign substance through the skin of the foot.

2. Machinists or mechanical workers employed in industries where metal filings or chips are underfoot are commonly subject to the entrance of these foreign particles.

3. Workers in plastic fibers or chips often develop infections from minute particles penetrating the skin.

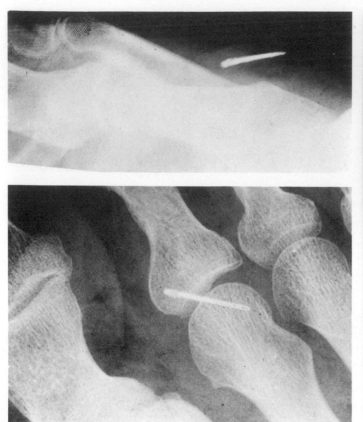
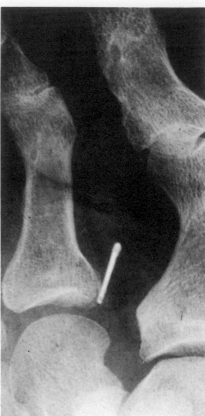

Fig. 193. Foreign body

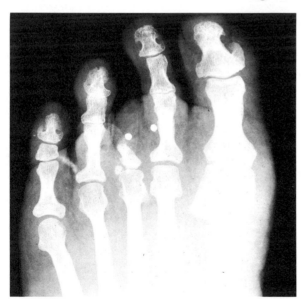

Fig. 194. Shrapnel in soft tissues from gunshot wound

4. Wood splinters may fall into the shoe and penetrate the skin.

5. Hair from pets may penetrate the unshod foot.

6. Hair linings in slippers often loosen and penetrate the skin.

7. Barbers, hairdressers, or workers in fine-wire articles develop painful tylomas. Reduction may reveal a hairlike particle perpendicular to the skin enveloped by a localized abscess. The locale of the foreign body usually appears yellow, gray, or brownish red, with surrounding redness and swelling. Pain is exquisite and localized.

8. Removal of the superficial excrescence usually reveals a dark spot with hemorrhagic extravasations or superficial seropurulent material. On its long axis in the center of this small necrotic area is a pinpoint, hairlike foreign body. Removal of this material often brings a surprise as to its length and depth of penetration. A residual ulceration or sinus remains to be treated.

9. It is not unusual to have an area of acute swelling, pain, redness, and heat without ap-

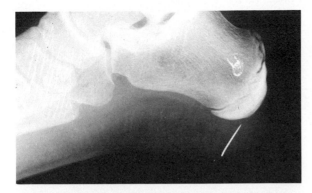

Fig. 195. Metallic density (foreign body)

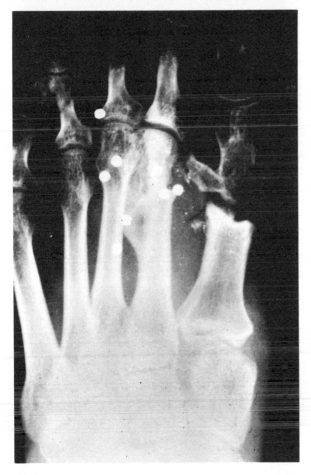

Fig. 196. Gunshot wound. Note dissolution of bone, displacement of fragment, and impacted fracture.

parent cause. Roentgenologic examination may show a radiopaque shadow of a foreign body that is deeper than the skin.

10. The diagnosis is dependent on history, clinical findings, and roentgenologic examina-tion

11. Special magnets and electromagnetic locators are used for the localization of foreign bodies.

ROENTGENOLOGIC INTERPRETATION
(Figs. 192-196)

1. Increased radiopacity will be demon-strated where certain foreign bodies exist.

2. The presence of subcutaneous glass or wood is difficult to recognize. Often metallic dyes in glass may produce roentgenologic vi-sualization.

3. Metallic density or density greater than soft-tissue density may be seen if the foreign body has penetrated the tissue.

4. Foreign bodies must be differentiated from accessory ossicles and calcareous degen-erations in the soft tissue.

BIBLIOGRAPHY

Anderson, K.J., Lecocq, J.F., and Clayton, M.L.: Athletic Injury to the Fibular Collateral Ligaments of the Ankle, Clin. Orthop. 23:146, 1962.

Esquerra Gomez, G., and Acosta, F.: Bone and Joint Le-sions in Leprosy, Radiology 50:619, 1948.

Ferguson, A.B.: *Roentgen Diagnosis of the Extremities and Spine.* New York: P.B. Hoeber, Inc., 1941.

Henderson, M.O.: Fractures, a Potential Source of De-formity and Disability, Collect. Papers, Mayo Clinic 34:582, 1942.

Hubey, C.A.: Sesamoid Bones of Hands and Feet, Amer. J. Roentgen. 61:500, 1949.

Jacobs, R.: Chronic Progressive Dislocation of Talo-navicular Joint, J. Bone Joint Surgery 46-B(2), 1964.

Kahan, R.: Talar Tilt Following Ankle Injury. J. Amer. Podiat. Ass. 49(1), 1959.

Lewin, P.: *The Foot and Ankle.* Philadelphia: Lea & Feb-iger Co., 1949.

Luck, J.V.: *Bone and Joint Diseases.* Springfield, Ill.: Charles C Thomas, 1950.

Moler-Christensen, V.: *Bone Changes in Leprosy* (trans. from the Danish), Copenhagen: Munksgaard, 1961.

Powell, H.D.: Extra Center of Ossification for the Medial Malleolus in Children, J. Bone Joint Surg. 43-B:107, 1961.

Purgett, D.L.: Surgical Correction for Dislocated Joint, Chiropody Rec. 21:52, 1938.

Ritvo, M.: *Bone and Joint X-ray Diagnosis.* Philadelphia: Lea & Febiger Co., 1955.

Rose, E.B.: Ainhum: A Case Report, J. Amer. Podiat. Ass. (June), 1958.

Schuster, O.N.: *Foot Orthopedics,* ed. 2. Albany, N.Y.: J.B. Lyon Co., 1939.

Sherwood, I.A.: Radiological Approach to the Subtalar Joint, J. Bone Joint Surg. 43-B(3), 1961.

Smillie, I.S.: *Osteochondritis Dissecans.* Edinburgh: Liv-ingston, 1960.

Weinmann, J.P., and Sicher, H.: *Bone and Bones.* St. Louis: C.V. Mosby Co., 1947.

Yale, I.: A Statistical Report on a Review of 1290 Foot Radiographs, J. Nat. Ass. Chiropodists 47:6, 1957.

11 HEREDITARY AND CONGENITAL ANOMALIES

Congenital and hereditary anomalies and deformities of the feet are not uncommon, and these must not be confused with the pathology that often results from trauma or the disease processes that disrupt normal development of bone. Many foot deformities can be traced to genetic origin or to birth defects due to a variety of biological dysfunctions, including toxic drugs and disease. Variations exist within the normal, so that abnormally short or long bones are the extremes of underdevelopment existing in dwarfism or overgrowth in gigantism.

The reader will recognize the seriousness of the problems presented in the illustrations. A challenge exists for a cooperative team approach to the treatment of these unfortunates by the geneticist, obstetrician, pediatrician, plastic surgeon, orthopedic surgeon, podiatrist, orthotist, psychologist, and social worker.

GENERAL CLINICAL ORIENTATION

Skeletal defects may occur in the feet when a complete bone or a part of bone fails to form in early fetal life. Hypoplasia or aplasia of bone may occur early. Furthermore, as Caffey (1946) states, "homologous parts of the two sides of the same skeleton may show considerable differences in development, and there may even be discrepancies in the maturational levels of different bones in a small structure."

At the stage of chondrification and subdivision of the skeleton, the failure of proper segmentation may be responsible for congenital malformations of the foot. Interphalangeal joints may be seen in a fused state with no evidence of a joint space where there is an undersegmentation of the bony anlage of the foot. Syndactylia is believed to be due to a faulty longitudinal segmentation of the phalanges.

Anomalous development of the mesoderm beginning early in fetal life may be the cause for arachnodactyly with its elongation of the feet and toes. The long bones are usually markedly elongated for the patient's skeletal age.

Abnormal transformation of mesenchymal bundles may result in excessive development of fibrous tissue which may be substituted for muscle fibers resulting in congenital dislocations and subluxations accompanied by dysplasias of bone (Fig. 197). Multiple dislocation as in arthrogryposis may result from extensive abnormal transformations of the mesenchymal bundles into fibrous tissue.

Arterovenous fistulas may result in overgrowth of muscle and bones.

The hereditary factor in some anomalies is pointed out by a study made by Cuevas-Sosa

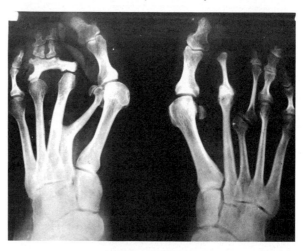

Fig. 197. Deformities from defective mesenchymal development.
1. Note elongation of metatarsals and some phalanges.
2. Faulty modeling of bones and abnormal development of phalanges.

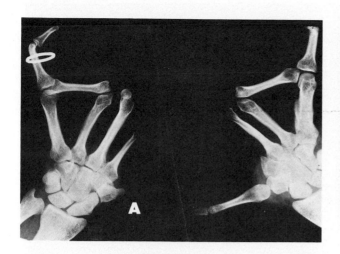

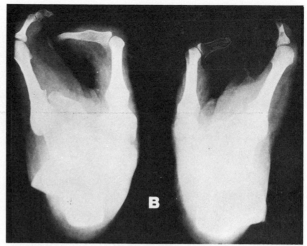

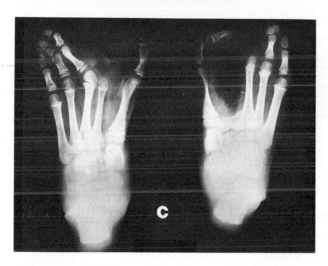

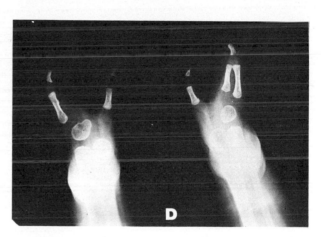

Fig. 198. Cleft foot. *A* and *B,* mother — age 21; *C,* daughter — age 6; *D,* daughter — age 19 months.

and Garcia-Segus (1970) of a seven-generation family pedigree with variable degrees of brachydactyly, characterized by hypoplasia of fingernails, absent middle phalanges in the fingers and in the lateral four toes. The thumbs and great toes were normal.

GENERAL ROENTGENOLOGIC INTERPRETATION

Undersegmentation (Figs. 198-200)
Oversegmentation (Figs. 201-207)
Aplasia (Fig. 208)
Synarthrosis (Figs. 209-210)
Synostosis (Fig. 211)

Multiple Ossification Centers (Fig. 212)
Brachydactylia (Fig. 213)
Supernumerary Bones (Figs. 214-217)

BIBLIOGRAPHY

Caffey, J.P.: *Pediatric X-ray Diagnosis.* Chicago: Year Book Publishers, 1946.

Cuevas-Sosa, A., Garcia-Segus, F.: Brachydactyly with absence of Middle Phalanges and Hypoplastic Nails. A New Hereditary Syndrome, J. Bone Joint Surg. 53-B: 101, 1971.

DeLorimier, A.A., Moehring, H.G., and Hannan, J.R.: Developmental and Systemic Conditions and Local Lesions in the Extremities, Vol. 1 of *Clinical Roentgenology.* Springfield, Ill.: Charles C Thomas, 1954.

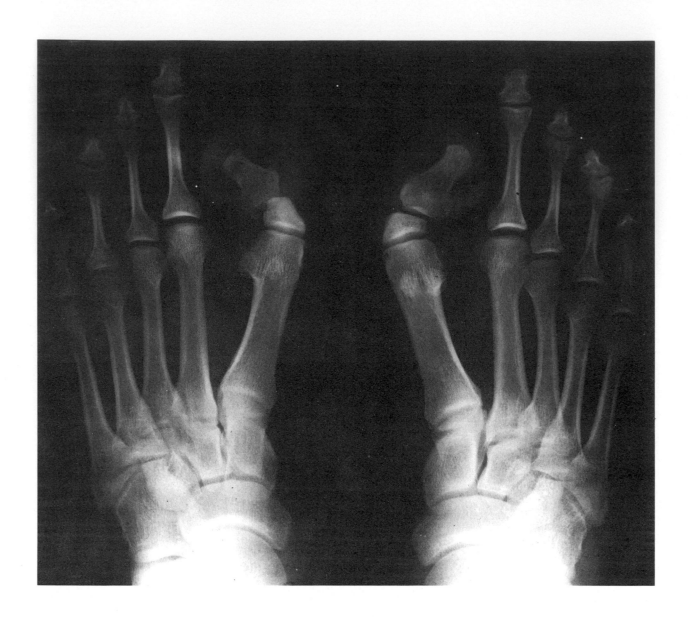

Fig. 199. Brachyphalangia of hallux
    1. Absence of middle phalanges of lesser toes
    2. Failure of proper development, promixal phalanges of hallux, bilateral.

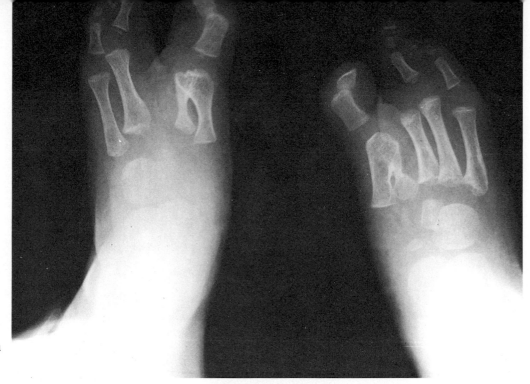

Fig. 200. Ecto-
dermal dysplasia
— severe claw-
foot deformities

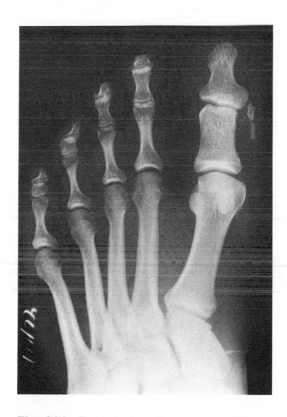

Fig. 201. Polyphalangia
   1. Rudimentary phalanges were found
encysted on surgical intervention. Complaint was a rather large hallux with in-
grown toenail.

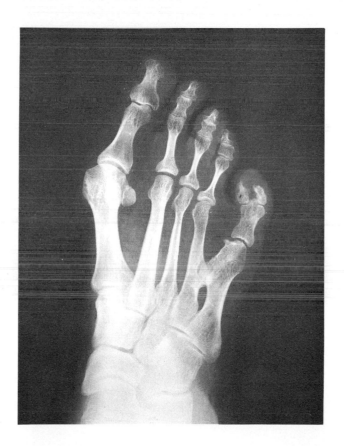

Fig. 202. Oversegmentation of fifth toe and synostosis
of fourth and fifth metatarsals. (Courtesy of C.E.
Krausz, D.P.M.)

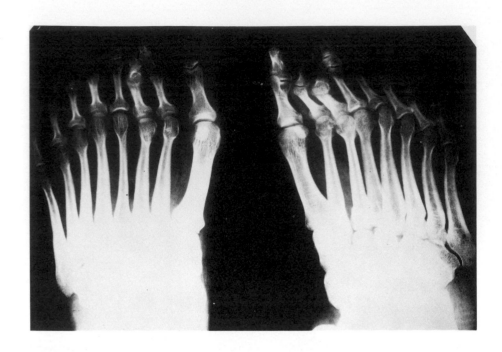

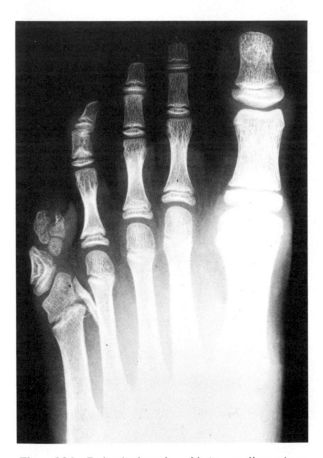

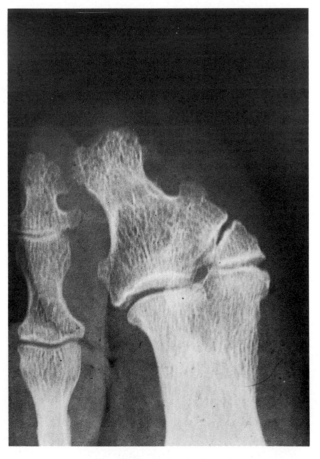

Fig. 203. Oversegmentation of toes, eight metatarsals, five cuneiforms. (Courtesy of Charles Turchin, D.P.M.)

Fig. 204. Polyphalangia. Note rudimentary metatarsal in fourth intermetatarsal space.

Fig. 205. Polyphalangia

160/HEREDITARY AND CONGENITAL ANOMALIES

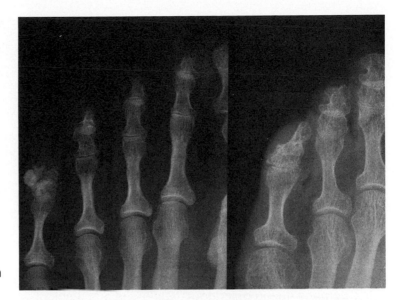

Fig. 206. Polydactylism

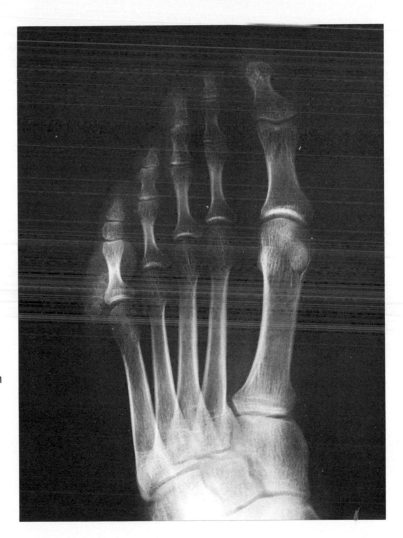

Fig. 207. Polydactylism

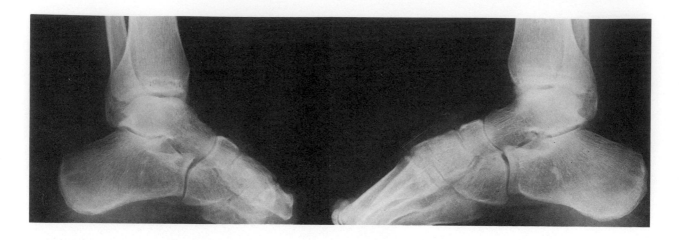

Fig. 208. Aplasia of the feet
1. Note lack of development of toes with evidence of short soft-tissue toe buds.
2. Complete fusion of left foot metatarsus.   3. Lack of development of phalanges.

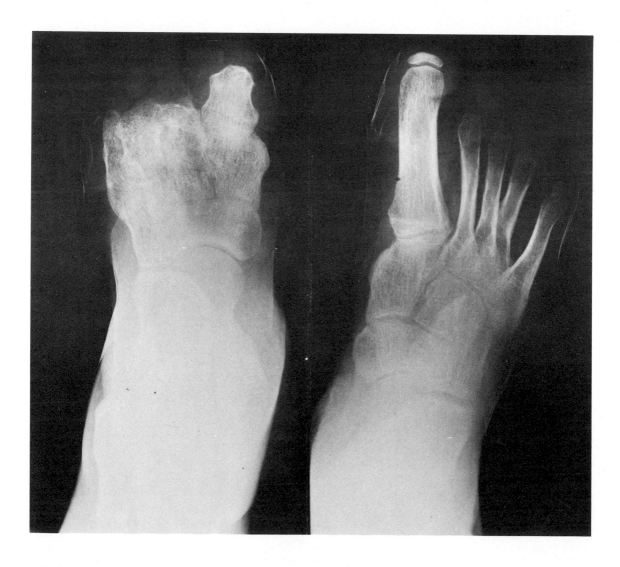

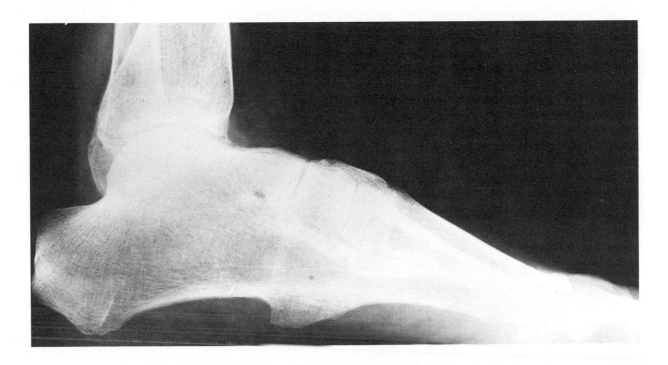

Fig. 209. Synarthrosis of tarsal and tarsal-metatarsal bones

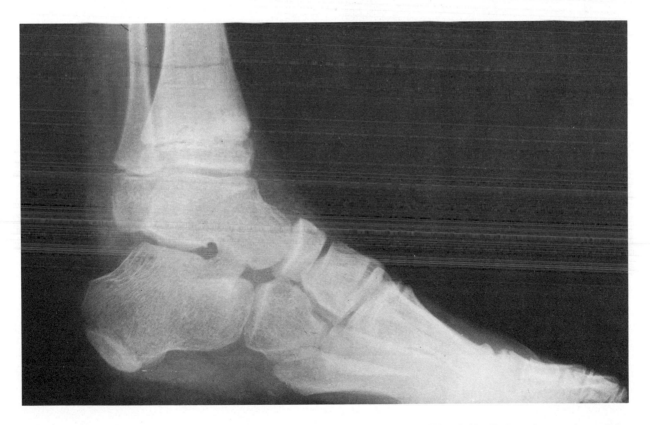

Fig. 210. Talocalcaneal coalition

HEREDITARY AND CONGENITAL ANOMALIES/163

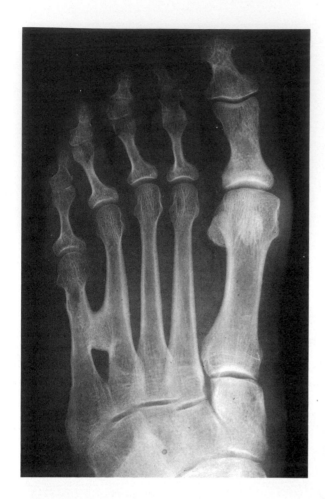

Fig. 211. Intermetatarsal coalition

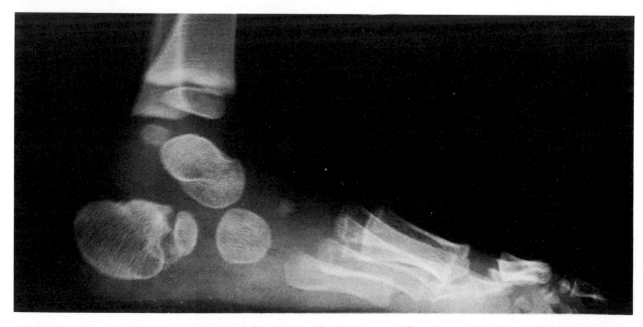

Fig. 212. Two centers of ossification for body of calcaneus. (Courtesy J.R. Thul, D.P.M.)

164/HEREDITARY AND CONGENITAL ANOMALIES

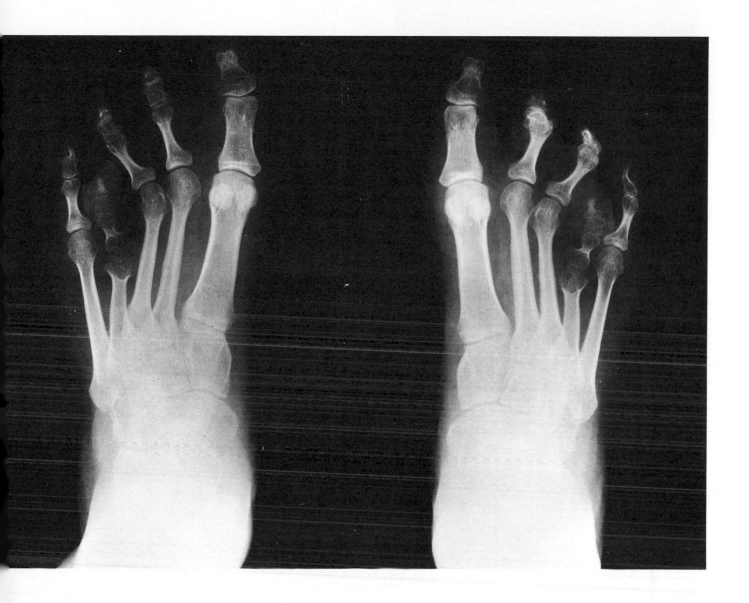

Fig. 213. Brachydactylia
   1. Bilateral and symmetrically short fourth metatarsal.
   2. Hereditary predisposition is noted with other members of the family exhibiting similar deformity.

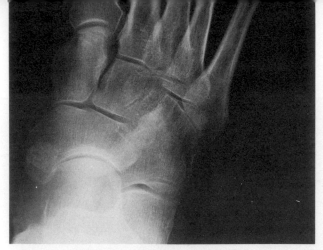

Fig. 214. Tibiale externum

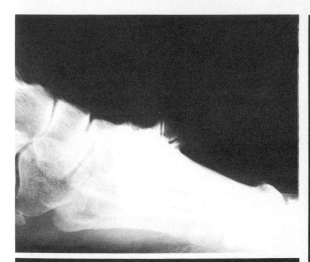

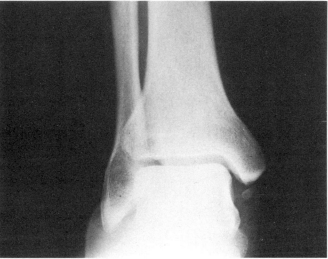

Fig. 216. Os tibiale

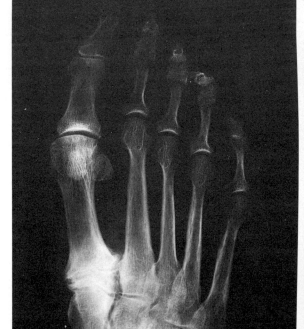

Fig. 215. Metatarsocuneiform wedge

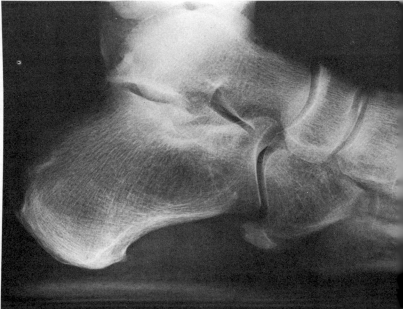

Fig. 217. Os peroneum

166/HEREDITARY AND CONGENITAL ANOMALIES

SECTION TWO

ROENTGENOLOGIC DIAGNOSIS OF FOOT PATHOANATOMY

12 ROENTGENOLOGY AND BIOMECHANICS

The interrelated disciplines of roentgenology and biomechanics are introduced in this chapter. Roentgen diagnosis of foot patho-anatomy provides a special assessment that may be correlated with biomechanical evaluations and related to clinical applications. Nomenclature is offered to establish a common basis for communication.

Clinical judgment benefits from roentgenologic and biomechanical assessment of the foot provided the information gleaned in each form of examination is placed in its proper perspective. A foot roentgenogram portrays only the osseous structure of the foot and is devoid of the other anatomical components that control its viability and functional capacity. Visualization from the roentgenogram of the bony arrangement of the foot should not reduce the estimate of its problems to such a simplistic architectural or mechanical concept that the total implication of all forces involving intrinsic anatomy and extrinsic vectors that contribute to the complete status of the foot is lost.

To achieve the ultimate in scientific foot care, the practitioner must have a thorough scientific knowledge of basic anatomic, roentgenologic, and biomechanical principles, concepts, and techniques to complete his armamentarium.

ORIENTATION

The biomechanics of the foot are complicated. Distribution of weight and stress forces is a primary foot function in standing and in gait. Many concepts have been advanced concerning the structural stability and function of the foot. As objective and clinical investigations advance, the importance of related concepts must be evaluated and those that are

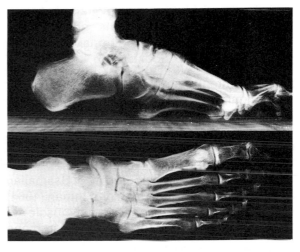

Fig. 218. Dissected foot under 50-kg pressure, muscles removed, ligaments intact, structural integrity maintained.

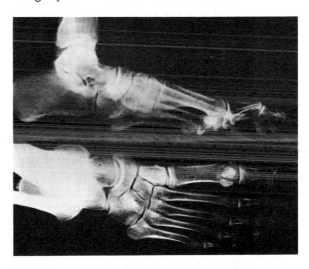

Fig. 219. The inferior calcaneonavicular ligament severed, the short calcaneocuboid ligament severed at the calcaneocuboid joint, and the long calcaneocuboid ligament severed *in toto*. Although midtarsal fault occurred, extreme foot collapse did not take place.

clinical measurement methods for quality, direction, and range of motion of the off-weight subject as well as by the use of stance correlations and charted on-weight roentgenograms and appraisals of gait proposes a different approach to understanding the etiological factors, topography, and morphology affecting body posture and foot function and integrity (Root, 1958).

26. The angle of gait for a given individual has been theoretically established as the amount of malleolar torsion present plus or minus the relative adduction or abduction of the whole foot to the body of the talus. Physical examination is used to determine malleolar torsion; charting of a dorsoplantar roentgenogram is used to establish interrelated values for the long axis of the calcaneus and the amount of tarsus abductus and metatarsus adductus (Sgarlato, 1965).

27. Determination of the axis of motion of the subtalar joint in an anatomic study indicated a total 17° deviation from the sagittal plane from posterolateral to anteromedial and a total 41° deviation from the transverse plane from posteroplantar to anterodorsal in the average foot. This study, based on Manter's original work, confirms Hick's hypothesis that the subtalar joint motion is hingelike affecting all three body planes (Root, Weed, Sgarlato, and Bluth, 1966). Foot motion in gait varies with the angulation of the axis of motion of the subtalar joint.

28. Tread impressions and photokinegrams are used in extensive studies of gait in locomotor problems as a method of obtaining individual case records. The tread impression is a simple procedure that provides a means for establishing the angle and base of gait more effectively than can be perceived by visual appraisal. Progress records are easy to obtain in this manner (Schuster, 1964).

29. Angular relationships of the talus and calcaneus in the developing foot were measured on 258 weight-bearing lateral roentgenograms of subjects 6 months to 18 years of age. Statistical study of these data indicates an age-dependent change for both inclination of the calcaneus and declination of the talus up to age 6. This finding supports the concept of ontogenic maturing of bone shape in this age range (Altman, 1968).

30. Each metatarsal head determines its own level and the weight it bears according to the amount of ray flexion present without dependence on its neighbors (Hicks, 1955).

The experimental investigations that have produced many of these theories have been limited to very special circumstances. Nevertheless, it is only through the tedious, painstaking time-consuming basic research of laboratory and clinical investigation that a truly scientific appraisal of the interrelated anatomy and function of the foot can be made.

Biomechanics of Stress

Throughout the roentgenologic interpretations there will be comments on stress reaction. This intangible force is a part of the clinical aspect of every case. Since it is the osseous system that transmits stress, the malformed bones that indicate faulty stress situations should be identified. Stunted growth of immature bone due to compression of epiphyses and change in shape of mature bone under persistent pressure are indications of the need for study of the roentgenographs for clues that indicate faulty forces of stress. Also the foot that is disorganized by subluxation and hypermobility loses its ability to distribute the forces of stress in normal pathways.

The framework of the foot is designed to deploy body weight to best advantage against gravity in stance and locomotion. A variety of mechanical principles are involved in these circumstances. Weight stress can only be transmitted through a solid substrate. It cannot jump across a gap. A properly aligned foot structure provides maximal efficiency for stress transmission. In stance, the posterior subtalar joint bears the brunt of stress distribution.

The investigations of stress distribution in the foot by Meldman (1950) strike at the dynamic aspect of stress transfer in foot locomotion. He describes the simultaneous forward and lateral pathways as a decussation in which forward forces from the talus move to the navicular and medial segment of the forefoot. The lateral forces are transmitted from the talus to the sustentaculum tali, to the calcaneocuboid articulation, and lateral segment of the forefoot, underpassing the forward stress movement as separated by the sinus tarsi. Roentgenologically, it becomes imperative that the sinus tarsi be visualized as an all-important functional component in the under-passing of stress and as an indicator of normal positions of the calcaneus and talus.

Zitzlsperger (1960) classifies the foot as a statically indetermined space framework and demonstrates an intricate meshwork of short-range and long-range stress pathways in a classical model and concept applying the rules and laws of analytical mechanics to anatomic specimens. Levy (1950) and Lewis (1964) reaffirm the importance of the propulsive function of the toes.

Relating Foot Form to Function

Many investigators have explored the inter-action of the osseous system with emphasis on the foot in gait. The establishment and confirmation of the theoretical axes of motion for the foot joints, the relative positions of and motion available in the major foot joints (Hicks, 1953) (Fig. 223 and Table 1), and the comprehensive study of the phases of gait (Mann and Inman, 1964) have significant bearing on the foot form as related to function. Several issues are of specific interest.

Elftman (1960) indicates that the midtarsal joint has dual axes, one for the calcaneocuboid joint and the other for the talonavicular joint. When these axes are parallel, as in the pronated foot, there is more freedom of motion. When these axes are in conflict, as in the supinated foot, the foot becomes more stable. Close and Inman (1953) found greater motion in the subtalar joint of the pronated foot than in the normal foot. Wright, Desai, and Henderson (1964) believe that the ankle joint and subtalar joint are interdependent and, in general, act as a single mechanism in walking. Mann and Inman (1964) conclude that the pronated foot requires greater intrinsic muscle activity to stabilize the midtarsal and subtalar joints than does the normal foot.

These pertinent concepts point up the fact that the normal foot presents a structural integrity that will sustain stability in stance and in gait, whereas the excessively pronated foot is destined to hypermobility because of a parallelism of the axes of joint motion that allows the foot to exceed the range of normal function. Roentgenologic examination of the foot in stance captures a visual record of the strength or weakness of the individual foot structures when the foot is most vulnerable.

The biomechanics of gait involves the action of muscles coordinated by a nervous system with abilities comparable to a computer. Elftman (1966) suggests that the nervous system can devise programs for complicated activities, store them for future use, and modify their implementation by feedback systems. The possible sophistication of its function is suggested by the foot action and body motion of the ballet dancer, but the execution of any manner of gait is complex. Ducroquet et al., (1968) uniquely orient walking gait into four phases, starting with the act of propulsion which they characterize as thrust, followed by oscillation or levitation of the independent limb, into the reception stage which measures, brakes, and regulates progression, and a final phase of unilateral support. Cineroentgenography is the ultimate method of recording bone motion in the foot during gait. Unfortunately, technical problems make it difficult to achieve roentgen motion pictures of gait and the value of the sequences that have been filmed are very limited.

In the normal phases of gait in the walking cycle (Figs. 224-229) the osseous structure is deployed through a range of joint motions that insure stability and balance throughout progression. The entire superimposed body weight is transmitted through the pelvis and leg to the ankle joint which permits movement in the sagittal plane and in the transverse plane. These movements are resolved in the subtalar and midtarsal joints.

Root et al. (1964) analyze the following phases and moments of joint motions: (1) heel contact — slight subtalar supination, (2) forefoot contact — subtalar pronation and midtarsal pronation, (3) midstance — resupination to neutral subtalar and midtarsal fully pronated position, (4) heel lift — stabilization of subtalar joint and midtarsal joints by supination and initiation of metatarsal flexion, (5) propulsion — forefoot segments, particularly the first metatarsal segment, the hallux and lesser toes, stabilize at initiation of propulsion, and (6) swing phase — foot slightly supinated in free swing.

Roentgenologic examination best addresses the problems of gait by diagnosing the imperfections in the osseous arrangements of the foot structure in the natural standing position that simulates the midstance phase of gait. Great care should be exercised in posing the patient in his natural base and angle of stance because this position coincides within acceptable limits with the foot position in the midstance phase. Standardization of these conditions is essential for providing uniform basic roentgenographic data for comparative study and evaluation. Standardized roentgenograms are used throughout this text. In the roentgenologic studies that follow, it will be obvious that form and function are undeniably interwoven

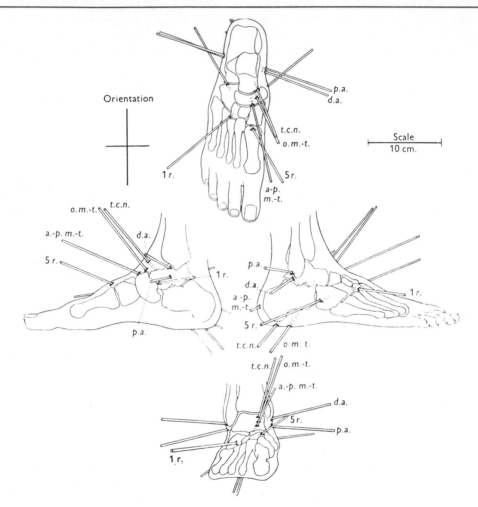

Fig. 223. Location of joint axes. The axes of all the foot joints (except those of the middle three rays) adapted from roentgenograms of the experimental foot. Foot in basic position of relaxed flat standing, the ankle being in a position of moderate extension, the talocalcaneonavicular and midtarsal joints at or near full pronation, the first ray at full extension-supination, and the fifth ray near to full flexion-supination. *d.a.,* dorsiflexion ankle axis; *p.a.,* plantar flexion ankle axis; *t.c.n.,* talocalcaneonavicular axis; *o.m.t.,* oblique mid-tarsal axis; *a.p.m.t.,* anteroposterior mid-tarsal axis; *1r.,* first ray axis; *5r.,* fifth ray axis. (Reprinted from "The Mechanics of the Foot: I. The Joints" by J.H. Hicks. J. Anat., 87:35, 1953, with kind permission of the author through the Cambridge University Press.)

TABLE 1. MOVEMENTS AND RANGES OF MOVEMENT

Joint	Description of movement	Range	Remarks
Ankle:			
(a) Dorsiflexion axis	Flexion with slight adduction and supination. Extension with slight abduction and pronation	50°	Work on other specimens and some normal young adults suggests that a more usual range is about 12° greater
(b) Plantarflexion axis	Flexion with slight supination. Extension with slight pronation		
Talo-calcaneo-navicular	Pronation-abduction-extension. Supination-adduction-flexion	24°	Other specimens and other methods show agreement to within 3°
Mid-tarsal:			
(a) The oblique axis	Pronation-abduction-extension. Supination-adduction-flexion	22°	
(b) The antero-posterior axis	Pronation with slight abduction-extension. Supination with slight adduction-flexion	8°	
First ray	Flexion-pronation. Extension-supination	22°	Other specimens and living subjects show agreement to within 8°
Third ray	Flexion. Extension	10°	
Fifth ray	Flexion-supination. Extension-pronation	10°	

Noto. These data are quoted from one selected specimen. The last column shows what variations may be expected.

(From "The Mechanics of the Foot: I. The Joints" by J.H. Hicks, J. Anat., 87:35, 1953 with kind permission of the author through the Cambridge University Press.)

---

into the static features on the roentgenogram.

Misconception Concerning "Foot Arches"

Although the foot framework presents the appearance of several arch conformations, the basic architectural and mechanical principles of arch support by fixed base pillars and keystone construction cannot be fully applied. When the plantar aponeurosis checks the span between the calcaneus and forefoot, some fixation of the foot framework by trusslike action takes place. However, in the static foot, stress distribution transcends the entire framework so that arch with keystone is an invalid simplification (Zitzlsperger, 1960).

The external conformation of the foot exhibits an arch contour on its medial border which is highly descriptive clinically. When structural collapse of the foot occurs, the arch conformation is obviously changed. It is unlikely that reference to the longitudinal arch will soon be eliminated from clinical language. However, we will limit our reference to arch shape in discussing conformation and in defining foot types to height of the foot framework.

NOMENCLATURE

Since clinical communication benefits from compatible terminology, the roentgenologic terms used in this text will be harmonized with contemporary anatomic terms into a common framework of reference. Unfortunately, there is confusion in the use of some anatomic terms and words that describe relative position of the osseous structures of the foot. The nomenclature of this revised text will seek to simplify some of the problems with the following terms.

1. The traditional reference plane for transverse position of the toes is not the same

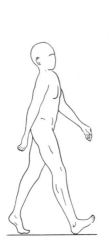
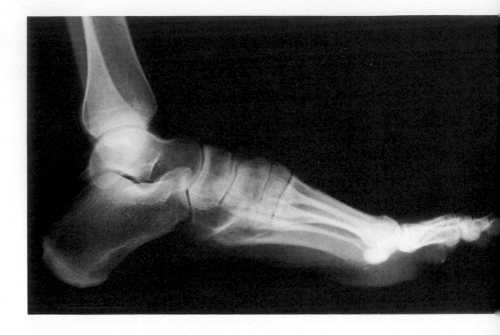

Fig. 224. Weight forces received through heel

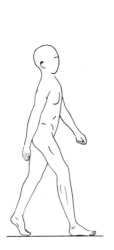
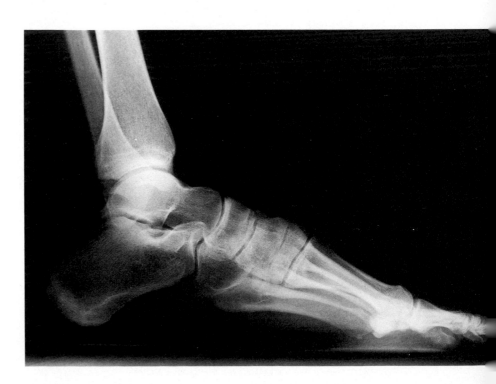

Fig. 225. Transmitting weight forces to forefoot

176/ROENTGENOLOGY AND BIOMECHANICS

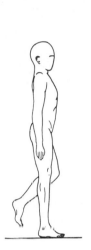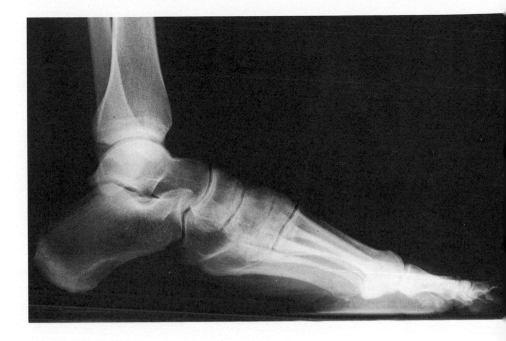

Fig. 226. Maximal stress on one foot

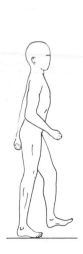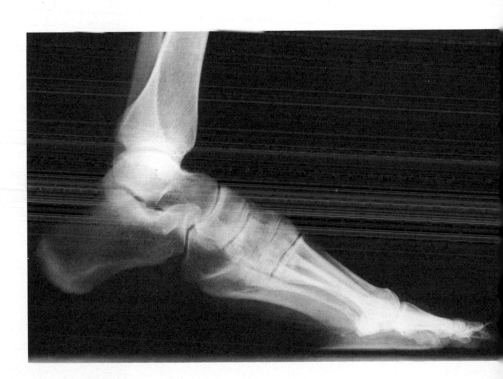

Fig. 227. Raising weight force at start of take-off

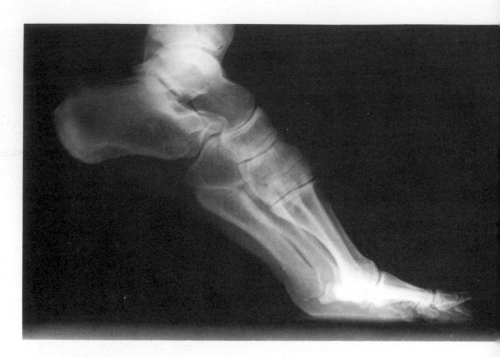

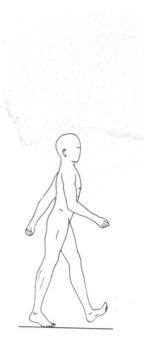

Fig. 228. All weight force on metatarsophalangeal joints and toes

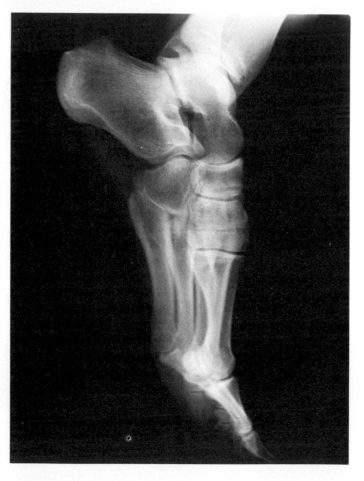

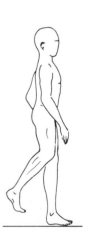

Fig. 229. Foot free while carried forward for next step

178/ROENTGENOLOGY AND BIOMECHANICS

as that for the rest of the foot. The midsagittal plane of the foot has been traditionally used as a plane of reference for the toes, while the median sagittal plane of the body was used as the plane of reference for the rest of the foot. Confusion arises when toes and the rest of the foot are being considered at the same time. Under this circumstance, the foot could be abducted and the hallux, if angulated in the same direction, would be adducted. To avoid this confusion, the midline of the body (median sagittal plane) will be used in this text as the standard of reference for the entire foot, a part of the foot, or a toe. Hence, hallux abductus is the position of the hallux when turned outward from the midline of the body.

2. Archaic usage of the terms "varus" and "valgus" relate to bending inward and outward. A very loose application of these terms has been traditionally used in reference to the knees, feet, and toes. The terms have often been erroneously used to describe a position in the transverse plane rather than one achieved by rotation in the frontal plane. This text will use the terms "varus" and "valgus" only to designate a position achieved by rotation in the frontal plane. Specifically, varus is a position in which the plantar surface is rotated toward the midline of the body and valgus is a position in which the plantar surface is rotated away from the midline of the body. Hence, hallux valgus describes only the position of the hallux when its plantar surface is rotated away from the midline of the body. The deformity hallux abductus valgus embodies two components, abduction and rotation. The entire foot or the forefoot may assume a rotated position of valgus or varus.

3. The terms "inversion" and "eversion" have widely accepted usage as meaning a tilting of the foot inward or outward. More precisely, these terms relate to rotation in the frontal plane. Inversion is a rotation of the plantar surface toward the midline of the body; eversion is a rotation of the plantar surface away from the midline of the body. As a designation of position, eversion is synonymous with valgus and inversion with varus, but only the appropriate forms of the verbs "invert" and "evert" may be used to describe movement. The Latin terms "varus" and "valgus" are only used to describe position, be it

structurally fixed or attained by rotation. Consequently, words derived from invert and evert are used in this text to describe rotation in a frontal plane.

4. Terms and definitions devised to serve special purposes must stand the criticism of the philogist. More importantly, older terms occasionally need refining and restricting to convey a better understanding of their intended meaning. This text will be careful in the usage of new terms and will review old definitions and revise where necessary.

Planes of Anatomic Reference

Weight-supporting plane: the horizontal substrate upon which the subject stands.
Median sagittal plane (midline of the body): the vertical plane that divides the erect body from front to back into equal left and right sides.
Sagittal plane: any vertical plane parallel to the median sagittal plane that divides the body or a part into medial and lateral segments.
Transverse plane: any horizontal plane that divides the body or a part into superior and inferior segments. The base upon which the subject stands is a transverse plane.
Frontal plane: any vertical plane that divides the body or a part into anterior and posterior segments.

Axes for Movements of the Foot or Part of Foot

Axis: a straight line about which a body may be considered to rotate. An axis may be directed obliquely and still qualify as the primary axis of reference.
Axis of joint motion: a theoretical line established by experimentation about which motion may occur for specific joints.
Transverse axis: a line about which there may be movement in the sagittal plane.
Vertical axis: a line about which there may be movement in a transverse plane.
Longitudinal axis: a line about which there may be movement in a frontal plane.

Terms of Anatomic Reference

Anatomic segment: a partial division of a foot at a selected level; *e.g.,* transverse divisions: hindfoot, midfoot, forefoot, metatarsal, toe segments; longitudinal divisions: medial forefoot segment, lateral forefoot segment, cuneometatarsal segment (metatarsal ray), toe segment.

Medial: refers to parts toward the midline of the body.

Lateral: refers to parts away from the midline of the body to the left or right depending on the side of reference.

Anterior: refers to a front part of the body.

Posterior: refers to a back part of the body.

Distal: refers to a front part of the foot.

Proximal: refers to a back part of the foot.

Superior: refers to an upper part of the foot.

Inferior: refers to a lower part of the foot.

Dorsal: refers to the superior surface of the foot.

Plantar: refers to the inferior surface of the foot.

Plantigrade: refers to a changed position of a bone or group of bones of the foot in the direction of the weight-supporting plane.

Abduction: distal part turned outward from the midline of the body.

Adduction: distal part turned inward toward the midline of the body.

Eversion: plantar surface rotated to face away from the midline of the body.

Inversion: plantar surface rotated to face toward the midline of the body.

Plantarflexion: plantar or distal aspect moved downward or away from anterior of leg.

Dorsiflexion: dorsal or distal aspect moved upward or toward anterior of leg.

Pronation: entire foot turned outward, rotated outward, and moved upward.

Supination: entire foot turned inward, rotated inward, and moved downward.

Subluxation: an incomplete displacement of one or more bones of a joint from its original position.

Hypermobility: an excessive range of movement in an otherwise stable joint.

Compensation: Adjustment of bone and joint position in response to an abnormal force. It may be either accommodative, in which the foot adapts to a minimal level of function, or corrective, in which the foot seeks to maintain a maximal level of function.

THE ROENTGEN IMAGE

The roentgen image of an anatomic structure embodies both geometric and roentgenologic phenomena. The greater the density of the structure, the less the amount of radiation that reaches the film and the clearer the processed area as contrasted with dark areas representing lesser densities. Any roentgenogram represents a summation of the varying densities of the superimposed structures, and it is not an image of a predetermined cross section. Rather, the image is like a finely detailed drawing recorded on film of a structure that has been compressed to a single flat plane. The trabecular architecture of the calcaneus is represented on a roentgenogram not as spongiose *per se* but as a summation of compressed striated patterns (Fig. 230).

Trabecular architecture shows how each foot bone is designed to withstand the stress of its individual function (Koch, 1917). Compressed trabeculae and the trabeculae of new periosteal bone formation are an indicator of bone reaction to the forces of weight-bearing stress and traction forces of ligaments, fascia, and muscle on bone (Wolff, 1870; Steindler, 1914). Trabecular patterns may cross over a joint to match similar striations in an adjacent bone (Hall, 1960, 1966). Mismatching in crossover trabecular pattern is a significant indicator of faulty biomechanics (Root and Weed, 1973). Henenfeld and Walkes (1961) evaluate bone resection in relation to the lines of force transmitted by trabecular trajectories and the extent of bone demineralization of the trabeculae. Carrel (1968) reviews the literature concerning trabecular patterns and advances the concept that solitary calcaneal bone cysts have a predilection for an area below the middle facet of the superior surface of the calcaneus that is relatively devoid of mineralized trabeculations.

The shape of the calcaneus is outlined by its cortex, and the sustentaculum tali is represented by a superimposed density. The relative positions of the bones of the medial and lateral segments of the foot are superimposed on a roentgenogram as a single plane of reference.

TABLE 2. RELATING ANATOMIC POSITIONS TO BIOMECHANICS

Position of Foot, Part of Foot, or Toe	Description of Position	Joint Involvement	Plane and Axis of Motion
Abduction	distal part turned outward from midline of body	midtarsal, tarsometatarsal	transverse plane vertical axis
Adduction	distal part turned inward toward midline of body	midtarsal, tarsometatarsal	transverse plane vertical axis
Eversion	plantar surface rotated to face away from midline of body	subtalar, midtarsal	frontal plane longitudinal axis
Inversion	plantar surface rotated to face toward midline of body	subtalar, midtarsal	frontal plane longitudinal axis
Plantarflexion	plantar or distal aspect moved downward or away from anterior of leg	ankle, intertarsal, tarsometatarsal, metatarsophalangeal	sagittal plane transverse axis
Dorsiflexion	dorsal or distal aspect moved upward or toward anterior of leg	ankle, intertarsal, tarsometatarsal, metatarsophalangeal	sagittal plane transverse axis
Pronation	entire foot turned outward, rotated outward, moved upward	transverse: midtarsal, tarsometatarsal frontal: subtalar, midtarsal sagittal: ankle, intertarsal, tarsometatarsal, metatarsophalangeal	tri-plane interrelated axes: vertical, longitudinal transverse
Supination	entire foot turned inward, rotated inward, moved downward	transverse: midtarsal, tarsometatarsal frontal: subtalar, midtarsal sagittal: ankle, intertarsal, tarsometatarsal, metatarsophalangeal	tri-plane interrelated axes: vertical longitudinal transverse

Consequently, it is necessary to have a second roentgenogram taken through a plane perpendicular to that of the first so that a perception of three-dimensional image may be obtained, since width, length, and height are present as roentgenographic images. Special roentgenographic views through tangential planes give additional perspective to provide more information about the structures.

The geometrics of roentgen image formation parallel the principles of shadow formation by light. The closer the part to the film, the more accurate the roentgen image; the farther removed from the film, the more magnified (Fig. 231). In a lateromedial view of the foot, the cuboid is actually enlarged in proportion to the image of the navicular which is in closer proximity to the film. Image fidelity is improved by greater object to roentgen source distance and by a small point of source. A fine focal spot tube and a long tube-film distance are to be desired where feasible. The central ray should be directed perpendicular to the flat plane of the part presented for roentgenography to insure accurate image formation. An obliquely directed ray distorts the image just as the shadow of an object is distorted if a point source of light were directed upon it from an oblique angle. Under all circumstances the rules for accurate image production (as listed in Chapter 24) should be followed. Standardized roentgen technique is absolutely necessary to provide roentgen images that present uniform geometric ap-

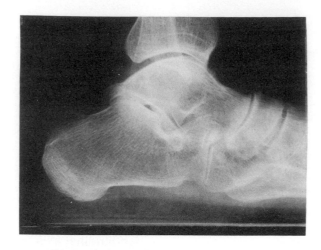

Fig. 230. Roentgenogram of foot demonstrating osseous trabecular architecture, cortical bone outlines, and sustentaculum tali represented by summation of superimposed densities.

pearances. The interpreter must master the intricate subtle profiles and densities that demonstrate bone shape and joint space. Foot roentgenographic technique is fully presented in the final section of this text. The present discussion will introduce the roentgen terminology.

Terms Used in Roentgenologic Anatomic Reference

Roentgen anatomy: anatomic structures visualized from the roentgenogram in their topographic and spatial relationships.

Roentgen pathoanatomy: anatomic structures visualized from the roentgenogram that have been altered in their topography or spatial relationships by a pathologic process or force.

Roentgen image: the portrayal of an anatomic structure on a roentgenogram by variable film densities.

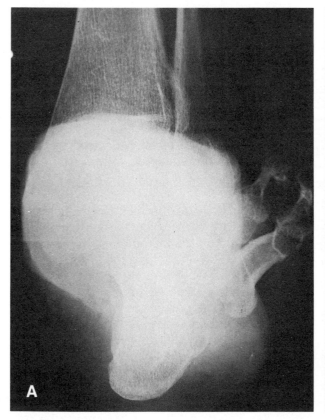
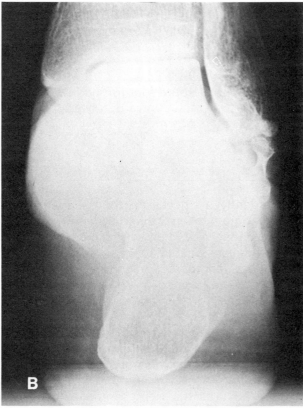

Fig. 231. Geometrics of roentgen image formation. A, anteroposterior view, heel toward film, shows normal bone size and fine detail; B, posteroanterior view, toes toward film, shows enlarged bone size and coarse detail.

TABLE 3. RELATING ROENTGEN VIEWS TO ANATOMIC PLANES

Anatomic Part	Roentgen View	Anatomic Plane
Foot, Toe, Ankle, Heel	Lateral	Sagittal
Forefoot, Toe, Heel	Dorsoplantar	Transverse
Ankle	Anteroposterior	Frontal
Foot	Oblique	Semi-transverse
Ankle	Oblique	Semi-frontal
Sesamoids, Metatarsophalangeal joint area, Heel	Axial	Frontal
Heel	Superoplantar	Transverse

Roentgen projection: the direction of the projected roentgen ray as related to the anatomic structure, described first by its surface of entry and second by its surface of exit; *e.g.,* dorsoplantar, lateromedial, superoplantar.

Roentgen view: a term used interchangeably to indicate (1) the plane of the anatomic structures visualized from the roentgenogram or (2) an orientation of the projection required to produce the required roentgenogram; *e.g.,* lateral, oblique, axial.

Terms Used in Anatomic Orientation of the Roentgenogram

Roentgen reference point: a point marked on a roentgen image (1) to designate a point of orientation for departure in measurements, (2) to connect with another reference point to establish a reference line, or (3) to use in connection with another reference point to establish a measured point of bisection.

Roentgen reference line: a line established by connecting two reference points not necessarily inherent in the anatomic roentgen image; *e.g.,* a line connecting an opaque point exposed on the film to another such point or to a selected anatomic reference point.

Angle: the figure formed by two lines diverging from a common point.

Polyhedral angle: the configuration formed by three or more planes having intersections that form a common vertex.

Roentgen reference angle: an angle formed by a line diverging from another roentgen reference line, such as the weight-supporting plane.

Degree of angulation: the amount of geometric divergence of an angle, commonly measured by a protractor.

Angle of inclination: the angle formed by a reference line for a bone or bones diverging upward from the weight-supporting plane.

Angle of declination: the angle formed by a reference line for a bone or bones diverging downward toward the weight-supporting plane.

Angle of medial deviation: the angle formed by a reference line for a bone or bones diverging from another reference line within the foot toward the midline of the body; *e.g.,* as applied to the talus in the talocalcaneal angle.

Angle of lateral deviation: the angle formed by a reference line for a bone or bones diverging from a reference line within the foot away from the midline of the body.

Note: Use a cleaning-fluid erasable skin or china marking pencil to indicate reference points or lines to avoid effacing roentgen images.

Special Reference Terms

Pitch: a term used to describe the angle subtended by the calcaneus with the weight-supporting plane; qualified by high or low.

Cyma: an architectural term designating a figure composed of united convex and concave curves; uniquely describes the midtarsal joint line as visualized from both lateral and dorsoplantar roentgen views (Gamble, 1937).

Talocalcaneal angle: an angle between bisectors of the talus and the calcaneus; this angle demonstrates the degree of deviation of the talus from the calcaneus and is commonly charted on the dorsoplantar view but may be charted on the lateral view.

Foot Bases and Angles Used in Roentgenologic Positioning

Base of stance: the transverse separation of the feet in natural standing position.

Angle of stance: the angle from the midsagittal plane assumed by each foot in natural standing position.

Base of gait: the transverse separation of the feet in walking.

Angle of gait: the angle from the midsagittal plane assumed by each foot in the midstance of walking.

ROENTGENOLOGIC INTERPRETATION OF FOOT BIOMECHANICS

The terms that have been defined are used to describe anatomic, biomechanical, and roentgenologic situations. Although the joints of the foot permit a combination of motions about a series of theoretical axes, a foot roentgenogram records only the fixed position of the bones, depending on the projected view. Consequently, the interpreter must visualize the total anatomic position by combining the features from each view. Analysis of this composition constitutes a roentgenologic interpretation of a phase of foot biomechanics.

The roentgenologic interpretation of osseous alignment of the foot with all its functional implications is predicated upon a thorough knowledge of the foot bones under normal and abnormal conditions and how they are visualized roentgenologically. This text will provide (1) basic descriptions that will identify each foot bone and its established alignment, (2) the integration of each foot bone into an organized joint structure or functional segment as visualized roentgenologically, and (3) the total foot alignment as completely articulated and represented as a roentgenologic entity. There will also be a discussion of methods of charting the foot roentgenogram as an additional means of studying alignment of the foot structure.

Roentgenologic descriptions that concern the structure in fixed position should not be confused with biomechanical descriptions that may be applied to a variety of structural situations, such as open- or closed-chain position.

BIBLIOGRAPHY

Altman, M.I.: Sagittal Plane Angles of the Talus and Calcaneus in the Developing Foot, J. Amer. Podiat. Ass. 58:463, 1968.

Basmajian, J.V., and Stecko, G.: The Role of Muscles in the Arch Support of the Foot. An Electromycographic Study, J. Bone Joint Surg. 45-A:1184, 1963.

Brantingham, C.R., Egge, A.S., and Beekman, B.E.: The Effect of Artificially Varied Surface on Ambulatory Rehabilitation with Preliminary EMG Evaluation of Certain Muscles Involved, J. Amer. Podiat. Ass. 53:733, 1963.

Burger, E.S.: Support of Body Weight, J. Amer. Podiat. Ass. 47:1, 1957.

Burger, E.S., Gabriel, G.R., and Oberheim, W.A.: Motion in Three Planes, J. Amer. Podiat. Ass. 62:250, 1972.

Carrel, J.M.: Roentgenologic Study of the Calcaneus in Relation to Disease Patterns, J. Amer. Podiat. Ass. 58: 55, 1968.

Close, J.R., and Inman, V.T.: The Action of the Subtalar Joint, Prosthetic Devices Research Project, University of California, Berkeley, Series 11, Issue 24, May 1953.

Close, J.R., Nickel, E.D., and Todd, F.N.: Motor-unit Action-potential Counts. Their Significance in Isometric and Isotonic Contractions, J. Bone Joint Surg. 42-A: 1207, 1960.

Close, J.R., and Todd, F.N.: The Phasic Activity of the Muscles of the Lower Extremity and the Effect of Tendon Transfer, J. Bone Joint Surg. 41-A:189, 1959.

Duchene, G.B.: *Physiology of Motion.* E.B. Kaplan (trans.-ed.). Philadelphia: J.B. Lippincott Co., 1949.

Ducroquet, R., Ducroquet, Jean, and Ducroquet, Pierre (with the collaboration of M. Saussey): *Walking and Limping.* Philadelphia: J.B. Lippincott Co., 1949.

Elftman, H.: The Transverse Tarsal Joint and Its Control, Clin. Orthop. 16:41, 1960.

Elftman, H.: Biomechanics of Muscle with Particular Application to Studies of Gait, J. Bone Joint Surg. 48-A: 363, 1966.

Frost, F.: Report of Scientific Committee, National Association of Chiropodists, 1948.

Gamble, F.O.: Research project, Professor Roentgenology, Temple University School of Chiropody, Philadelphia, 1947.

Gratz, C.M.: Tensile Strength and Elasticity Test of Human Fascia Lata, J. Bone Joint Surg. 13:334, 1931.

Gratz, C.M.: Biomechanical Studies of Fibrous Tissues Applied to Fascial Surgery, Arch. Surg. 34:461, 1937.

Hall, M.C.: The Trabecular Pattern of the Normal Foot, Clin. Orthop. 16:15, 1960.

Hall, M.C. (with the assistance of D.S. Kinoshita): *The Architecture of Bone.* Springfield, III.: Charles C Thomas, 1966.

Harford, G.E.: Personal assistance. Research project. Professor Anatomy, Temple University School of Chiropody, Philadelphia, 1947.

Henenfeld, M., and Walkes, M.H.: Bone Resection in Relation to Trabecular Patterns, J. Amer. Podiat. Ass. 51:255, 1961.

Hicks, J.H.: The Mechanics of the Foot. I. The Joints, J. Anat. 87:345, 1953.

Hicks, J.H.: The Mechanics of the Foot. II. The Plantar Aponeurosis and the Arch, J. Anat. 88:25, 1954.

Hicks, J.H.: The Mechanics of the Foot. IV. The Action of Muscles on the Foot in Standing, Acta Anat. 27:180, 1955.

Hicks, J.H.: Three Weight-bearing Mechanisms of the Foot. In Evans, F.G. (ed.), *Biomechanical Studies of the Musculo-skeletal System,* pp. 161-191. Springfield, III.: Charles C Thomas, 1961.

Hlavac, H.F.: Differences in X-ray Findings with Varied Positioning of the Feet, J. Amer. Podiat. Ass. 57:465, 1967.

Howorth, B.: Dynamic Posture in Relation to the Feet, Clin. Orthop. 16:74, 1960.

Huxley, J.S.: *Man Stands Alone.* New York: Harper and Bros., 1941.

Jones, R.I.: The Human Foot. An Experimental Study of Its Mechanics, and the Role of Its Muscles and Ligaments in the Support of the Arch, Amer. J. Anat. 68:12, 1941.

Keith, A.: The History of the Human Foot and Its Bearing on Orthopedic Practice, I.I.O. Thomas Memorial Lecture, 1928.

Koch, J.C.: The Laws of Bone Architecture, Amer. J. Anat. 21:177, 1917.

Lake, N.C.: *The Foot,* ed. 4. Baltimore: The Williams & Wilkins Co., 1952.

Lapidus, P.: Misconception about Springiness of Longitudinal Arch, Arch. Surg. 46:410, 1943.

Levy, B.: An Appliance to Induce Toe Flexion, J. Nat. Ass. Chiropodists 40:24, 1950.

Mann, R., and Inman, V.F.: Phasic Activity of Intrinsic Muscles of the Foot, J. Bone Joint Surg. 46-A:469, 1964.

Manter, J.T.: Movements of Subtalar and Transverse Tarsal Joints, Anat. Rec. 80:397, 1941.

Meldman, E.C.: New Aspects of Foot Dynamics in Practical Application, Transcript of Lecture, Region 3, Chiropody Science Conclave, 1950.

Mommaerts, H.M.: Fundamental Aspects of Muscle Function, J. Bone Joint Surg. 41-A:1313, 1959.

Murray, M.P., Drought, A.B., and Kory, R.C.: Walking Patterns of Normal Men, J. Bone Joint Surg. 46-A:335, 1964.

Perkins, G.: Pes Planus or Instability of Longitudinal Arch. President's Address, Proc. Roy. Soc. Med. 41:31, 1948.

Rampsberger, A.G.: *Philosophies of Science.* New York: Appleton-Century-Crofts, Inc., 1942.

Root, M.L.: An Approach to Foot Orthopedics, J. Amer. Podiat. Ass. 54:115, 1964.

Root, M.L., and Weed, J.H.: Personal communication, 1973.

Root, M.L., Weed, J.H., Sgarlato, T.E., and Bluth, D.R.: Axis of Motion of the Subtalar Joint, J. Amer. Podiat. Ass. 56:149, 1966.

Rothbart, B.A.: Nomenclature and Its Importance in Modern Podiatry, J. Amer. Podiat. Ass. 62:298, 1972.

Schuster, R.D.: Gait Analysis in Rehabilitation, J. Amer. Podiat. Ass. 54:99, 1964.

Schwartz, R.P., Heath, A.L., Morgan D.W., and Towns, R.C.: A Quantitative Analysis of Recorded Variables in the Walking Pattern of "Normal" Adults, J. Bone Joint Surg. 46-A:324, 1964.

Schwartz, R.P., Heath, A.L., and Wright, J.N.: Electrobasographic Method of Recording Gait, Arch. Surg. 27:926, 1933.

Sgarlato, T.E.: The Angle of Gait, J. Amer. Podiat. Ass. 55:645, 1965.

Sgarlato, T.E. (ed.): *A Compendium of Podiatric Biomechanics.* San Francisco: College of Podiatric Medicine, 1971.

Shenesh, A.: *Cineradiographic Observations of a Reflex Contracture of the Arch of the Foot During Walking,* Rept. No. 327, Army Medical Research Laboratory, Fort Knox, Jan. 15, 1958.

Smith, J.W.: Muscular Control of the Arches of the Foot in Standing. An Electromyographic Assessment, J. Anat. 88:152, 1954.

Steindler, A.: *Mechanics of Normal and Pathological Locomotion in Man.* Springfield, III.: Charles C Thomas, 1935.

Weinstein, F.: Foot Orthopedics. In Weinstein, F. (ed.), *Principles and Practice of Podiatry,* p. 205. Philadelphia: Lea & Febiger, 1968.

Whitney, A.K.: The Podokinetograph. A Device for Recording Foot Movements During One Foot Balance, J. Amer. Podiat. Ass. 54:111, 1964.

Whitney, A.K.: Podokinetics and Gait. In Weinstein, F. (ed.), *Principles and Practice of Podiatry,* p. 299. Philadelphia: Lea & Febiger, 1968.

Whitney, A.K.: *Orthopedic Examination Procedure.* Philadelphia: Pennsylvania College of Podiatric Medicine, 1970.

Willis, T.A.: The Function of the Long Plantar Muscles, Surg., Gynec., Obstet. 60:150, 1935.

Wolff, J.: Ueber die innere Architektur de Knochens, Virchow Arch. Path. Anat. 50:389, 1870.

Wright, D.G., Desai, D.M., and Henderson, W.H.: Action of the Subtalar and Ankle Joint Complex During the Stance Phase of Walking, J. Bone Joint Surg. 46-A:361, 1964.

Wright, D.G., and Rennels, D.C.: A Study of the Elastic Properties of Plantar Fascia, J. Bone Joint Surg. 46-A: 482, 1964.

Zitzlsperger, S.: The Mechanics of the Foot Based on the Concept of the Skeleton as a Statically Indetermined Space Framework, Clin. Orthop. 16:48, 1960.

NORMAL FOOT STRUCTURE 13

The structural and functional integrity of the foot is reflected in the roentgenographic appearance of the mature foot in stance. Bones of strong shape are aligned together in proper positions for structural stability and function in the normal foot. Deficiencies of bone shape and alignment identify the abnormal foot. Standardized lateral and dorsoplantar views in stance are required to demonstrate these.

Variations in body type and racial strain account for different kinds of feet, such as long, thin feet; short, broad feet; heavy-boned feet;

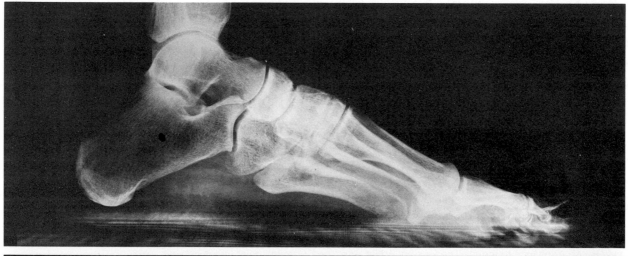

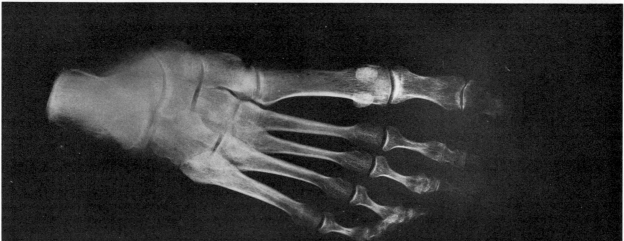

Fig. 232. Normal foot. Cardinal features: sinus tarsi is apparent; midtarsal joint line is a continuous cyma; forefoot has straight alignment.

and light-boned feet. Feet may vary in the height of the arch of their skeletal framework, and the inclination of the calcaneus is an index of this height. In spite of these variations, a normal foot is strikingly uniform in its roentgenologic features and may be easily identified (Fig. 232).

The structurally strong normal foot can take a great amount of use and abuse without breakdown. A person with a normal foot may wear unreasonable footwear and still have no significant foot problems, whereas a person with an abnormal foot is soon in trouble with incompatible footwear. An athlete may subject a normal foot to exceptional stress and retain a foot structure within normal limits. To cite a dramatic example with the permission of the party involved, Jesse Owens was a winner of four gold medals for jumping and running in the 1936 Olympics. Roentgenograms taken of his feet in 1973 (Fig. 233) show a normal structural alignment.

NORMAL FOOT DEFINITION

A normal foot is a mobile framework of individual bones of correct conformation that are aligned for maximal structural stability and functional efficiency.

The foot functions in two major capacities: (1) in gait and (2) in stance. Normal foot position in gait is achieved at the midstance phase. Normal foot position in stance is achieved with the feet in natural base and angle of stance.

For the present study, the foot is divided into segments that have meaningful alignment and that perform reciprocal functions. Each bone in the segment is described, and bone-to-bone alignment of the articulations of the segment are also described. These criteria are fundamentally significant. A minimum of reference lines and angular indexes will be used. A later chapter gives detailed roentgenographic charting. As each segment is presented for roentgenologic interpretation, brief clinical comments will be offered. Emphasis will be placed on the pathways of stress and on mobility and stability. This approach directs attention to the clinical foot rather than to an immobile charted roentgenographic image. In-

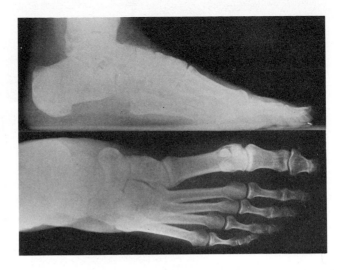

Fig. 233. Roentgenogram taken in 1973 of foot of Jesse Owens, 1936 Olympic winner of four gold medals for jumping and running. Note normal sinus tarsi, normal midtarsal joint, parallel talus, ontogenically long neck and head of talus, and slightly adducted lesser metatarsals. (Roentenogram courtesy of M.J. Kates, D.P.M., and reproduced with kind permission of Jesse Owens.)

deed, the roentgen image is fixed, but from it the functional capacity of the foot may be interpreted. A talus closely bound to the calcaneus speaks out that it is stable and not hypermobile. To read out a clinical import with validity requires a comprehensive understanding of foot biomechanics. The concepts of bone-to-bone motion and foot-to-floor position are essential. The measurement of off-weight joint motion needs comparison with a measurement of weight-loaded position. The on-weight supported foot roentgenogram shows positional changes, evidence of ligament weakness, structural abnormalities, and compensations otherwise unattainable by any other diagnostic medium (Fig. 234).

Mastery of the differentiation between the overlapping images of the foot bones on the roentgenogram is aided by having a foot skeleton at hand while studying the roentgenogram. Tracings of bone outlines from roentgenograms are shown as diagrams in illustrations to assist with interpretation. Too often the roentgenogram has been accused of falsi-

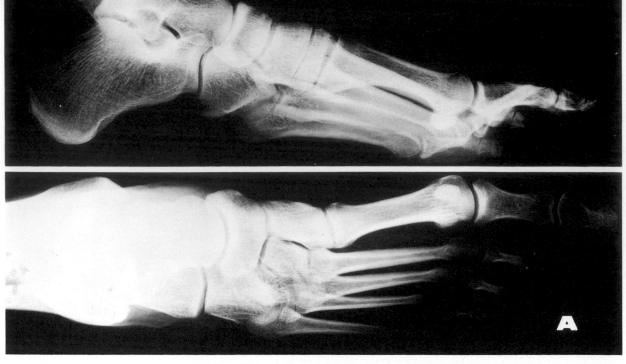

Fig. 234. Off-weight and on-weight foot roentgenograms. *A,* Non-weight-supported foot presents false appearance of normalcy; *B,* Same foot in weight-supported stance shows a faulty foot. Sinus tarsi is not visible, midtarsal cyma line broken, and forefoot abducted.

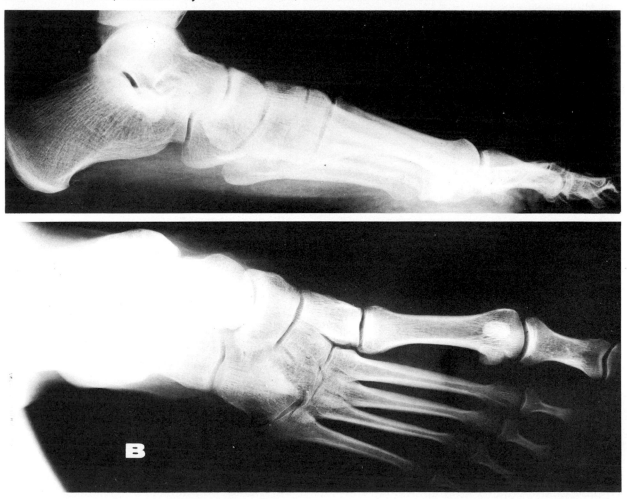

188/NORMAL FOOT STRUCTURE

fying when it is the ability of the examiner to read the truth portrayed that is at fault. Study of the subtalar joint of a skeleton specimen, although devoid of soft-tissue constituents, dramatically demonstrates the considerable amount of space involved in the sinus tarsi and its oblique direction, so that its appearance on the roentgenogram becomes very significant. Examination of the surfaces of apposing articular facets indicates the capacity for motion in a joint. The space in the sinus tarsi is indicative of the room available for malposition in hypermobile abnormalities. A motion of the talus that is seldom considered is its posterior glide and pivot on the subtalar calcaneal posterior facet and its upward rise anteriorly from the subtalar sustentaculum tali and the anterior process of the calcaneus.

GENERAL ROENTGENOLOGIC INTERPRETATION

Standardized relationships of roentgen projection, film-foot position, and the natural posture of the patient in base and angle of stance are the bases of roentgenograms presented for the study of roentgen features of the normal and abnormal foot in later chapters. Each foot is roentgenographed individually so that the roentgen projection may be accurately centered to avoid geometric distortion of the bony topography. Dorsoplantar and lateral views are basic to the study. Special projections may be used for additional information.

The basic bone shape outlines that may be visualized on the roentgenogram need to be mastered so that each bone may be identified and the spatial relationships of the foot bones can be established (Fig. 235). As each of the major foot bones is presented in the following roentgenologic interpretation a detailed description of its shape and relative position will be given.

HINDFOOT, SUBTALAR, AND MIDTARSAL JOINT ORGANIZATION

It is axiomatic that the form and integrity of the foot are practically assured if the bones of the subtalar and midtarsal joints are of normal shape and alignment.

The hindfoot consists of the calcaneus and talus articulated by the subtalar joint. The hindfoot is articulated with the navicular and cuboid bones by the midtarsal joint. Normal ontogenic maturity provides bones of acceptable shape in relative positions for proper joint conformation.

TALUS

The position of the talus is the key to the interpretation of major foot faults and foot types because of its strategic mobility.

The talus is a passive bone which has no muscle attachments and maintains its position through influence of leg bones and the calcaneus. It moves according to the design of articular surfaces within the limitations of ligaments that permit some up and down, side to side, and fore and aft motion. In pronation, the talus adducts, plantarflexes, and everts. In supination, the talus abducts, dorsiflexes, and inverts.

The talus transmits all of the stress of body weight through normal pathways if properly articulated. Normally, most of the stresses react in the large posterior subtalar articulation. The sustentaculum tali acts as a stabilizing post for the talus and provides the substrate to carry stress to the calcaneocuboid articulation. The anterior facet of the calcaneus and the calcaneonavicular ligaments together with the substantial sustentaculum tali support the anterior surface of the talus.

Talar Shape (Sagittal plane — lateral view; Fig. 235)

1. The talus presents a complete profile of the head, neck, and body with distinguishing features for each part.

2. The head of the talus extends from the dorsum of the talonavicular joint in a mild curve to the plantar aspect of this joint. It then curves in a posterior direction until it meets the junction of the neck and body, which is the sulcus tali. (The sulcus tali and sulcus calcanei together form the sinus tarsi.) *It is the plantar curve of the talus that forms the facet that articulates with the sustentaculum tali.* The total density of the sustentaculum tali presents an outline not to be confused with the facet area for the talus.

3. Dorsally, the neck of the talus is visualized as a short depression in the profile where

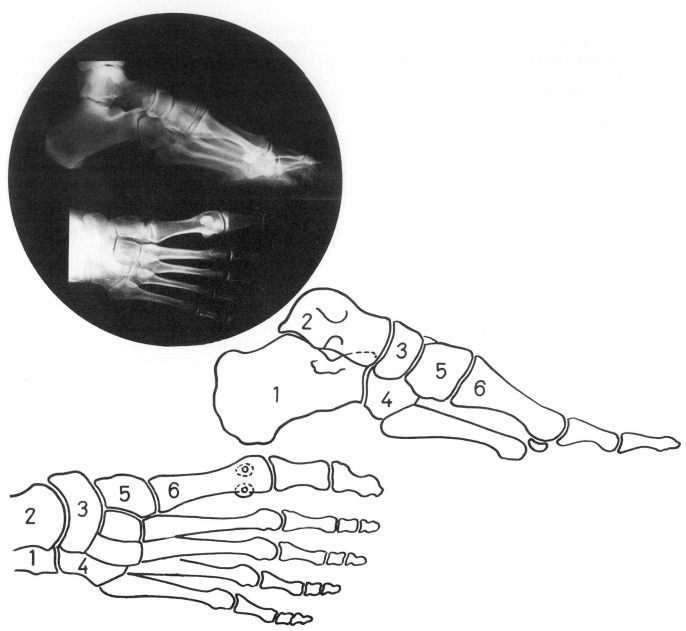

Fig. 235. Roentgenologic features of dominant shapes prevailing in foot bones.

1. Calcaneus: (a) rounded posterior tuberosity, (b) rounded plantar tuberosities, (c) substantial-sized sustentaculum tali, (d) sustentaculum tali parallel with transverse plane of subtalar joint, and (e) moderate-sized anterior process.

2. Talus: (a) rounded crown of body, no flattening or excessive posterior tubercle, (b) definite neck shape of talus is not excessively long, and (c) substantial-sized head of talus is rounded.

3. Navicular: (a) rectangular shape, approximately the same width on both medial and lateral aspects in the dorsoplantar view; and (b) no excessive tuberosity to extend prominently on medial border of foot.

4. Cuboid: smoothly rounded plantar tuberosity with no excessive molding.

5. Medial cuneiform: anterior margin should be practically perpendicular to the long axis of the bone so that the base will set square in articulation with the first metatarsal.

6. First metatarsal bone: basal articular margin perpendicular to the long axis of the bone to set square with the internal cuneiform.

it meets the trochlear aspect of the talus.

4. The body of the talus presents a convexly curved trochlear surface on the dorsum. The lateral process appears on the plantar aspect as a triangular-shaped area of increased density with the apex seemingly over the posterior aspect of the sustentaculum tali; however, it is situated in the wide lateral area of the sinus tarsi.

5. The posterior process of the talus is visualized as a projection; however, this process is as wide as the total posterior subtalar articulation, and it transmits a major proportion of the stress reactions.

Talar Shape (Transverse plane — dorsoplantar view; Fig. 235)

1. The curved distal profile of the head of the talus shows a distinct margin on both sides where it meets the sloping sides of the neck that extend posteriorly to the body of the talus. The leg structures obscure the rest of the talus.

2. The head and neck of the talus may be bisected by drawing a line across the head from the medial junction at the neck to the lateral junction of the neck and marked by a reference point at the bisection. A line drawn perpendicular from this point bisects the head and neck of the talus.

3. The set of the head and neck of the talus is oblique to the body of the talus. This angulation is structural, however, when the talus adducts, it involves a positional change, and the angulation is increased from a roentgen impression.

Talar Shape (Frontal plane — special anteroposterior view, patient standing, heel and ankle toward vertical film; see Fig. 434, Chapter 24)

1. The tibiotalar surface of the trochlea is flat.

2. The lateral surface of the talus presents a sloping facet for articulating with the fibula.

3. Unfortunately, the oblique set of the head and neck of the talus cannot be visualized on a conventional roentgenogram. A planigram of the weight-supporting foot can only be achieved with special equipment and technique.

Talar Position (Sagittal plane — lateral view)

1. A line drawn from the posterior talocalcaneal joint passing through the reference point at the superior surface of the sinus tarsi is essentially parallel with the weight-supporting plane. This line represents the relative position of the body of the talus (Fig. 236).

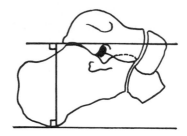

Fig. 236. Body of the talus normally parallel with the weight-supporting plane

2. The angle of declination of the talus relates to the position of the neck and head of the talus relative to the weight-supporting plane. A framework of reference is obtained by drawing a reference line from the superior articulation of the head of the talus with the navicular to the inferior articulation of the head of the talus with the calcaneus. From the point of bisection, a line is drawn perpendicular extending proximally through the neck and head to bisect the talus. The same line is extended distally to meet the weight-supporting plane, and the angle formed is the angle of declination of the talus. This angle decreases with supination and increases with pronation.

Talar Position (Transverse plane — dorsoplantar view)

1. In normal position, the head of the talus is closely bound to the calcaneus and is superimposed over the anterior portion of the calcaneus (Fig. 237). When pronation occurs, there is less overlap; in supination, there is greater overlap.

2. With adequate penetration, the outline of the sustentaculum tali may be visualized under the talus and the length of the inferior calcaneonavicular ligament determined as the distance from this process to the navicular. It is

not possible to roentgenograph the true proportions of the sustentaculum tali, calcaneus, and navicular bones of the subtalar articulation in the dorsoplantar view because of the superimposed talus and ankle structure. Only a roentgenogram of a dissected foot (Fig. 238) can show the true proportions.

3. It is the medial inclination of the neck of the talus that gives this impression that the talus appears to be in an eccentric position on the calcaneus because it rests in part on the sustentaculum tali. However, the body of the talus is practically parallel with the midline of the hindfoot. There are many variations in the angle between the talar head and the body, and some are ontogenic.

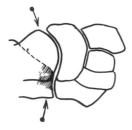

Fig. 237. Talus normally bound closely to anterior process of calcaneus

4. For practical purposes a 15° ±5° angle of medial deviation from the hindfoot is considered a normal relationship between the head and neck of the talus and the calcaneus. A line is drawn across the widest dimension of the head of the talus and bisected. From this point, a line is extended to meet the long axis of the hindfoot. The angle formed is the *angle of medial deviation of the talus,* or the *talus-long foot axis angle.* The long axis of the hindfoot is a line drawn from the center of the calcaneus distally through a point at the junction of the medial aspect of the calcaneocuboid joint. This line may be extended to represent the long axis of the foot, and in a normal foot usually falls between the second and third metatarsal heads. Altered positions of forefoot or hindfoot disturb this relationship. Abnormal bone shapes can distort the framework of reference (Fig. 239).

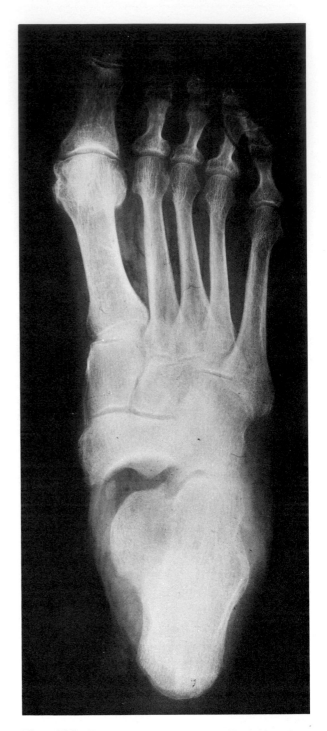

Fig. 238. Roentgenogram of dissected foot specimen with talus removed, showing total subtalar joint with true proportions of sustentaculum tali, calcaneus, and navicular bones. (Dissection, courtesy of G. Elmer Harford D.P.M.; roentgenogram, courtesy of Leon E. Kehr D.P.M.; specimen, courtesy of Pennsylvania College of Podiatric Medicine.)

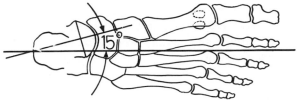

Fig. 239. Long axis of talar neck normally deviated 15° ±5° from the long axis of the foot extended from the long axis of the hindfoot

Talar Position (Frontal plane — special anteroposterior view, patient standing, heel and ankle toward vertical film; see Chapter 24, Fig. 436)

1. The tibiofibular articulation with the superior aspect of the talus is visualized, and the trochlear margin is parallel with the weight-supporting plane.

CALCANEUS

The position of the calcaneus is of prime importance in maintaining normal foot alignment. The calcaneus is responsive to tibial motion through its articulation with the talus. The placement of the foot and its movements in gait are resolved by calcaneal position in the hindfoot. The prime movers of the body in locomotion, the triceps surae, terminate in their attachment to the posterior aspect of the calcaneus and influence its position. The plantar fascia and the principal intrinsic muscles of the foot as well as the triceps surae and the tendons passing from other leg muscles regulate calcaneal position. When weight is borne, the calcaneus must transmit most of it through its plantar tuberosity contact areas.

"As the heel goes so goes the foot" is a valid truism. Even compensations for forefoot problems are referred to the calcaneus for accommodation.

Calcaneal Shape (Sagittal plane — lateral view; Fig. 235)

1. A calcaneus of normal shape provides adequate support for the talus by the posterior subtalar facet, the sustentaculum tali, and the superior anteromedial facet. Facets are represented by a line at the articular contact area.

a. The posterior subtalar facet presents a slope that extends from the superoposterior border of the calcaneus downward to the plantar apex of the outline of the talus. An angle formed by this slope and a line drawn along the posterosuperior margin of the calcaneus is proposed as an index of calcaneal shape found in high-arch to low-arch framework. The more acute the angle, the higher the framework (see Chapter 17, Fig. 338).

b. The sustentaculum tali varies in shape. It may be an abruptly terminated process differentiated from the anterior part of the calcaneus by a canalized notch, or it may be a sloping process that extends to the laterodistal margin of the calcaneus. The abruptly terminated process with little slope is the less supportive. The sustentaculum tali facet should be visualized by matching it with the plantar aspect of the talus distal to the apex outline. The total shape of the entire sustentaculum tali is represented by an oblong area of increased density extending distally below the apex of the plantar aspect of the talus.

c. The superior anteromedial facet is not a constant finding, even in normal feet. The facet is difficult to differentiate roentgenographically from the distal margin of the facet of the sustentaculum tali. However, when present, it provides additional support to the talus.

2. A calcaneus with a long anterior portion beyond the sustentaculum tali is more likely to have a facet for support of the talus than one with a short anterior portion.

3. The anterior portion of the calcaneus extends dorsally and overlaps the plantodistal margin of the talus. It should be realized that this "calcaneal beak" is on the laterosuperior margin of the anterior portion of the calcaneus adjacent to the lateral border of the cuboid. The overlapped appearance is not indicative of support for the talus nor is it an indicator of talar plantarflexion. The anterior portion is an anatomical process that rises above the cuboid joint and is subject to fracture.

4. A calcaneus that has reached ontogenic maturity is purported to be a longer bone than one less developed. This length includes the anterior portion.

5. The distal aspect of the calcaneus articulates with the cuboid and is variable in

shape. Normally, it presents a straight joint surface. Abnormally, the joint surface is curved to articulate with a cuboid that has a hooklike process.

Calcaneal Position (Sagittal plane — lateral view)

1. The angle of inclination of the calcaneus establishes the height of the foot framework. The angle is formed by the weight-supporting plane and a line drawn from this plane through the anteroplantar margin of the calcaneal tuberosity to the plantar margin of the anterior portion of the calcaneus.

    a. Range of calcaneal inclination: low, 0°-10°; medium, 10°-20°; high, 20°-30° (Fig. 240).

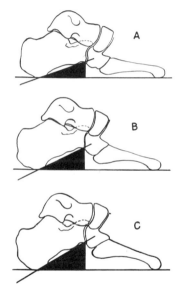

Fig. 240. Calcaneal pitch indicates height of foot framework: *A*, low pitch, 0° - 10°; *B*, medium, 10° - 20°; and *C*, high 20° +

    b. Normally, both feet have similar calcaneal inclinations.

    c. A difference in calcaneal inclination between the feet may be determined by comparison of the two feet.

    d. Normal subtalar and midtarsal joints are indicative of an unaltered calcaneal inclination.

2. The posterior subtalar joint space may be visualized when the calcaneus is in normal position.

3. An increased summation of densities of the medial tuberosity is visualized above the lateral tuberosity when the calcaneus is in normal position. This is lost on eversion (Fig. 241).

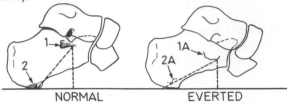

Fig. 241. Indications of calcaneal position. *Normal position: 1,* density of sustentaculum tali sharply defined, and *2,* density of lateral tuberosity defined. *Everted position: 1A,* broad, lower, indefinite outline of sustentaculum tali, and *2A,* density of lateral tuberosity lost.

4. The sustentaculum tali is defined by an increased summation of densities when the calcaneus is in normal position. This is lost on eversion (Fig. 241).

Calcaneal Position (Transverse plane — dorsoplantar view)

1. Only the anterior portion of the calcaneus is readily visualized in this view. In normal position, a short margin of the lateral border of the calcaneus is essentially parallel with the long axis of the hindfoot. When the calcaneus is abducted or adducted, the line will vary accordingly.

2. The distal margin of the normal calcaneus presents a straight line from its lateral border to the junction of the notch or slope of the sustentaculum tali. This line corresponds to the calcaneocuboid joint. The extension of this line represents the transverse division of the foot into forefoot and hindfoot.

3. A point at the junction of the medial aspect of the calcaneocuboid joint is a reference point from which a line may be drawn to the center of the calcaneus to represent the long axis of the hindfoot. Variations in the shape of the anterior portion of the calcaneus and the sustentaculum tali make it difficult to ascertain the medial margin of the calcaneocuboid joint. It is best to follow the proximal margin of the cuboid as a guide.

Calcaneal Position (Frontal plane — special posteroanterior view, patient standing, toes toward vertical film. See Fig. 502, Chapter 25)

In normal alignment, the calcaneus is essentially vertical under the fibular side of the talus. In valgus position, it is everted and lateral to the fibular side of the talus.

Calcaneal Position (Frontal plane — special anteroposterior view, patient standing, heel in contact with vertical film, forefoot elevated on a block of balsa wood; see Fig. 430, Chapter 24)

1. This view gives a good profile of the posteroplantar aspect of the calcaneus showing the position of the weight-supporting contour of the plantar tuberosity and the concavity of the medial border rising to the sustentaculum tali.

2. The body of the calcaneus is dramatically portrayed situated under the fibular side of the talus in normal alignment.

3. The tibiotalar articulation and tibiofibular articulations are so demonstrated that the relative position of the calcaneus is easily established. The natural shape of the calcaneus tends to be convex on the lateral border simulating an appearance of inversion.

SUBTALAR JOINT

Congruity of the subtalar joint is insured by normal positions of the talus and calcaneus. Roentgen visualization of this vital articulation is portrayed most significantly by the seating of the talus in relation to the sinus tarsi (Fig. 242).

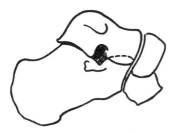

Fig. 242. Visible sinus tarsi indicates proper seating of talus. A key feature.

Anatomically, the subtalar joint is divided into two separate encapsulated joint cavities. The posterior joint cavity is situated between the posterior facets of the talus and calcaneus. The anterior joint cavity lies between the medial calcaneal facet of the sustentaculum tali and the medial facet of the head of the talus, between the anterior facet of the calcaneus and the anterior facet of the talus, and the distal aspect of the anterior cavity lies between the facets of the talus and navicular and the plantar calcaneonavicular ligament. The two cavities are virtually separated by the sinus tarsi which is filled mainly by the powerful talocalcaneal interosseous ligament, masses of fat, and a bursa. Clinically, the range of mobility of the talus is controlled by the ligamentous integument and the space available in the sinus tarsi. The separate joint cavities indicate the dual role that the subtalar joint has in distributing stress posteriorly through the body of the talus and anteriorly through the head of the talus. (See Fig. 238.)

Roentgen identification of the subtalar joint is made from the following criteria:

POSTERIOR TALOCALCANEAL ARTICULATION (SAGITTAL PLANE — LATERAL VIEW; FIG. 235)

The posterior talocalcaneal joint space is evenly distributed from the posterior aspect of the joint where it slopes distally and plantarly to the plantar apex of the body of the talus.

SINUS TARSI (SAGITTAL PLANE — LATERAL VIEW; FIG. 242)

1. This very important roentgen landmark appears as an oval area of decreased density above the sustentaculum tali where the neck of the talus joins the body at its inferior surface.

2. The roentgenologic appearance is, in reality, only a small cross section of the oblique subtalar canal which permits an overpass of stress from the talus to the navicular and an underpass of stress from the calcaneus to the cuboid.

3. Complete visualization indicates a level subtalar joint, a properly seated talus, and a calcaneus in normal position.

MEDIAL TALOCALCANEAL
ARTICULATION (SAGITTAL PLANE —
LATERAL VIEW; FIG. 235)

The sustentaculum tali permits the medial facet of the calcaneus to articulate with the plantar facet on the head of the talus. The joint space between these facets is visualized where it slopes from the plantar apex of the body of the talus to the junction of the superimposed anterosuperior process of the calcaneus. This joint space is just distal to the sinus tarsi.

ANTERIOR TALOCALCANEAL
ARTICULATION (SAGITTAL PLANE —
LATERAL VIEW; FIG. 235)

This joint space can only be seen in the absence of an anterosuperior process of the calcaneus which usually superimposes and obliterates its visualization.

NAVICULAR

Navicular Shape (Sagittal plane — lateral view; Fig. 235)

1. The profile of the navicular is concave at the proximal margin articulating with the talus.
2. The plantar margin slopes downward and distally.
3. The dorsal margin slopes distally parallel with the distal part of the talus until it meets the level of the second cuneiform where it dips abruptly plantarward until it meets the posterior margin of the first cuneiform.
4. The distal margin is convex where it articulates with the first cuneiform.
5. The dip in the dorsal margin of the navicular is a significant roentgen landmark because it permits identification of the base-upward triangle representing the second cuneiform bone.

Navicular Shape (Transverse plane — dorsoplantar view; Fig. 235)

1. The navicular presents an oblong profile somewhat narrower laterally than medially, but it is not wedge shaped. There is sometimes a tuberosity extending medially.
2. The posterior margin is concave to ar-

ticulate with the rounded head of the talus.
3. The distal margin is convex and is divided by two ridges to provide articulation for the three cuneiforms.
4. The extreme posterolateral margin overlies the cuboid, which is the site of articulation.
5. If a frontal plane view were possible, the navicular profile would curve from a high point laterodorsal to a low point medioplantar.

Navicular Position (Sagittal plane — lateral view; Fig. 235)

1. The facets of the navicular and talus should match at their dorsal margin.
2. The dorsal margins of the navicular and talus should be parallel.
3. The profiles that have been described as shape indicate a normal position of the navicular.

Navicular Position (Transverse plane — dorsoplantar view)

1. Normally, at least 75% of the talar head should articulate with the navicular (Fig. 243).

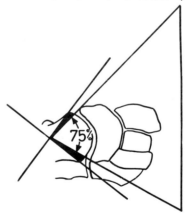

Fig. 243. At least 75% of talar head normally articulates with navicular

2. The articular facets for the cuneiform bones indicate a normal position when the first and second cuneiforms are clearly shown in articulation with corresponding metatarsal bases and only a little of the third naviculo-cuneiform joint is visible. The reverse order is present when the navicular is everted.
3. The navicular transverse axis is perpendicular to the long axis of the hindfoot.

CUBOID

Cuboid Shape (Sagittal plane — lateral view; Fig. 235)

1. The profile of the cuboid is more triangular than cuboid.

2. The calcaneocuboid margin of the cuboid may vary from a straight line to a convex one.

3. The plantar tuberosity of the cuboid also varies from a moderate curve to an extended protuberance.

4. The distal articulation of the cuboid with the fourth metatarsal has the shape of its cuboid facet.

5. Although there is an overlapping shadow from the first cuneiform, the articulation of the cuboid with the third cuneiform can usually be visualized.

Cuboid Shape (Transverse plane — dorsoplantar view; Fig. 235)

1. The entire shape of the cuboid is discernible, although there is some overlap of the third cuneiform and navicular where they articulate with the cuboid.

2. The calcaneocuboid margin is essentially straight and parallel with the transverse axis of the foot. In variants in which the joint is extremely saddle shaped, the line curves. However, from lateral margin to medial margin a line may still be drawn that will be essentially parallel with the transverse axis.

Cuboid Position (Sagittal plane — lateral view; Fig. 235)

1. The cuboid has a closely bound articulation with the calcaneus through facets of almost equal size that allow little joint movement.

2. Normal calcaneal position indicates correct cuboid alignment.

3. The facets of the calcaneus and cuboid should match at their plantar margins (Fig. 244).

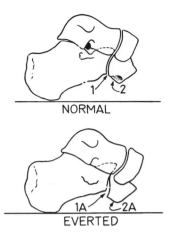

Fig. 244. Indications of cuboid position. *Normal position: 1,* plantar facets of calcaneocuboid joints are even, and *2,* peroneal groove defined. *Everted position: 1A,* uneven articulation of facets, and *2A,* density of peroneal groove lost.

4. The distal articulation of the cuboid with the fourth metatarsal has the shape of its cuboid facet.

5. Joint space between calcaneus and cuboid should be uniform.

6. When the calcaneus lowers in pitch, the cuboid follows.

Cuboid Position (Transverse plane — dorsoplantar view; Fig. 235)

1. The lateral facets of the calcaneus and cuboid should match.

2. The joint space between calcaneus and cuboid should be uniform.

3. The lateroposterior facet of the cuboid should match the laterodistal facet of the calcaneus. When the calcaneus is everted, it is difficult, though not impossible, to define this point of articulation.

SIGNIFICANT ROENTGENOLOGIC FEATURES OF NORMAL HINDFOOT, SUBTALAR AND MIDTARSAL JOINT ORGANIZATION (FIGS. 245 and 246)

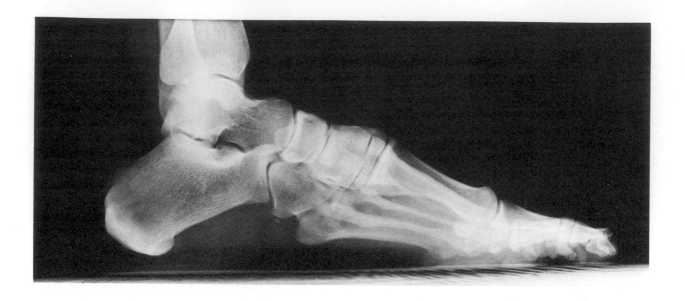

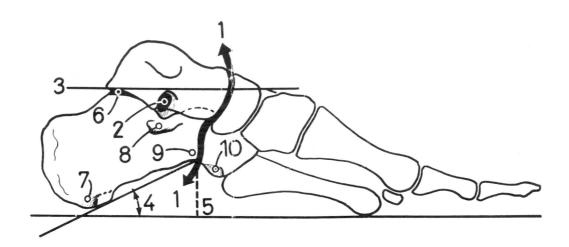

Fig. 245. Roentgenologic features of normal hindfoot, subtalar, and midtarsal joint, *lateral view*

1. Midtarsal joint line is a continuous cyma.
2. Sinus tarsi is visible.
3. Body of talus is parallel with weight-bearing plane (posterior talocalcaneal joint through superior surface of sinus tarsi).
4. Calcaneal inclination of both feet should be uniform.
5. Calcaneal inclination is an index of height of foot framework.
6. Space at posterior aspect of subtalar joint indicates a level calcaneus.
7. Plantar tuberosities of calcaneus are visualized by summation of densities.
8. Sustentaculum tali is defined as a dense area under sinus tarsi.
9. Cuboid articular facet is evenly aligned with calcaneus articular facet.
10. Peroneal groove of cuboid is delineated by added density.

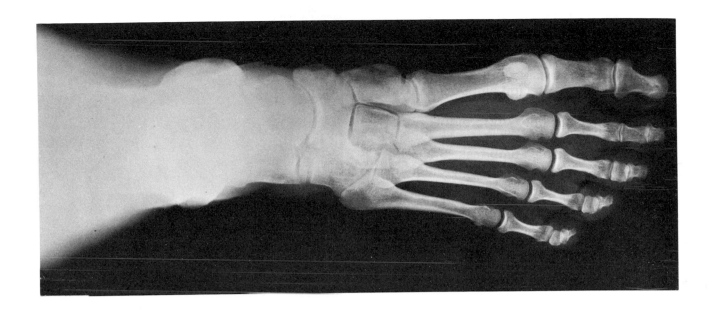

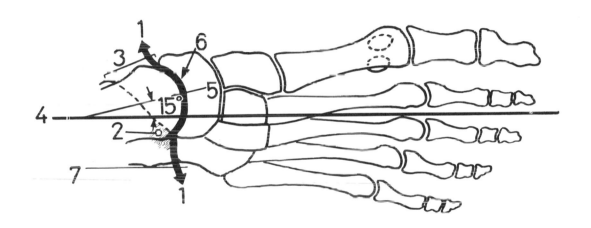

Fig. 246. Roentgenologic features of normal hindfoot-subtalar-midtarsal joint organization, *dorso-plantar view*

1. Midtarsal joint line is a continuous cyma.
2. Head of talus is closely bound to anterior process of calcaneus.
3. Length of plantar calcaneonavicular ligament; appraise from sustentaculum tali to navicular.
4. Long axis of the hindfoot is from center of calcaneus through medial junction of calcaneocu-boid joint. Long axis of the foot is an extension of the long axis of the hindfoot.
5. Medial deviation of talus from long axis of foot 15° ± 5°.
6. Seventy-five percent of head of talus should articulate with navicular.
7. Lateral border of calcaneus at its anterior portion lies parallel with long axis of foot.

be used to control both hindfoot and forefoot balance. Check calcaneal position in axial view to appraise hindfoot posting.

NAVICULOCUNEIFORM FAULT SYNDROME

Although a frequent sequel to midtarsal fault, naviculocuneiform fault represents a basic foot weakness and may be diagnosed as a major fault syndrome. It usually occurs in long feet with a maximal stress at this articulation (Fig. 278). Weakness of the tibialis anticus muscle or a variation of its insertion may also contribute to the problem.

The profound structural changes that originate from hindfoot and midtarsal faults are extended to the tarsal region into two anatomically oriented divisions, although stress pathways transcend such compartmentalization as naviculocuneiform fault with involvement of the medial forefoot segment and calcaneocuboid fault with involvement of the lateral forefoot segment. The transverse tarsometatarsal articulation is also involved.

ROENTGENOLOGIC INTERPRETATION

Naviculocuneiform Articulation

1. The lateral view defines the important roentgenologic features.

2. There is a sagging depression at the naviculocuneiform articulation.

3. The anterior margin of the navicular pivots downward as it follows the maldirection of the talus.

4. The posterior margins of the cuneiforms pivot downward producing depression of the articulation.

5. Joint space is closed at the dorsum and open at the plantar aspect.

6. Because the first cuneiform rotates medially, the second cuneiform is visualized as more of it is exposed as an inverted triangle with base upward.

7. The superior margin of the articulation between the first cuneiform and the first metatarsal becomes prominent and is frequently the site of exostotic formation and shoe irritation.

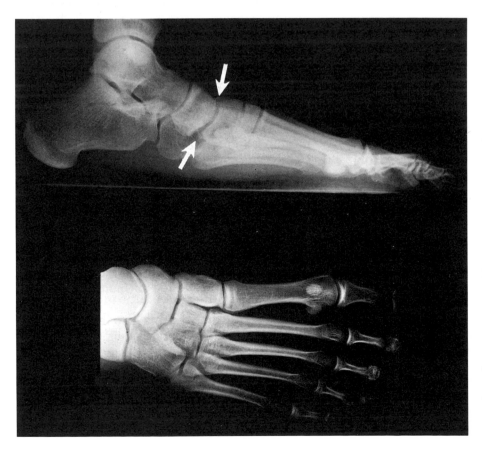

Fig. 278. Naviculocuneiform fault. Depression on dorsal aspect, gap at plantar aspect of naviculocuneiform joint. Lowering of medial forefoot segment *(lateral view).* Hypermobility gap between medial and middle cuneiforms *(dorsoplantar view).*

ROENTGENOLOGIC FEATURES OF
NAVICULOCUNEIFORM FAULT
SYNDROME (Fig. 279).

ACQUIRED FAULTS OF MEDIAL FOREFOOT SEGMENT

Subtalar, midtarsal, and naviculocuneiform faults may be contributory. The dorsoplantar view defines the roentgenologic features of the transverse plane and, by indirect evidence, the frontal plane. The lateral view shows sagittal plane features. Axial views may be used to explore frontal plane positions of sesamoids and metatarsal heads.

1. Entire medial segment buckling reactions (zigzag foot). As the talar head pushes the navicular forward, medially, and downward, a buckling reaction takes place at the cuneiform articulations due to the flowing back of counterforces from contact areas of the first, second, and third metatarsal heads (Fig. 280).

a. The first cuneiform everts and instead of its being normally aligned parallel to the midline of the foot tends to buckle into abduction. The base of the first metatarsal also abducts and everts, which diverts the transverse position of the shaft into adduction. The foot presents a zigzag line from talus to navicular, to first cuneiform, to first metatarsal base, to metatarsal head.

b. The second cuneiform and base of second metatarsal shift laterally, and the shaft of the second metatarsal adducts. The second toe slightly abducts.

c. The third cuneiform abducts, as demonstrated by its articulating member, the third metatarsal, which shifts laterally at its base and deviates the shaft and head into adduc-

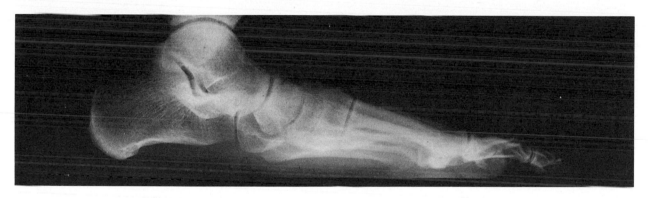

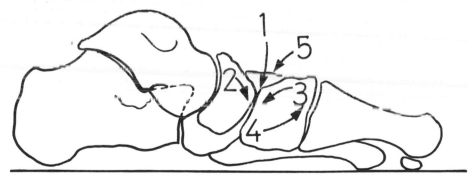

Fig. 279. Roentgenologic features of naviculocuneiform fault. *Lateral view.*

1, Depression of naviculocuneiform joint.

2, Navicular pivoted downward at anterior border.

3, Medial cuneiform pivoted downward at posterior border.

4, Anterior border of medial cuneiform pivoted upward throwing the first metatarsal base into prominence.

5, In extreme cases, middle cuneiform is visualized as an inverted triangle rising above the articulation.

tion. The third toe abducts markedly when this malalignment occurs and is observed clinically as a separation of the second and third toes when the patient stands.

2. First metasarsal segment hypermobility gap (cuneiform split).

a. In the dorsoplantar view, eversion of the first cuneiform opens a gap between the first cuneometatarsal and second cuneometatarsal joints. This condition has been described by Morton (1935) as hypermobility; others refer to it as cuneiform split.

b. In severe and extreme eversion of the first cuneometatarsal from the second cuneometatarsal joint, the gap is closed from a roentgenologic visualization because the plantar aspect of the joint is closed. However, the experienced observer will identify the bone margins by their cortices which indicate the existing gap.

3. Depression of the first metatarsal segment. When the first metatarsal segment (first ray) is depressed at its proximal aspect, a lower angle of declination of the segment occurs in response on weight bearing to an excessive range of dorsiflexion of the segment. The depression is visualized in the lateral view.

The dorsoplantar view of a depressed first metatarsal will appear comparatively longer at the metatarsophalangeal joint level than an

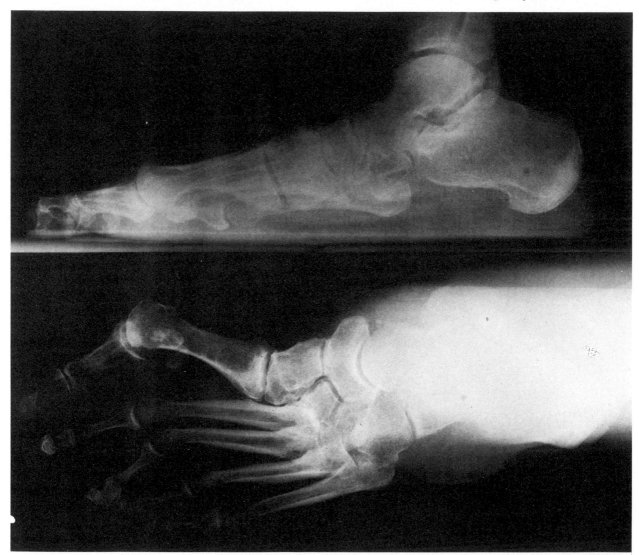

Fig. 280. Medial segment buckling reactions — midtarsal fault (zigzag foot with hallux abductus valgus)

elevated first metatarsal. When sesamoid bones appear comparatively displaced posteriorly the metatarsal is depressed, whereas in distal displacement of the sesamoids the metatarsal is elevated. On- and off-weight views are required.

ROENTGENOLOGIC FEATURES OF MEDIAL FOREFOOT SEGMENT INVOLVEMENT (Fig. 281)

CLINICAL CORRELATION AND MANAGEMENT

1. Long thin feet frequently produce naviculocuneiform fault due to excessive stresses that develop in the long arch span.

2. Where roentgenologic evidence of gaping joints exists, these areas are usually painful on palpation when the patient is standing.

3. When naviculocuneiform fault syndrome is the major syndrome, the typical Shaeffer-type longitudinal appliance will be beneficial because it undergirds the joint and bones at fault.

4. Secondary involvement of the medial forefoot segment indicates the need for extensive rehabilitative programs with appropriate physiotherapeutic measures and adhesive retention tapings.

5. It is a mistake to use an appliance for calcaneal control on this foot type unless the fault is secondary to midtarsal fault.

6. Naviculocuneiform fault secondary to midtarsal fault requires realignment of the hindfoot as well as the forefoot segment.

7. Design of any appliance must consider the reapportionment of stress to better advantage.

CALCANEOCUBOID FAULT SYNDROME

Continuation of malalignment from the calcaneus involves the calcaneocuboid articulation and the lateral forefoot segment. Instances occur, usually in feet of high arch shape, where the fault is found specifically. Although clinicians frequently designate a foot condition in this area as a "dropped cuboid," actually a specific downward displacement is

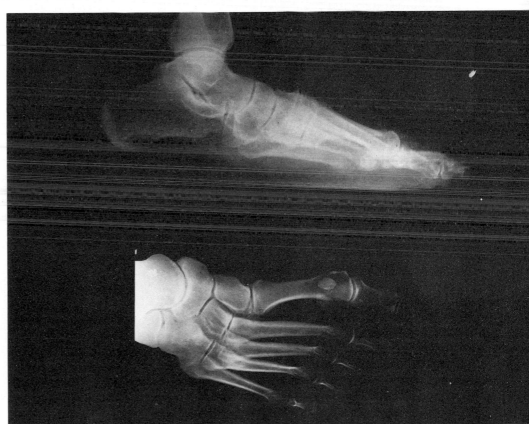

Fig. 281. Roentgenologic features of medial forefoot segment involvement

1. Medial segment buckling reactions (zigzag foot).

2. First metatarsal segment hypermobility gap (cuneiform split).

3. Depression of first metatarsal segment, posterior sesamoids (dorsiflexed first ray).

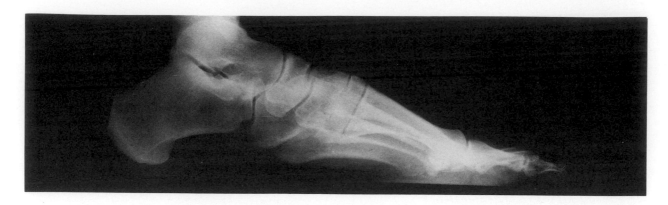

Fig. 282. Calcaneocuboid fault — dropped cuboid

rare (Fig. 282). Rather, the cuboid rotates on its long axis, tightly bound with the calcaneal movement. The individual integrity of the various ligament bands determines how the bone will behave under stress and several variations in position are possible.

ROENTGENOLOGIC INTERPRETATION

1. As the calcaneus lowers in pitch, the cuboid follows (lateral view).

2. The cuboid rotates on its long axis with the eversion of the calcaneus.

3. The plantar tubercle of the cuboid loses the roentgenologic density of the peroneal groove as it rotates.

4. The twisting stress that develops, coupled with the breaking stress as it is forced downward, may open a gap at the dorsal aspect of the joint and close the plantar aspect.

5. In some instances, the cuboid moves to a position under the anterior process of the calcaneus, especially in cases of extremely high foot framework (Fig. 283).

6. In rare cases, the cuboid is displaced in a direct downward movement.

ROENTGENOLOGIC FEATURES OF CALCANEOCUBOID FAULT SYNDROME (Fig. 284)

ACQUIRED FAULTS OF LATERAL FOREFOOT SEGMENT (Fig. 285)

1. Rotation of the cuboid alters the position of the bases of the fourth and fifth metatarsal bones.

2. Although the base of the fourth metatarsal overlaps the fifth by approximately 50% in the normal foot, calcaneocuboid fault reduces the overlap to as little as 10%.

3. The fifth metatarsal rotates on its long axis so that the base appears broadened, the shaft bowed, and the obliquity of the metatarsal's articulation with the cuboid is reduced.

4. Both fourth and fifth bases open a

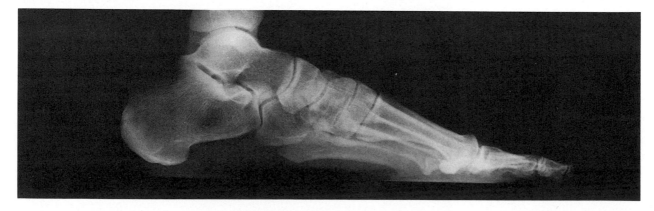

Fig. 283. Calcaneocuboid fault — cuboid under anterior process of calcaneus

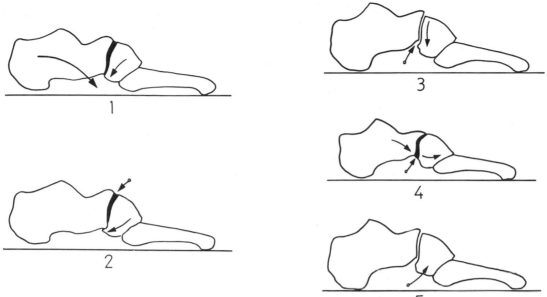

Fig. 284. Roentgenologic features of calcaneocuboid fault. *Lateral view.* 5

1, Cuboid is forced downward with change in pitch of calcaneus.

2, Cuboid sometimes moves under anterior process of calcaneus.

3, Rarely, cuboid drops with articular space even but articulating margin lowered at its plantar aspect.

4, Sometimes dorsal aspect of joint is closed and plantar aspect is open due to weakness of calcaneocuboid ligaments.

5, Calcaneocuboid fault with lateral segment involvement. Cuboid lowered and everted. Gap at base of fourth metatarsal as it articulates with fifth metatarsal. Broadening of base of fifth metatarsal caused by rotation.

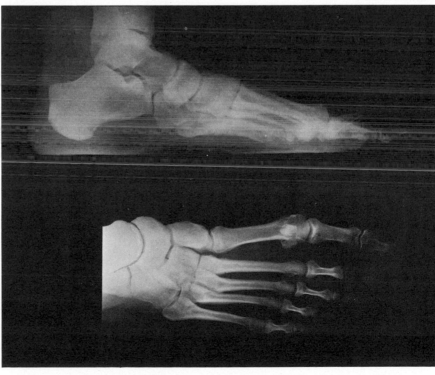

Fig. 285. Calcaneocuboid fault with lateral segment involvement. Cuboid lowered and everted. Gap at base of fourth metatarsal as it articulates with fifth metatarsal. Broadening of base of fifth metatarsal caused by rotation.

ACQUIRED FOOT FAULT SYNDROMES/229

widened articulation with the cuboid. New-man (1940) describes this as hypermobility of the fifth metatarsal segment.

ROENTGENOLOGIC FEATURES OF LATERAL FOREFOOT INVOLVEMENT: DORSOPLANTAR VIEW (Fig. 286)

Clinical Correlation

1. The rotation of the cuboid greatly lessens the ability of this bone, together with the fourth metatarsal, to accommodate the transfer of forces from the medial forefoot segment. This reduces foot action from a well-integrated mechanism into two separate and relatively independent structural segments with loss of efficiency.

2. The position of the cuboid in this fault syndrome is frequently the site for manipula-tive effort. It is a valid movement that attempts to press the bone upward and laterally from the plantar aspect. However, mobilization is of little avail unless remedial measures are taken to reposition the calcaneus.

3. Hypermobility of the fifth metatarsal segment identified clinically indicates a need for appraisal of the total foot situation.

4. Rotation of the fifth metatarsal places the fifth toe in a position which makes it liable to adductovarus deformity and thereby fore-runs a joint condition.

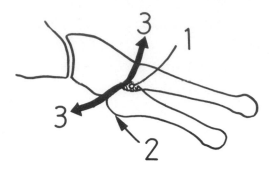

Fig. 286. Roentgenologic features of involve-ment of lateral forefoot segment. *Dorsoplantar view.*

1. Fourth metatarsal base overlaps fifth less than 50%.

2. Base of fifth metatarsal appears broad-ened due to rotation.

3. Increased joint space between fourth and fifth metatarsals with cuboid results in hyper-mobility and laxness.

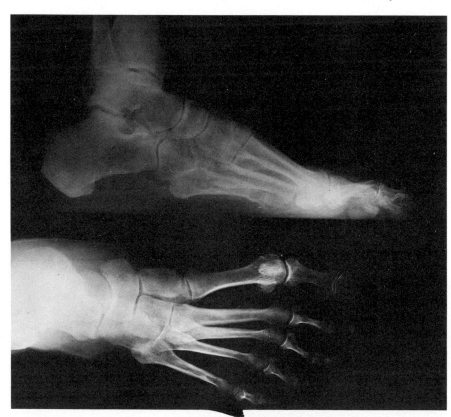

Fig. 287. Normal hindfoot and midtarsal joint. Medium inversion with adduction of second and third metatarsal shafts. Buckling of third toe. Slight hypermobility of first cuneiform and second cuneiform bones.

ACQUIRED FAULTS OF THE TRANSVERSE TARSOMETATARSAL ARTICULATIONS (Fig. 262)

The bases of the metatarsals articulate with the cuneiforms and the cuboid bone. Transversely, these bones articulate in a curve dorsally convex from medial to lateral border of the foot, called the transverse tarsometatarsal articulation or arch. The dorsoplantar view shows changes that may occur in these articulations.

1. Normally, metatarsal bases overlap and the joint margins of the cuneiforms and cuboid are obscured.

2. As the forefoot everts and abducts, a spreading of the tarsometatarsal joints occurs and space is visualized between the second and third cuneiforms and the overlap of metatarsal bases is diminished.

3. With severe and extreme eversion, valgus rotation of the first metatarsal segment occurs and the first cuneiform may underlap the second cuneiform

4. When all three acquired fault syndromes are involved with extension to both medial and lateral forefoot segments, the transverse tarsometatarsal articulation is flattened and may become completely disorganized (Figs. 287 and 288).

MALALIGNMENT OF TOTAL FOREFOOT

The forefoot is the structure distal to the midtarsal joint. It includes the lesser tarsal bones and the medial and lateral forefoot segments with their toes. The medial and lateral forefoot segments articulate at the third cuneiform-cuboid joint and the third-fourth metatarsal joint.

Abduction and adduction are the major forefoot malalignments demonstrated by the dorsoplantar roentgenogram. The angle formed by the calcaneocuboid joint line and a line extended from the lateral border of this joint to the distal extreme of the head of the talus represents the forefoot angle. If the forefoot angle is increased abduction is present, abduction of the lesser tarsus is increased; if it is decreased, adduction is present (Fig. 261-262).

Some of the features of metatarsal malalignment have here been presented on a segmental basis and are given in more detail in the chapter on metatarsal disorders

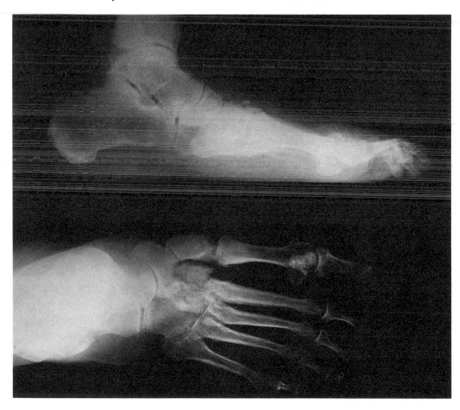

Fig. 288. Same case as Fig. 287, 5 years later. Midtarsal fault. Naviculo-cuneiform fault. Complete disorganization of transverse tarsal articulation and medial and lateral forefoot segments.

Hypertrophy and Atrophy of Metatarsal Bones (Fig. 300)

1. One of the most dramatic demonstrations of Wolff's law of functional adaptation in bone is shown in the hypertrophy of the shaft in instances of excessively long metatarsal bone that takes the weight-force impost during gait. The cortical walls are increased in thickness and the entire volume of the bone is heavier. Adjacent members are of normal width in the dorsoplantar view.

2. Atrophy results from a lack of work load. A single metatarsal rarely abstains from substantial function. Even a short first carries enough burden to retain its form except in excessive shortness or malfunctioning position. Couched members, such as the fourth, are likely to be diminutive.

3. When adjacent members are of equal length, hypertrophy of the second metatarsal may have occurred prior to a now present elongation of the foot due to midtarsal fault.

Impingement Factors (Refer to Figs. 302 and 303)

1. Foot collapse with adducted position of metatarsal shafts causes impingement.

2. Juxtaposition of two metatarsal heads is common in metatarsals of uniform length.

3. Intermetatarsal bursitis is a frequent problem when metatarsal heads are squeezed together by a tight shoe.

4. Nerve impingement causing Morton's neuralgia is a sequel to juxtaposition of bony elements in some feet.

5. The dorsoplantar view indicates impingement factors.

6. Ligamentous restriction may bind metatarsals into impingement. This may be checked by clinical palpation.

Abnormalities of Shape of Metatarsal Heads (Fig. 301)

1. Heavy-boned individuals sometimes have metatarsal heads which create crowding situations with impingement.

Adducted Position of Metatarsal Bones (Fig. 302 and 303)

1. The sequence of alignment altered by foot collapse presents a syndrome affecting

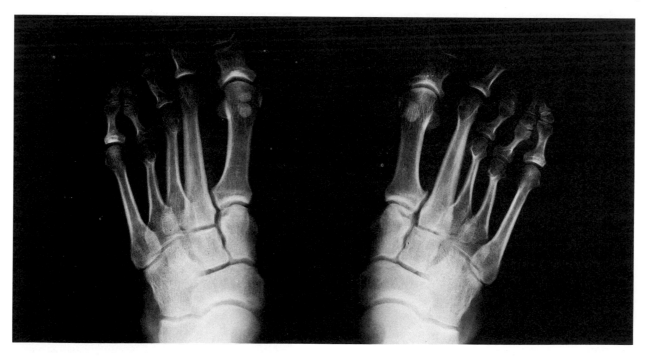

Fig. 300. Short third and fourth metatarsals. Hypertrophy of second metatarsals. Atrophy of third and fourth metatarsals.

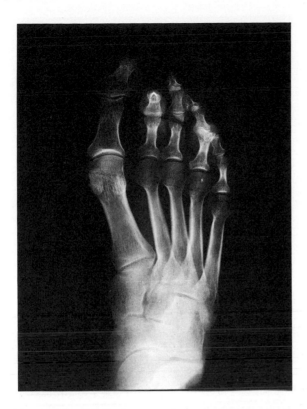

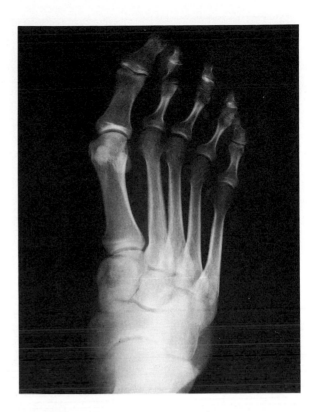

Fig. 301. Club-shape abnormalities of the metatarsal heads. Impingement through juxtaposition of uniform metatarsal length. Note hammertoe deformity of second toe.

Fig. 302. Adducted position of the metatarsal bones with impingements. Mild adductus displacement of second and third metatarsal shafts with juxtaposition of metatarsal heads and lateral deviation of third toe secondary to medium midtarsal fault and contraction of toe extensor tendons.

the metatarsal-toe relationship (zigzag foot) (Fig. 280).

a. When the second and third metatarsal are diverted into an adducted position and rotate on their long axes, impingement of the second and third metatarsal heads is created. Also, there is excessive pressure on the lateral plantar condyles which may cause intractable plantar heloma.

b. Spreading of the second and third toes occurs as the third toe abducts and its metatarsal member adducts.

c. As the foot elongates by derangement, the toe extensor tendons cannot elongate in the same proportion and the toes are drawn back and off axis.

d. The dorsal interossei stabilize the second toe against immediate lateral deviation by insertions on both sides of the base of the proximal phalanx.

e. The third toe is diverted into abduction because there is only a single insertion on the

lateral side of the proximal phalangeal base.

f. Additionally, torsion of the third cuneiform contributes to rotation and adduction of the third metatarsal.

2. Clinically, a spread of the second and third toes is often a guide sign that indicates major internal foot derangement.

3. The adducted foot presents several shafts in varus position. The parabola from the first to the fifth metatarsophalangeal joint is acute. Clinically this foot often overrides the outside of the shoe with attendant excrescence problems. Pigeon-toed gait is usually present. (See chapter on pes adductus.)

Abducted Position of Metatarsal Bones

1. In the severely abducted foot, the first

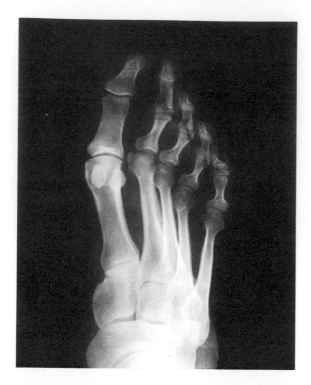

Fig. 303. Adducted position of the metatarsal bones with impingements. Adductus displacement of second, third, and fourth metatarsal shafts with juxtaposition of metatarsal heads, alteration of length pattern, and lateral deviation of toes secondary to adducted foot.

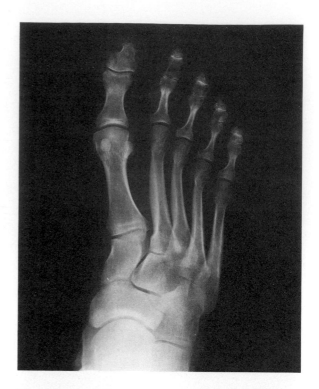

Fig. 304. Abducted bowing of the metatarsal bones. Compensatory adduction of forefoot.

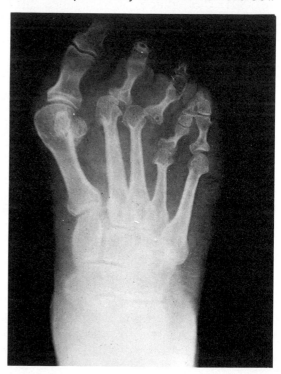

Fig. 305. Metatarsophalangeal subluxations secondary to hallux abductus valgus and short fourth metatarsal

metatarsal may rotate into abduction and the lesser metatarsals follow.

2. The fifth metatarsal frequently assumes abduction in calcaneocuboid fault.

3. Abducted bowing of a metatarsal may occur when stress from outflare gait persists. It is rare (Fig. 304).

Metatarsophalangeal Joint Luxation, Subluxation, and Associated Toe Contractions (Figs. 305 and 306)

1. The most common symptom-producing problems of metatarsal disorder consist of joint disorganization of varying degrees with associated toe contraction.

2. Painful metatarsal bursitis, nerve impingement, tissue inflammation, and skin excrescences are usually present in some degree.

3. Roentgenologically, loss of joint space is visualized.

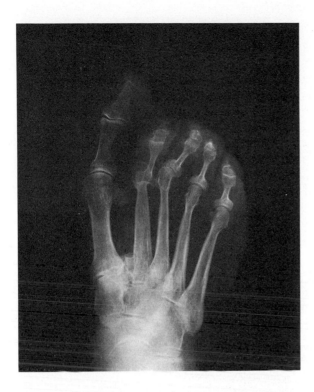

Fig. 306. Metatarsophalangeal subluxations. Complete subluxation of second metatarsophalangeal joint. Partial subluxation of third metatarsophalangeal joint. Secondary to trauma. Note base of second metatarsal. No hallux abductus valgus.

4. Side-to-side luxation occurs in hallux abductus valgus. Trauma may be a factor.

5. Simple subluxations are the result of the contracted extensor digitorum longus from protracted wearing of high-heeled shoes.

6. Complicated subluxations occur in cavus feet, poliomyelitic deformities, and neurotrophic joint resorption.

7. Fibular deviation of toes due to incompetence of the short flexors of the toes, plantar interossei, and lumbricales occurs as a pathognomonic feature of rheumatoid arthritis.

8. When toes are contracted, they are not effective in gait take-off; consequently, friction and stress points are received in the adjacent metatarsal head area and are another reason for intractable helomata.

Metatarsus Latus (Fig. 307)

1. Laxity of the transverse metatarsal liga-

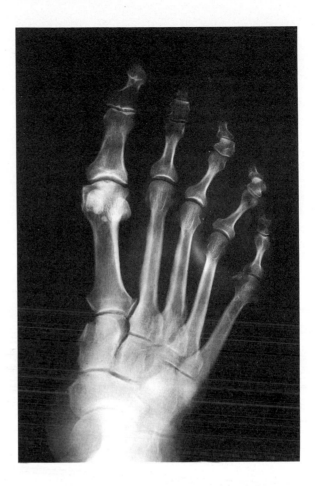

Fig. 307. Metatarsus latus. Laxity of transverse metatarsal ligament and general foot flaccidity.

ments and associated musculature permits extreme splaying of metatarsal segments.

2. Clinically, the flaccidity of this foot is difficult to fit properly with shoes. Several surgical procedures aim at binding the bones in closer proximity.

Pathology of Metatarsophalangeal Area (Figs. 308 and 309)

1. The destructive ravages of various forms of arthritis produce extensive metatarsal disorders.

   a. Rheumatoid arthritis — joint disorganization.

   b. Degenerative arthritis — restricted joint motion.

   c. Infectious arthritis — acute inflammation and effusion.

    d. Gouty arthritis — articular weakness due to urate salt-loaded bones and limitation due to pain and swelling.

    e. Minimal traumatic arthritis — insidious degenerative process.

    2. Osteochondritis of second metatarsal with deformity of its head results in restricted motion and excessive stress problems. Any lesser metatarsal may become involved.

    3. Osteomyelitis and malignancy occur infrequently. Secondary invasion from synovioma has been recorded.

    4. Every case of clinical metatarsal problem warrants roentgenographic examination to exclude pathology.

CLINICAL CORRELATION

    1. The roentgenologic study should reveal

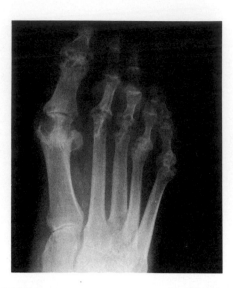

Fig. 308. Gouty arthritis in advanced stage presents a weakened and painful structure.

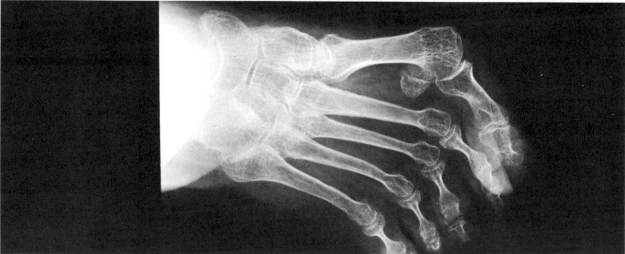

Fig. 309. Advanced rheumatoid arthritis. Complete disorganization of metatarsophalangeal joints.

the structural factors involved in the case, and this information should be used to decide the type of accommodative appliance to be used and the plan for rehabilitation treatment.

2. The roentengologic findings should be correlated with kinetic factors of gait and weight impost. Other clinical manifestations, such as skin excrescences, should also be considered, particularly the intractable plantar heloma.

3. The torsion of the tibia should be studied as a factor in directing the weight distribution. The torsion varies with subtalar and midtarsal fault.

4. Muscle groups should be evaluated to determine imbalance, such as, for example, a contracted calf group as a factor in creating unyielding flexion at the ankle during gait, resulting in excessive pressure in the metatarsophalangeal area.

5. Neuritis associated with peripherovascular disease, diabetes, and other diseases should be considered when evaluating metatarsal insufficiency after the roentgenologic study has been completed.

CONSERVATIVE MANAGEMENT

1. Irregularity of the metatarsal length pattern requires compensation. The leverage arm of the short member or members is extended by a platform placed under the head of the deficient member. Appliances designed in this manner may be made of felt until the proper correction is obtained and later duplicated in Celastic or leather.

a. Although a short metatarsal may require an extended platform, the total foot situation must be considered and all the modifications necessary for the total foot problem should be incorporated in the same appliance.

b. Atrophy of a metatarsal shaft indicates that is has not participated in the work load and needs compensation.

2. Impingement factors exemplify some change in the total structure of the foot, and normal alignment may only be achieved through total rehabilitation of the foot structure and gait. Simple devices, such as spot metatarsal lifts under the specific metatarsal involved, may offer some relief but will fall short of effecting complete correction.

3. Club-shaped abnormalities need little more than adequate accommodation in the shoe.

4. Adducted position of the metatarsal bones due to pes adductus must be treated accordingly. When it is because of internal derangement of the foot caused by foot collapse, the usual rehabilitation for that condition must be instituted.

5. Abducted bowing of the metatarsal bones is rare, and a specific evaluation of the problem must be made to correct it.

6. Metarsophalangeal joint subluxations and associated toe contractions are conditions which present the most common manifestation of metatarsal disorder and in extreme cases the most devastating problem found in this area.

MILD.

a. Mild forms of subluxation are provoked by habitual use of high-heeled shoes which disturbs muscle balance and weight distribution. Use of proper footgear during the greater part of the day is essential.

b. Comprehensive muscle rehabilitation through stretching, use of electrical contractile currents, and toe-grasping exercises are beneficial.

c. The conventional metatarsal pads have little effect and their use is an outdated approach.

ADVANCED. Advanced forms of subluxation with toe contraction require orthodigital devices for their correction

a. Felt or plastic purchase crests placed underneath the affected toes to encourage use of the toe-flexing muscles are very effective in overcoming the contracted extensor muscles and permitting the subluxation to be reduced.

Even the severe cases due to rheumatoid arthritis are benefited, and where it does not materially reduce the subluxation, the balance and stability of the foot are improved by giving the short toe flexors, plantar interossei, and lumbricales an opportunity to act.

In the arthritic foot, where disorganization of the joint permits the long toe flexors to act in a detrimental manner, the use of the purchase crest will neutralize this effect.

b. Molded inlays are satisfactory provided adequate modification is insured to accommodate the severely dislocated metatarsophalangeal joint by pocketing the depressed metatarsal head or heads.

c. Dynamically molded inlays may be created by applying an appropriate liquid latex-filler mix in the shoe and having the patient walk-in the accommodations needed to compensate for the deficiencies. Another method is to use a pressure-sensitive inner sole foundation that will record pressure areas so that proper crests and other compensations may be added at the appropriate places.

d. Placement of accommodations for intractable helomata is critical, and Hymes has devised a method for checking their locations. First, the lesion is outlined with fine steel suture wire attached by tape. An inner sole pattern of the shoe is made and drawn on a paper envelope loaded film-holder. This is cut to shape in the darkroom, and the edges sealed with light-opaque tape. The inner sole-shaped film-holder is slipped into the shoe, the patient dons the shoe, and a roentgenogram is made which shows the locations in functional position.

e. When joint destruction has occurred or in cases where other measures fail, the metatarsal bar attached to the sole of the shoe transfers weight across the shafts of all the metatarsal bones and creates a fulcrum on an unaffected area for the take-off in walking.

f. The use of molded shoes in which a crest is incorporated under the toes creates a special foot environment that is conducive to good toe action and relieves metatarsal head pressure. The toes are held in a position of flexural contact which is better than the uninhibiting flat surface provided by the inner sole of the conventional shoe.

The molded shoe completely encloses the foot and toes, and accommodation on an individual basis may be accomplished. The combination of better foot accommodation and opportunity for intrinsic muscle action provided by the molded shoe should sublimate metatarsal disorder. The heavy sole commonly applied offers a further advantage in protecting the foot from the harshness and irregularity of present-day walking surfaces.

7. When pathology involves the metatarsophalangeal elements and ambulation is possible, there is some value to accommodative footgear and devices to disperse weight forces from the metatarsophalangeal area posteriorly to the shafts and tarsal area. Metatarsal bars on the outside of the shoes are used and soft sponge material is utilized in specific padding under the metatarsophalangeal joints.

8. Insufficient adipose tissue under the metatarsophalangeal area may require artificial padding to supplement the deficiency.

9. The author has devised an appliance that resolves many of the metatarsal disorders. It consists of a rigid hindfoot correction with a dynamically self-molding forefoot extension that distributes stress on an equalizing basis. The forepart extension consists of a top cover of lightweight leather and a bottom cover of suede which extends to the full outline of the innersole. Between top cover and bottom cover, a layer of controlled, nonhardening, latex-ground cork filler is sewed. This material adjusts to pressure and molds toe crests, depressed metatarsal heads, etc. perfectly. Innersoles to compensate for shearing stress are effective; e.g., Plastazote or Spenco's Neoprene.

10. Orthotics of plastic posted to accommodate the degree of varus or valgus of the forefoot are highly effective in achieving controlled gait and forefoot balance.

SURGICAL RELEVANCE

1. The intractable plantar heloma associated with excessive impost on metatarsal heads requires surgical intervention. Selective osteotomy procedures of metatarsal bones to decrease plantarflexion are indicated for relief of excessive contact pressures and intractable plantar lesions.

2. Surgical reconstruction of the intractable arthritic case of metatarsal insufficiency is frequently the only feasible way of overcoming all the associated problems. Resection of the involved metatarsal heads and surgical straightening of the toes into an improved position are the usual procedures.

3. Metatarsus latus involves an idiopathic flaccidity of the foot which is difficult to control. Joplin's surgical procedure to provide an artifical metatarsal binding by threading a tendon through holes in the shafts of the metatarsals to achieve reconstruction is effective.

BIBLIOGRAPHY

Addante, J.B.: Metatarsal Osteotomy as an Office Procedure to Eradicate Intractible Plantar Keratosis, J. Amer. Podiat. Ass. 60:397, 1970.

Amberry, T.R.: Foot Surgery, in *Principles and Practice of Podiatry,* F. Weinstein (ed.). Philadelphia, Lea & Febiger, 1968.

Austin, D.W.: New Concepts of the Etiology and Treatment of Helomata, J. Nat. Ass. Chiropodists 40:2, 1950.

Barany, J.W., and Greene, J.W.: The Force-platform: An Instrument for Selecting and Training Employees, Amer. J. Psychol. 74:121, 1961.

Barany, J.W., and Whetsel, R.G.: Construction of a Portable Force Platform for Measuring Bodily Movement, Report to National Science Foundation, Grant No. GI 7738, Aug. 1962.

Billig, H.E.: Condylectomy for Metatarsalgia, J. Int. Coll. Surg. 25:220, 1956.

Brown, J.E.: Functional and Cosmetic Correction of Metatarsus Latus (Splay Foot), Clin. Orthop. 14:166, 1959.

Bunkhead, H.R.: The Diagnosis and Treatment of Forefoot Disturbances, J. Nat. Ass. Chiropodists 44:9, 1954.

Clayton, M.L.: Surgery of the Lower Extremity in Rheumatoid Arthritis, J. Bone Joint Surg. 45-A:1517, 1963.

Demp, P.H.: A Mathematical Model for the Study of Metatarsal Length Patterns, J. Amer. Podiat. Ass. 54:107, 1964.

Elftman, H.: A Cinematic Study of the Distribution of Pressure in the Human Foot, Anat. Rec. 59:481, 1934.

Gamble, F.O.: Orthopedic Weight Distribution Foot Imprint Radiograph, J. Nat. Ass. Chiropodists 42:8, 1952.

Harris, R.I., and Beath, T.: *Army Foot Survey,* Ottawa: National Research Council of Canada, 1947.

Henenfeld, M.: Pathogenesis of Forefoot Disease, J. Nat. Ass. Chiropodists 43:3, 44:4, 1953.

Hlavac, H.F., and Schoenhaus, H.: The Plantar Fat Pad and Some Related Problems, J. Amer. Podiat. Ass. 60: 151, 1970.

Holbrook, W.P., Hill, D.F., and Stephens, C.A.L., Jr.: *Manual of Rheumatic Disease.* Chicago: The Year Book Publishers, Inc., 1950.

Jones, R.L.: The Functional Significance of the Declination of the Axis of the Human Talocalcaneonavicular Joint, Anat. Rec. 88:12, 1944.

Joplin, R.J.: Surgical Procedure for Correction of Splayfoot, Metatarsus Primus Varus and Hallux Valgus, J. Bone Joint Surg. 32-A:779, 1950.

Kelikian, H.: Hallux Valgus, *Allied Deformities of the Forefoot and Metatarsalgia.* Philadelphia: W.B. Saunders Co., 1965.

Krausz, C.E.: Survey of 5,644 Nail Disorders, 1942-1963, Personal communication, Philadelphia, Pa., 1964.

Lewis, M.R.: *Roentgen Foot Diagnosis.* Chicago: Von Schill Memorial Press, 1952.

McGlamry, D.E., Kitting, R.W., and Butlin, W.E.: Prominent Lesser Metatarsal Heads — Some Surgical Considerations, J. Amer. Podiat. Ass. 59:303, 1969.

McGlamry, D.E., Kitting, R.W., and Butlin, W.E.: Plantar Condylectomy, Current Modification of Technique, J. Amer. Podiat. Ass. 59:345, 1969.

McGlamry, D.E., Kitting, R.W., and Butlin, W.E.: Osteoplasty of Head or Osteotomy of Shaft, J. Amer. Podiat. Ass. 59:394, 1969.

Morton, D.J.: *The Human Foot.* Morningside Heights N.Y. Columbia University Press, 1935.

Morton, D.J.: *Human Locomotion and Body Form.* Baltimore: The Williams & Wilkins Co., 1952.

Nutt, J.J.: Functions of Mediotarsal Joint — Their Disturbance a Cause of Flatfoot, Amer. J. Surg. 32:53, 1936.

Root, M.L.: An Approach to Foot Orthopedics, J. Amer. Podiat. Ass. 54:115, 1964.

Sansone, R.E.: The X-ray Evaluation of Forefoot Imbalance due to Alteration of the Metatarsus Parabola, Lecture, American Society Chiropodical Roentgenology, 1940.

Sansone, R.E.: Forefoot Imbalance due to Alteration of the Metatarsus Parabola, North Amer. Chiropody Jour. 47:220, 1957.

Sansone, R.E.: Strip Padding for Weight Stress Distribution and Redirection, J. Amer. Podiat. Ass. 60:193, 1970.

Schuster, O.: Personal correspondence, Sept. 1946.

Schwartz, R.P., Heath, A.L., Misiek, W., and M. Wright, J.N.: Kinetics of Human Gait: The Making and Interpretation of Electrobasographic Records of Human Gait; The Influence of Rate of Walking and the Height of Shoe Heel on Duration of Weight-bearing on the Osseous Tripod of the Respective Feet, J. Bone Joint Surg. 17-A:343, 1954.

Seeburger, R.H.: Surgical Implants of Alloyed Metal in Joints of the Feet, J. Amer. Podiat. Ass. 54:391, 1964.

Stess, R.M.: A Surgical Approach to Advanced Rheumatoid Arthritis of the Forefoot, J. Amer. Podiat. Ass. 62:259, 1972.

Tarara, E.: Personal communication, 1965.

Zitzlsperger, S.: The Mechanics of the Foot Based on the Concept of the Skeleton as a Statically Indetermined Space Framework, Clin. Orthop. 16:48, 1960.

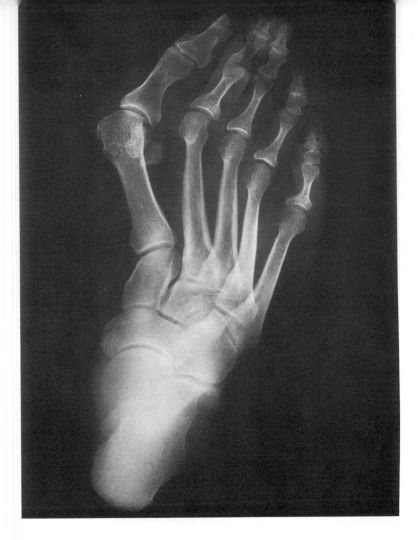

Fig. 323. Hallux abductus valgus, severe

1. Abducted hallux (55°). Subluxed metatarsophalangeal joint.

2. Valgus of hallux, underlap of subluxed second metatarsal.

3. Adduction of first metatarsal (20°). Adducted lesser metatarsals. Hypermobile gap at first metatarsal segment.

4. Distal metatarsal articulation exposed (55%).

5. Medial sesamoid lateral to crista area.

6. Cratering of eburnated medial epicon-cyle, sagittal groove, first metatarsal head.

3. Deviation of metatarsophalangeal joint.

4. Eburnation, medial epicondyle, first metatarsal head.

5. Medial prominence of metatarsal head, distal articulation exposed 20% to 30%.

6. Relative lateral displacement of sesamoid bones (Position 3, Fig. 318).

7. Adduction of first metatarsal, intermetatarsal angle 12°-18°.

Severe Hallux Abductus Valgus (Fig. 323)

1. Positional abduction of hallux, 30°-45°.

2. Hallux assumes valgus position, may underlap second toe.

3. Subluxation of the metatarsophalangeal joint.

4. Excessive eburnation and erosion of medial epicondyle, first metatarsal head.

5. Medial prominence of metatarsal head, distal articulation exposed 30% to 45%.

6. Exhibition of sagittal groove on distal articulation of metatarsal head.

7. Relative lateral displacement of sesamoid bones (Position 4 or 5, Fig. 318), osteochondrosis of medial sesamoid.

8. Adduction of first metatarsal, intermetatarsal angle 15°-25°.

9. Axial rotation of first metatarsal, either varus or valgus.

Extreme Hallux Abductus Valgus (Fig. 324)

1. Positional abduction of hallux, greater than 45°.

2. Hallux in extreme valgus position, may underlap more than one subluxed toe.

3. Subluxation of metatarsophalangeal joint.

4. Cratering of eburnated medial epicondyle, first metatarsal head, from pressure erosion.

5. Medial prominence of metatarsal head characterized as a gross protrusion, distal articulation over 45% exposed.

6. Exhibition of sagittal groove on distal articulation of metatarsal head, head may be flattened.

7. Displacement of sesamoid bones into interspace (Position 5, Fig. 318).

8. Osteochondritis of sesamoid bones; exostotic formation may occur on sesamoids.

9. Extreme adduction of first metatarsal, intermetatarsal angle may be greater than 25°.

10. Axial rotation of first metatarsal, usually in valgus because of extreme pronation and subluxation of entire foot. Metatarsal may not be rotated because of wide intermetatarsal angle stabilizes it in the transverse plane.

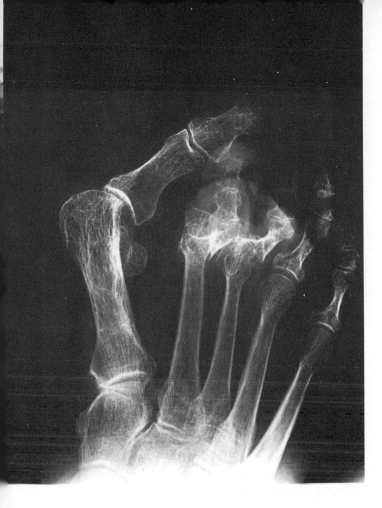

Fig. 324. Hallux abductus valgus, extreme

1. Abducted hallux (65°). Subluxed metatarsophalangeal joint.

2. Valgus of hallux minimal. Subluxed second and third toes.

3. Adduction of first metatarsal (16°). Hypermobile gap at first metatarsal segment.

4. Distal metatarsal articulation exposed (75%).

5. Medial and lateral sesamoids turned to valgus position in the interspace at a posterior location.

6. First metatarsal head unusually rounded and medial epicondyle atrophic.

CONSERVATIVE MANAGEMENT

The biomechanics of hallux abductus valgus are complex. Two extremes in foot type may develop the abnormality as a secondary complication, and each must be treated according to its basic type. The subluxation of a pronated equinus or compensated forefoot varus foot which creates push-off and roll-off forces on the hallux of a hypermobile dorsiflexed first metatarsal in valgus position is a primary problem to be controlled by a properly balanced orthotic foot appliance. The adducted foot or forefoot valgus of the inverted cavus foot needs an orthotic appliance that relieves the structural instability and the tendency for muscle imbalance that plantarflexes and creates a varus of the first metatarsal leading to abduction of the hallux. Even the foot in normal alignment may have a broad spread of the forefoot that may develop hallux abductus valgus from shoe distortion. In this foot type, the first metatarsal seldom has axial rotation in the frontal plane and neither valgus nor varus position is assumed. Advice concerning footwear, stockings, and gait are important in this foot type.

Specific measures may be directed toward alleviating the acute symptoms associated with hallux abductus valgus. The following therapy is directed toward relative degrees of deformity:

1. Bursitis and excrescence formation are the lesions that result from excessive friction and pressure upon the medial aspect of the metatarsal head. The excrescence may be reduced operatively. Adequate protection and padding should be instituted immediately. The bursitis may be relieved by negative galvanism, an astringent medication, parenteral injection of steroids, or ultrasonic radiation.

2. Mild deformity in which there is a normal basal articulation of the first metatarsal responds to traction, rotation exercise, strengthening of the abductor hallucis and flexor brevis digitorum through exercise and electrical muscle stimulation, and proper shoes.

3. Moderate deformity may be improved by the application of protective devices and by the same routine treatment given mild deformities. In addition, day slings and night splints may be employed.

4. Severe deformity defies conservative corrective measures and must be accommodated by special shoes or modified by surgical intervention.

SURGICAL RELEVANCE

Before surgical intervention, it is imperative for the surgeon to evaluate thoroughly the roentgenological and biomechanical status of the entire foot, and proper measures should be instituted to insure structural and functional

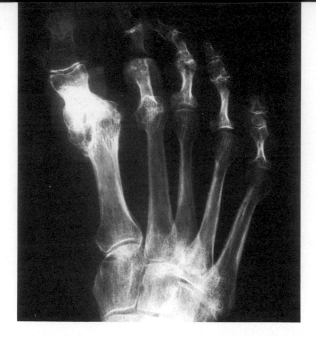

Fig. 325. Iatrogenic disaster from hallux abductus valgus surgery

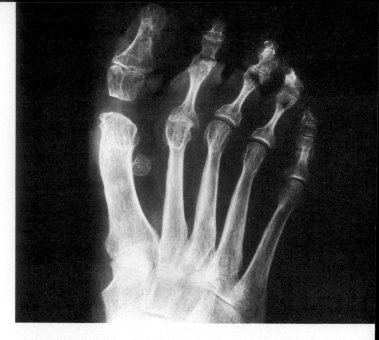

Fig. 326. Excellent result from Keller procedure in hallux abductus valgus surgery. However, second toe abnormality should have been repaired; it required surgery later.

foot competence if surgical correction is to be maintained. Precise surgical judgment must be exercised in choice of procedure and techniques to be employed in the correction of hallux abductus valgus deformity. The significance of every roentgen feature listed should be determined for the individual patient. The degree of deformity indicated by various angles and positions of the osseous elements should be gauged against active and passive ranges of foot motion. The interrelationships of specific pathoanatomy must be appraised to insure desired results. The iatrogenic problems that are not uncommon in hallux abductus valgus surgery are mute evidence of inept surgical assessments (Bonney and Macnab, 1952) (Fig. 325). Postsurgical roentgenograms are essential (Fig. 326).

The number of procedures that have been devised for the correction of hallux abductus valgus are interminable. Many have been given eponyms from their originators. The student of foot surgery is well acquainted with the step-by-step techniques for performing the major named procedures that have stood the test of time and proper application. Current literature offers modifications which enhance many older procedures. The reader is referred to the bibliography at the end of this chapter.

Weil (1972) divides surgical procedures into five basic categories: (1) simple exostectomy, (2) simple exostectomy with soft-tissue correction, (3) arthroplasty, (4) osteotomy, and (5) arthrodesis. Elaborate and detailed multiple

surgical applications are sometimes needed to cope with complex levels of deformity and total foot limitations. Weil lists the following accessible osteotomy procedures: Akin, closing abductory wedge osteotomy (A.A.S.O.), opening abductory wedge osteotomy (O.A.W.O.), double osteotomy (D.O.), and de rotational angulational transpositional osteotomy (D.R.A.T.O.). Silastic implants and tendo achillis lengthening (T.A.L.) are frequently utilized. It is the judicious use of such procedures that is necessary for successful results.

The roentgenogram is useful in charting and measuring the shape and amount of wedge to be delivered in an osteotomy (Sgarlato, 1971; Kroeker and Sokoloff, 1973). The validity of measurements depends on the geometric accuracy of the roentgenographic image of the involved bone. Correct standardized positioning technique is essential for a valid image. It is always wise to measure bone length in two views to test for true roentgenographic images. A plantarflexed metatarsal may give the false impression of shortness. The lateral view provides the sagittal plane of the first metatarsal and demonstrates its angle of inclination. Appropriate measurements for surgically raising and lowering this position may be taken from this view. Mastery of the appearance of the shape of the metatarsal shaft and base in the dorsoplantar view will be of material value in assessing its axial rotation. This view is of even more importance than an axial view in frontal plane. It is the key for selecting procedures to correct congenital metatarsus primus adductus and the reduction of positional adduction. The metatarsocuneiform relationships are also assessed from the dorsoplantar view.

Physical criteria to be correlated with the roentgenogram that the surgeon always evaluates include the medical history with emphasis on arthritis, age as related to bone age and development, sex as a determining factor in the size of bone structures, and occupation, activity, weight, and footgear as factors that influence the integrity of the structure. Proper evaluation of these criteria is fundamental to making a competent surgical determination.

HALLUX ADDUCTUS (HALLUX VARUS)

The ideal foot with the first metatarsal posed at a normal divergence should present its hallux in moderate adduction, thereby presenting a strong forefoot. Unfortunately, this type of foot and hallux is not common due to the insidious deformation from shoes.

An excess adduction of the hallux has been observed in an individual wearing a flexible, extreme inflare shoe for many years. Occasionally, poor reconstructive surgical judgment for hallux abductus results in hallux adductus.

ROENTGENOLOGIC INTERPRETATION (Fig. 327)

The hallux assumes an adducted or straight alignment with the first metatarsal shaft.

CLINICAL CORRELATION

The functional hallux adductus requires an inflare last shoe. Hallux adductus due to poor operative results needs the same type of shoe accommodation provided surgical repair is not feasible.

HALLUX FLEXUS

Hyperflexion of the interphalangeal articulation of the hallux is secondary to overactivity of the flexor hallucis longus muscle. This is due to a compensatory effort to stabilize a structurally weakened foot or the lack of flexion of the adjacent second toe. Muscle imbalance due to neuromuscular disease of poliomyelitis, muscular sclerosis, or spastic paralysis is a frequent offender. Rheumatoid arthritis may also produce the deformity.

A flexion deformity of the first metatarsophalangeal joint with resulting hyperostosis

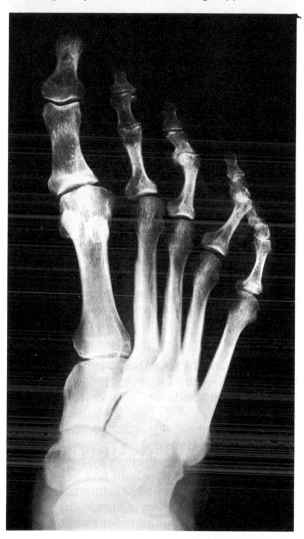

Fig. 327. Hallux adductus. Normal bone shapes enter metatarsocuneiform articulation. This foot has been shod in a flexible, inflare last a lifetime. Note unusual bone condensation of second and third metatarsal shafts caused by stress pattern. Third, fourth, and fifth toes are distorted in coping with gait. Midtarsal fault persists.

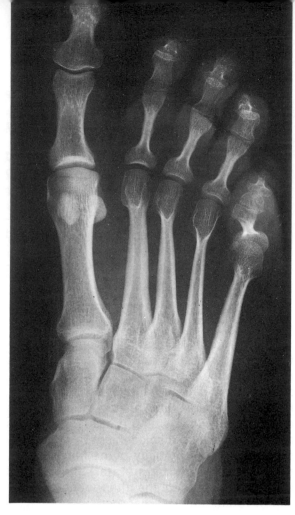

Fig. 332. Minimi digiti quinti adductus with subluxation adduction of fifth toe. Subluxation of fifth metatarsophalangeal articulation. This neutralizes to some extent the prominent metatarsal head with hyperostotic formation on the lateral border that is a typical finding.

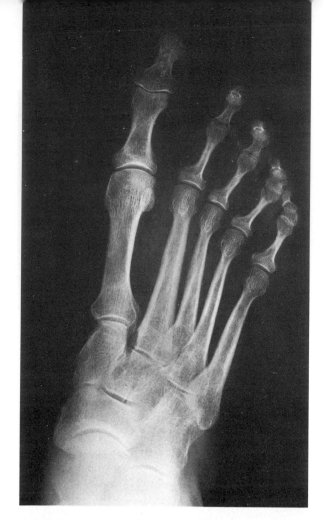

Fig. 333. Sesamoid lesion. Absence of medial sesamoid. Note hypertrophy of second metatarsal shaft.

tarsal.

2. Budin recommends traction splints and a rubber band sling to draw the toe into correct alignment. Additionally, he suggests taping the fifth metatarsal into proper position if it has become rotated.

3. Protective padding is indicated.

4. Surgical intervention is indicated in severe cases. Lantzounis (1940) describes a periosteocapsuloplasty for correction of congenital subluxation of the fifth toe. Anderson (1971) resects the metatarsal head and uses a modified toe webbing procedure.

5. Amputation of the fifth toe is seldom advisable because loss of the fifth toe invites problems at the head of the fifth metatarsal and about the fourth toe.

SESAMOID LESIONS

The sesamoid bones associated with the flexor hallucis longus tendon are frequently displaced in hallux abductus, and excessive weight is borne on the medial sesamoid resulting in osteochondrosis. Normal articular movement with the metatarsal head is obstructed and painful sesamoiditis occurs. In some instances, the sesamoid bone may become fragmented. Secondary lesions of the underlying epidermis consist of neurovascular tyloma as a result of the irregular counterpressure from the irregular sesamoid bone.

Bipartite sesamoid bones may be congenital in origin. If displaced, they too become symptomatic. Absence of a sesamoid has been noted, and in this case, faulty weight distribution may be expected.

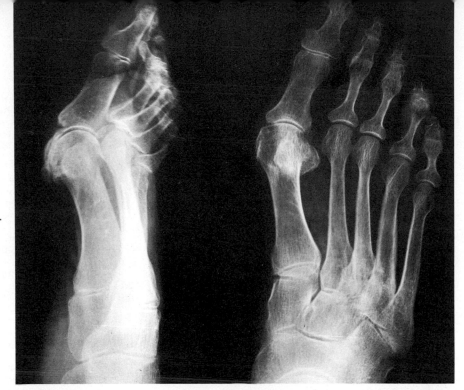

Fig. 334. Sesamoid lesion. Osteochondrosis medial sesamoid secondary to malposition in hallux abductus (valgus).

ROENTGENOLOGIC INTERPRETATION (Figs. 333 and 334)

1. In osteochondrosis, the dorsoplantar view demonstrates irregular enlargement of the sesamoid.

2. Diminution of joint space between the sesamoid and the head of the metatarsal can be visualized in an axial view of the sesamoid.

3. A fractured sesamoid bone may be differentiated from a bipartite sesamoid by the following means. In the fractured bone there is an irregular, serrated line of cleavage with sides that match and a lack of cortical density along the fracture line, while the bipartite bone demonstrates smooth contours of the division and the cortical density is uninterrupted throughout.

CLINICAL CORRELATION

1. Appropriate physiotherapy, such as ultrasonic radiation, should be used to relieve the sesamoiditis.

2. An appliance should be applied with support along the shaft of the first metatarsal, deep cupping for the sesamoid area, and a metatarsal platform under the lateral metatarsals to transfer the weight load away from the traumatized sesamoid area. Balanced orthotics are effective.

3. Metatarsal shoe bars are effective in relieving sesamoid lesions.

4. Sesamoid lesions sometimes develop in the highly arched foot because the sesamoid bones move under the metatarsophalangeal joint junction. Pes cavus management is indicated.

BIBLIOGRAPHY

Anderson, B.V.: Combination Surgery for Overlapping Fifth Digit, J. Amer. Podiat. Ass. 61:137, 1971.

Beck, E.L.: An Evaluation of the DuVries Modification of the McBride Hallux Abducto Valgus Correction. J. Amer. Podiat. Ass. 61:445, 1971.

Berntsen, A.: De l'Hallux Valgus. Contribution a son étiologie et a son traitement, Revue d'Orthopedie, 3e serie, 17:101, 1930.

Bhangoo, H.S. and Haines, R.W.: Feet in Uganda, The Chiropodist 28:39, 1973.

Bonney, G., and Macnab, I.: Hallux Valgus and Hallux Rigidus, J. Bone Joint Surg. 34-B:366, 1952.

Budin, H.A.: *Principles and Practice of Orthodigita.* New York: Strathmore Press, 1941.

Carey, R.D.: Reduction of Severe Hallux Valgus and Hallux Limitus: Dow Corning Silastic Finger Joint Prosthesis, J. Foot Surg. I.1, 1971.

Charlesworth, F.: *Chiropody, Theory and Practice,* ed. 3. London: The Actinic Press, 1949.

Clarke, J.J.: Hallux Valgus and Hallux Varus, Lancet 1:609, 1900.

Conley, D.A., Jr.: Personal communication, Tulsa, Okla.

Ebisue, J.M.: The First Ray Axis and the First Metatarsophalangeal Joint. An Anatomical and Pathomechanical Study, J. Amer. Podiat. Ass. 58:160, 1968.

Ewald, P.: Die Aetiologie des Hallux Valgus, Dtsch. Ztschr. Chir. 114:90-103, 1912.

Gamble, F.O.: *Applied Foot Roentgenology.* Baltimore: The Williams & Wilkins Company, 1957.

Gibson, J., and Piggott, H.: Osteotomy of the Neck of the First Metatarsal in the Treatment of Hallux Valgus. A Follow-up Study of Eighty-two feet, J. Bone Joint Surg. 44-B:349, 1962.

Greenberg, H.H.: Plantar Digital Tenotomy for Underlapping and Contracted Toes, J. Amer. Podiat. Ass. 56:65, 1966.

Haines, R.W., and McDougall, A.: The Anatomy of Hallux Valgus, J. Bone Joint Surg. 36-A:272, 1954.

Hara, B.: Surgical Judgment. In *Modern Therapeutic Approaches to Foot Problems.* Scientific papers presented at the 60th Annual Meeting of the American Podiatry Association. Mount Kisco, N.Y.: Futura Publishing Company, Inc., 1973.

Hardy, R., and Clapham, J.C.R.: Observations on Hallux Valgus Based on a Controlled Series, J. Bone Joint Surg. 33-B:376, 1951.

Hardy, R., and Clapham, J.C.R.: Hallux Valgus (Letter to the Editor), Lancet, Aug. 23:387, 1952.

Harris, R.I., and Beath, T.: *Army Foot Survey.* Ottawa: National Research Council of Canada, 1947.

Harrison, M.H.M., and Harvey, F.J.: Arthrodesis of the First Metatarsophalangeal Joint for Hallux Valgus and Rigidus, J. Bone Joint Surg. 45-A:471, 1963.

Henderson, R.S.: Os Intermetatarseum and a Possible Relationship to Hallux Valgus, J. Bone Joint Surg. 45-B:117, 1963.

James, C.S.: Footprints and Feet of Natives of the Solomon Islands, Lancet 237:1390, 1939.

Kalcev, B.: Hallux Valgus (Letter to the Editor), Lancet :937, 1952.

Kaplan, E.G.: A New Approach to the Surgical Correction of Overlapping Toe, J. Amer. Coll. Foot Surg. 3:12, 1964.

Kaplan, E.G.: Discussion of Hara, Ben, Surgical Judgment, In *Modern Therapeutic Approaches to Foot Problems.* Scientific papers presented at the 60th Annual Meeting of the American Podiatry Association. Mount Kisco, N.Y.: Futura Publishing Company, Inc., 1973.

Kelikian, H.: *Hallux Valgus, Allied Deformities of the Forefoot and Metatarsalgia.* Philadelphia: W.B. Saunders Company, 1965.

Kempf, C.F.: Personal communication, 1956.

Kroeker, R.: X-rays and Biomechanical Preoperative Evaluation of the Surgical Patient. Seminar, New Mexico Podiatry Ass., Albuquerque, 1973.

Lantzounis, L.A.: Congenital Subluxation of the Fifth Toe and Its Correction by a Periocapsuloplasty and Tendon Transplantation, J. Bone Joint Surg. 22:147, 1940.

Lapidus, P.W.: "Dorsal Bunion": Its Mechanics and Operative Correction, J. Bone Joint Surg. 22- :627, 1940.

Lapidus, P.W. The Author's Bunion Operation from 1931 to 1959, Clin. Orthop. 16:119, 1960.

Levy, B.: An Appliance to Induce Toe Flexion on Weight Bearing, J. Nat. Ass. Chiropodists 40:6, 1950.

Locke, R.K.: Locke Syndrome, Curr. Chiropody 1:9, 1952.

Maldin, R.A.: Axial Rotation of the First Metatarsal as a Factor in Hallux Valgus, J. Amer. Podiat. Ass. 73:85, 1972.

McCain, L.R.: The "Sesamoid Ligament" and Its Employ in the Suturing of the Keller Bunionectomy Procedure, J. Amer. Podiat. Ass. 59:479, 1969.

McGlamry, D.E., and Feldman, M.H.: A Treatise on the McBride Procedure; A Review of the McBride Publications on Hallux Valgus Correction with Observations on Rationale of the Original Procedure and the Current Modifications, J. Amer. Podiat. Ass. 61:161, 1971.

McGlamry, E.D., Kitting, R.M., and Butlin, W.E.: Hallux Valgus Repair with Correction of Coexisting Long Hallux, J. Amer. Podiat. Ass. 60:86, 1970.

McGlamry, E.D., Kitting, R.M., and Butlin, W.E.: Keller Bunionectomy and Hallux Valgus Correction, J. Amer. Podiat. Ass. 60:161, 1970.

Meade, J.C.: The Physiological Approach to Hammer Toe Surgery, J. Amer. Coll. Foot Surgeons 3:12, 1964.

Mitchell, L., Fleming, J.L., Allen, R., Glenney, C., and Sanford, G.A.: Osteotomy-Bunionectomy for Hallux Valgus, J. Bone Joint Surg. 40-A:41, 1958.

Moeller, F.A.: Biomechanics and Its Relationship to Foot Surgery. In *Conservative vs. Surgical Management of Foot Disorders.* Scientific papers presented at the 59th Annual Meeting of the American Podiatry Association. Mount Kisco, N.Y.: Futura Publishing Company, Inc., 1972.

Morton, D.J. *The Human Foot.* Morningside Heights, N.Y.: Columbia University Press, 1935.

Ogden, M.D.: Observations of barefoot peoples of New Guinea and New Hebrides, personal communication, 1971.

Piggott, H.: The Natural History of Hallux Valgus in Adolescence and Early Adult Life, J. Bone Joint Surg. 42-B:749, 1960.

Polokoff, M.J.: *Orthodigita.* Paterson, N.J.: Privately published, 1950.

Robin, C.R.: Joplin's Sling Operation in Adolescent Hallux Valgus, J. Amer. Podiat. Ass. 51:260, 1961.

Root, M.L.: An Approach to Foot Orthopedics, J. Amer. Podiat. Ass. 54:115, 1964.

Runting, E.G.V.: *Practical Chiropody.* London: Faber, 1935.

Schoenhaus, H., Rotman, S., and Meshon, A.L.: A Review of Normal Inter-metatarsal Angles, J. Amer. Podiat. Ass. 63:88, 1973.

Schuster, R.O.: Modifications in the Construction of the Levy Mould, J. Nat. Ass. Chiropodists 40:33, 1950.

Seeburger, R.H.: Surgical Implants of Alloyed Metals in Joints of the Feet, J. Amer. Podiat. Ass. 54:391, 1964.

Sgarlato, T.E.: Transplantation of the Flexor Digitorum Longus Muscle Tendon in Hammertoes, J. Amer. Podiat. Ass. 60:383, 1970.

Sgarlato, T.E.: *A Compendium of Podiatric Biomechanics.* San Francisco: California College of Podiatric Medicine, 1971.

Simmonds, F.A., and Menelaus, M.B.: Hallux Valgus in Adolescents, J. Bone Joint Surg. 42-B:761, 1960.

Smith, D.S.: The Surgical Treatment of Hallux Abducto Valgus. In *Conservative vs. Surgical Management of Foot Disorders.* Scientific papers presented at the 59th Annual Meeting of the American Podiatry Association. Mount Kisco, N.Y.: Futura Publishing Company, Inc., 1972.

Sokoloff, T.H.: Biomechanical Implications of Foot Surgery. In *Conservative vs. Surgical Management of Foot Disorders.* Scientific papers presented at the 59th Annual Meeting of the American Podiatry Association. Mount Kisco, N.Y.: Futura Publishing Company, Inc., 1972.

Sokoloff, T.H.: Preoperative Evaluation of the Surgical Patient. Seminar, New Mexico Podiatry Ass., Albuquerque, 1973.

Straus, W.L.: Growth of the Human Foot and Its Evolutionary Significance, Contrib. Embryol. 19:93, 1927.

Thomas, F.B.: Keller's Arthroplasty Modified. A Technique to Ensure Post-operative Distraction of the Toe, J. Bone Joint Surg. 44-B:356, 1962.

Turvey, J.W.J.: Hallux Valgus (Letter to the Editor). Lancet, :243, 1952.

Weil, L.S.: Surgical Correction of Hallux Abducto Valgus. In *Conservative vs. Surgical Management of Foot Disorders.* Scientific papers presented at the 59th Annual Meeting of the American Podiatry Association. Mount Kisco, N.Y.: Futura Publishing Company, Inc., 1972.

Wilson, C.L.: A Method of Fusion of the Metatarsophalangeal Joint of the Great Toe, J. Bone Joint Surg. 40-A:384, 1958.

Wilson, J.N.: Oblique Displacement Osteotomy for Hallux Valgus, J. Bone Joint Surg. 45-B:552, 1963.

17 CONGENITAL PES PLANUS AND RELATED DEFORMITIES

Congenital pes planus is a plantigrade foot type exhibiting a characteristic osseous architecture that varies from that of the acquired form of structural failure. Roentgenograms are needed to differentiate the congenital type from the acquired form. While the acquired faulty type of hypermobile pes planus is often painful and disabling, in many cases the congenital type is not painful and is disabling only to the extent that the foot lacks mobility and resilence and may precipitate faulty gait and posture problems (Fig. 335). This foot type may be compensated to attain ultimate efficiency.

Although congenital pes planus is a comparatively innocuous foot type, its alignment is related to a major clubfoot deformity, talipes equinovalgus. Components of this defor-

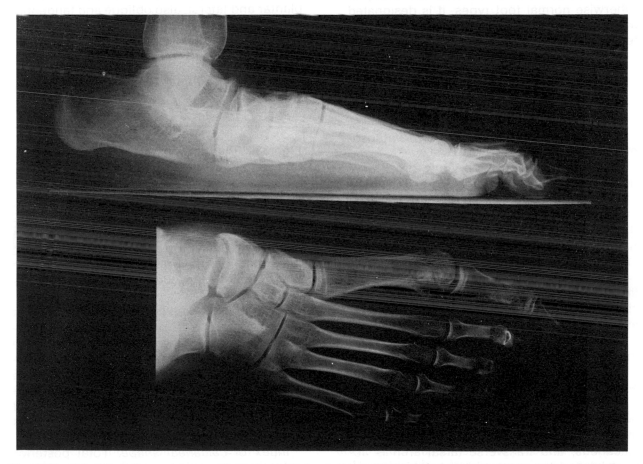

Fig. 335. Congenital pes planus. Severe medial rotation of talus. Pseudonormal midtarsal joint line. Head of talus flattened. Tarsal articulation spread. Fifth metatarsal loosely articulated. Straight compensated forefoot.

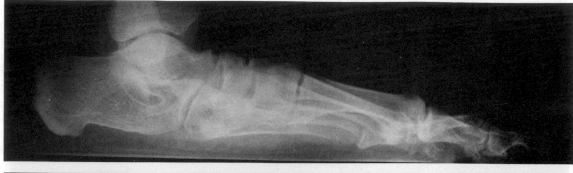

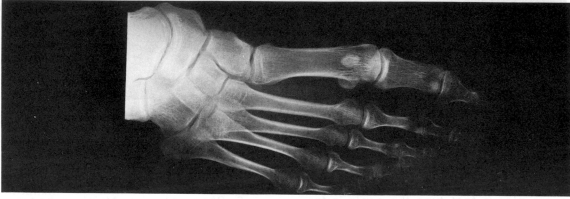

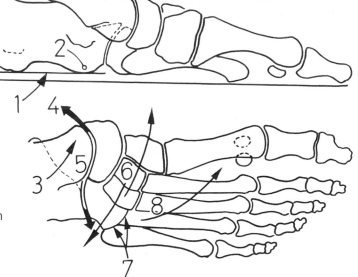

Fig. 339. Roentgenologic features of congenital pes planus

1, Plantigrade calcaneus
2, Anterior portion of calcaneus condensed and convex
3, Medial rotation of talus
4, Pseudonormal midtarsal joint line
5, Head of talus flattened
6, Tarsal articulation spread
7, Fifth metatarsal loosely articulated
8, Forefoot compensated into adduction

2. If compensation has developed early in childhood, the forefoot will be abducted by rotating the leg. In these cases, the metatarsophalangeal segments assume an adducted position in spite of the eversion of the hindfoot.

This adduction of the forefoot bones, while not apparent outwardly, is demonstrated roentgenographically.

ROENTGENOLOGIC FEATURES OF CONGENITAL PES PLANUS (Fig. 339).

Differential Diagnosis

The crux of a differential diagnosis between an extreme acquired foot collapse and a con-

TABLE 5. DIFFERENTIAL DIAGNOSIS OF CONGENITAL AND ACQUIRED PES PLANUS

	Acquired Foot Collapse	Congenital Pes Planus
Calcaneal position	Assumes a pitch of 10° or better with the weight-bearing plane	Lies at a pitch of less than 10° with the weight-bearing plane and usually parallel to it
Shape of calcaneus	Concave from plantar tuberosities to anterior process	Markedly convex and condensed from the plantar tuberosities to the anterior process
Midtarsal joint	Altered joint line. Talus juts forward	Pseudonormal joint line. Medial displacement of the talus

genital pes planus is gained through a careful study of the position and shape of the calcaneus, plus a careful evaluation of the midtarsal joint (Table 5).

ACQUIRED COMPLICATIONS OF CONGENITAL PES PLANUS

Through the course of a lifetime, the congenital pes planus receives more or less constant abuse. However, in spite of the mechanical disadvantage under which this foot functions, it maintains its typical pattern surprisingly well.

Adduction, although it may be considered an added defect, occurs as a compensatory change and, in reality this altered alignment is distinctly a better functioning one.

Some features of midtarsal fault may augment the congenital pes planus and indicate a further weakening of the ligamentous integument. Forward displacement of the talus and alteration of the normal midtarsal joint line are exemplified to a mild degree since there is little chance for this fault to develop in a foot lying on so low a plane.

Peroneal muscle spasm is a frequent complication of congenital pes planus. Deformities associated with anterior poliomeyelitis, spastic paralysis, muscular dystrophy, joint disease, and trauma represent another group of acquired complications contributing to congenital pes planus.

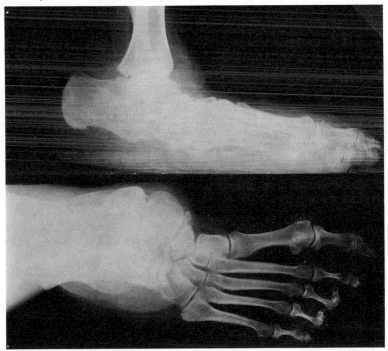

Fig. 340. Extreme congenital pes planus. Posterior portion of calcaneus at higher pitch than anterior part. Rocker-bottom plantar foot contour.

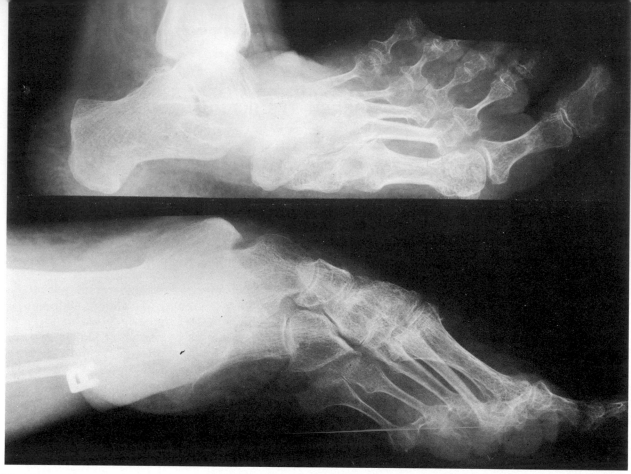

Fig. 341. Acquired talipes equinovalgus. Lateral view: declined and everted calcaneus; plantarflexed talus; navicular, cuneiform and first metatarsal totally plantigrade; lesser metatarsals and toes elevated placing the forefoot plane in valgus position. Dorsoplantar view: talus severely adducted; entire forefoot abducted; medial forefoot segment bones overlapping and lateral forefoot segment loosely articulated at cuboid joint indicate the frontal plane forefoot valgus position.

ROENTGEN INTERPRETATION OF CONGENITAL COMPLICATIONS AND FORMS OF DEFORMITY RELATED TO CONGENITAL PES PLANUS (Figs. 340 and 341)

1. *Talipes equinovalgus* — ankle equinus, subtalar valgus, forefoot abductovalgus (all components of clubfoot).

2. *Talipes equinus* — plantarflexed foot at ankle joint, unaffected subtalar joint and forefoot. Walks on forefoot.

   a. Ankle equinus block, compensated: subtalar valgus, forefoot dorsiflexed at midtarsal joint, talus plantarflexed, talar trochlea flattened. Extreme pes planus.

   b. Short gastrocnemius, compensated: subtalar and midtarsal pronation. Extreme plantarflexion and abduction of talus. Cuboid is abducted and plantarflexed. Rockerbottom plantar foot contour.

3. *Pes calcaneovalgus* — a total foot involvement with calcaneus in valgus position with forefoot dorsiflexed and abducted. Appraise neonatal or as early as possible. Simulate posture roentgenographic views by holding infant in position.

4. *Vertical talus* — talus plantarflexed to a vertical position and the navicular is dislocated dorsally above the talus. Calcanecuboid subluxation often occurs.

5. *Subtalar valgus* — the entire foot assumes an everted plane.

6. *Tarsal coalitions* — anomalies with a bar bridging either the calcaneonavicular or talocalcaneal joints are responsible for rigid planus and secondary peroneal spasms.

7. *Peroneal spastic flatfoot* — foot retained in planus due to spastic peroneus brevis and tertius muscles with no tarsal coalitions.

8. *Neurological flatfoot* — anomalies at birth attributable to spina bifida and other defects of spinal and cerebral neurogenic origin.

CLINICAL CORRELATION

The serviceability of the untreated congenital pes planus depends on an early forefoot adduction compensation that will permit parallel gait and freely functioning knees.

Problems to Be Considered

1. A straightforward, shuffling gait is the outcome when the foot is in compensated adduction, whereas a flailing gait with outturned feet and excessive motion at the midtarsal joint occurs in the basic pes planus deformity.

2. The non-elastic gait leads to minimal traumatic arthritic changes that are profound and may be painful in late adult life.

3. The possible development of acquired faults, as mentioned previously, must be considered.

4. Peroneal spasm and kindred soft-tissue problems are likely to develop. The calf group of muscles is invariably shortened in this foot type by means of the span to its attachment in the posterior aspect of the foot at the ankle.

5. The rotation of the calcaneus tends to push the heel counter over the lateral side of the shoe. The weight forces, carried medially on the foot, break down the medial border and shank of the shoe.

CONSERVATIVE MANAGEMENT

The foot should receive as much accommodative support as its flexibility will permit.

1. Reinforced shoes with corrective modifications may be all that can be tolerated.

2. The Whitman plate may be acceptable for the child with flexible feet.

3. Cupped heel seat Whitman plates are indicated for the adult.

4. Strongly constructed shoes will be needed to undergird any supportive device.

5. Gait training is essential.

6. Infant feet should be corrected by casts followed by splints.

SURGICAL RELEVANCE

Symptomatic complications of the congenital pes planus that prevent an acceptable function for this foot type, such as short calf muscle group, tarsal coalitions, and outright subluxation of talus and navicular (vertical talus), require surgery. Corrective surgical procedures are usually performed during childhood. Rarely, surgery is directed toward reconstructing the adult congenital pes planus, except tendo achillis lengthening release procedures.

BIBLIOGRAPHY

Alverez, H., and Caldeyro, R.: Contractability of the Human Uterus Recorded by New Methods, Surg. Gynec. Obstet. 191:1, 1950.

Arey, L.D.. Developmental Anatomy, ed. 6. Philadelphia: W.B. Saunders, 1950.

Bardeen, C.R.: Morphogonosis of the Skeletal Systems. In Keibel, F. (ed.), Manual of Human Embryology, Vol. 1. Philadelphia: J.B. Lippincott, 1910.

Bechtol, C.O., and Mossman, H.W.: Club-foot and Embryological Study of Associated Muscle Abnormalities, J. Bone Joint Surg. 32-A:827, 1950.

Congenital Defects. Papers and Discussions Presented at the First Inter-American Conference on Congenital Defects. Philadelphia: J.B. Lippincott Co., 1963.

Ganley, J.V.: Calcaneo-valgus Deformity in Infants, J. Podiat. Med. 57:12, 1972.

Giannestras, N.J.: Foot Disorders — Medical and Surgical Management. Philadelphia: Lea & Febiger, 1967.

Gordon, G.C.: Congenital Deformities. Edinburgh: E. & S. Livingston, Ltd., 1961.

Grice, D.S.: The Role of Subtalar Fusion in the Treatment of Valgus Deformities of the Feet. In Instruction Course Lectures, The American Academy of Orthopoedic Surgeons, Vol. 16, pp. 127-150. St. Louis: The C.V. Mosby Co., 1959.

Haveson, S.B.: Congenital Flatfoot Due to Talonavicular Dislocation (Vertical Talus), Radiology 72:19, 1959.

Herndon, C.H., and Heyman, C.H.: Congenital Convex Pes Valgus, J. Bone Joint Surg. 15-A:406, 1963.

Leavitt, D.G.: Subastragaloid Arthrodesis for the Os Calcis Type of Flat Foot, Amer. J. Surg. (new series) 59:501, 1943.

Patten, B.M.: Human Embryology, ed. 2. New York: The Blakiston Co., 1953.

Pollock, J.H., and Carrell, B.: Subtalar Extra-articular Arthrodesis in the Treatment of Paralytic Valgus Deformities, J. Bone Joint Surg. 46-A:533, 1954.

Snaglie, J.K., and Roby, H.R.: Bilateral Peroneal Spastic Flat Feet Associated with Congenital Fusion of the Navicular and Talus. A Case Report, J. Bone Joint Surg. 43-A:1237, 1961.

Tachdjian, M.O., Congenital Convex Pes Valgus, Symposium on Current Pediatric Problems, Orthopedic Clinics of North America, vol 3, no. 1, March 1972.

Tanz, S.S.: The So-called Tight Heel Cord, Clin. Orthop. 16:184, 1960.

PES ADDUCTUS 19

Pes adductus is a congenital foot type in which the forefoot is adducted, the hindfoot usually inverted, and the metatarsal bones turned on their long axes into adductovarus (Fig. 345). This foot type presents problems of pigeon-toed gait, lateral instability, excrescences under fifth metatarsal, overriding of lateral side of the shoe, and a hallux adductus position easily displaced into hallux abductus-valgus.

ORIENTATION

Etiologically, pes adductus deformity is simi-lar to talipes equinovarus in alignment except the components are of mild degree and there is no major congenital bone deformity. It may escape notice beyond infancy until it becomes symptomatic with a pigeon-toed gait.

Acquired adduction of the forefoot may be present in the compensated midtarsal fault, the pes valgoplanus foot, or the pes cavus foot originating from poliomyelitis or other neuromuscular disease.

In the young subject, hallux adductus frequently accompanies the normal adducted position of the first metatarsal and may give the impression of metatarsus adductus. Although a

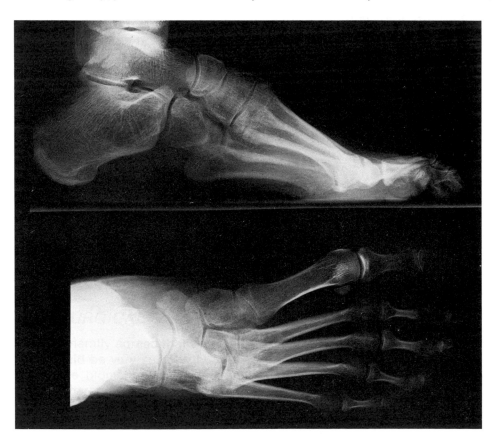

Fig. 345. Pes adductus. Inversion of hindfoot. Adduction of forefoot.

divergence of 5.8° of the first metatarsal is normal at birth, if the divergence is greater than 8.0° it is of clinical significance. It is the metatarsus adductus that attracts the greatest attention in cases of pes adductus.

Metatarsus adductus is frequently overlooked in infancy. Kite (1963) claims that not until between 6 weeks and 6 months, when the persistent action of the anterior tibial muscle creates forefoot deformity, is it first noticed.

Palmer (1964) has recently presented a study which indicates that primary talipes equinovarus should not be considered a single entity but should be divided into two groups: (1) partially or totally nonhereditary with a negative family history, predominance of younger mothers, an increased male-female ratio, and no significant recurrence risk, and (2) hereditary with sex ratio and maternal age curve similar to those of a control population and a recurrence risk of almost 10%. Probably an autosomal dominant trait is responsible.

An abnormal insertion of the abductor hallucis tendon to the medial side of the base of the proximal phalanx of the great toe attributes to hallux adductus (varus) and metatarsus adductus (varus) according to Thomson (1960). He recognizes two types: (1) primary and (2) secondary, associated with congenital equinovarus deformity.

In a review of 300 cases of metatarsus adductus (varus), Jacobs (1960) found 10% of the cases had hip dysplasia indicating that congenital malformation of the hip plays an important role in varus deformities.

The hindfoot inversion component of talipes equinovarus has been classified by LeNoir (1971) into two types: type I, in which the cuboid is rotated around the distal calcaneus, and type II, in which the cuboid is not rotated. The first type, which is more resistant to correction, occurred in 25% of 480 idiopathic feet. The second type occurred in 16% of this series.

ROENTGENOLOGIC INTERPRETATION

The two standard projections, dorsoplantar and lateral, are required. Roentgenograms of the infant's foot are valuable in diagnosis and the study of the results of corrective procedures.

Hindfoot

ROENTGENOGRAPHIC APPRAISAL OF INVERSION

1. The talus is closely bound to the anterior process of the calcaneus. If there is a 50% overlap, inversion may be assumed.

2. Overlapping of the navicular over the cuboid, the cuboid over the base of the fifth metatarsal, and the lesser cuneiforms over the cuboid is demonstrated.

3. There is superimposition of the bases of the metatarsals.

4. Adductovarus position of the metatarsals is in proportion to the degree of inversion.

5. On the lateral projection, there is exaggeration of the size of the opening of the sinus tarsi with the talus sitting high on the subtalar joint and the medial forefoot segment rising above the cuboid level.

Forefoot

1. Normal alignment of metatarsophalangeal segments is disturbed with first, second, third, and fourth metatarsal shafts assuming an adducted position. The fifth is usually practically straight but in extreme conditions may be adducted.

2. The metatarsophalangeal length-pattern ratio is materially altered, usually 1:2:3:4:5. The greater the adduction and hindfoot inversion, the longer the first metatarsal will appear and the more the joint-line parabola will taper toward the fifth metatarsal.

3. There is a high incidence of a massive atavistic internal cuneiform in the pes adductus foot. It has been the author's observation not only is the distal margin of the internal cuneiform slanted to direct the first metatarsal into adducted position but of greater importance the massive size of the cuneiform carries the metatarsocuneiform articulation forward and abets the inclination to adduction deformity of the entire forefoot (Fig. 346).

ROENTGENOLOGIC FEATURES OF

PES ADDUCTUS (Fig. 347)

22 THE FOOT ROENTGENOGRAM

The foot roentgenogram should be evaluated by its diagnostic quality, which depends on film detail, density, contrast, and image fidelity. Guide lines are offered for film improvement. Exposure charts are given to assist in producing good foot roentgenograms.

DIAGNOSTIC QUALITIES OF A GOOD FOOT ROENTGENOGRAM (Fig. 376)

The rule by which the diagnostic quality of a roentgenogram should be judged is that every element under examination must be clearly and accurately visualized. It is the responsibility of the physician to evaluate systematically the qualities represented in the film with an understanding of the factors that influence them.

TABLE 7

ABSORPTION COEFFICIENTS

Water: 2.506 λ^3	Blood: 2.61 λ^3
Protein: 1.78 λ^3	Pus: 2.67 λ^3
Fat, human: 1.135 λ^3	Sinew (connective
Muscle, lean: 2.57 λ^3	tissue): 2.37 λ^3
Nerves: 3.12 λ^3	Fatty tissue: 1.37 λ^3
Bone cortex: 13.24 λ^3	Chemical glassware
Cartilage: 2.70 λ^3	(jena): 15.05 λ^3
Fingernail: 2.57 λ^3	Sandstone or quartz:
	10.25 λ^3
	Iron: 107.7 λ^3

The doctor interprets black, gray, and white graphic representations into a visualization of tissue elements. His ability to interpret these representations depends on his knowledge of their significance based on experience in the study of normal and pathologic roentgen anatomy. The relative thickness and degree of density of the tissues is a significant factor. A study of the absorption coefficients of certain substances chosen from a table prepared by Barnes and McLachlan from Zuppinger's cal-

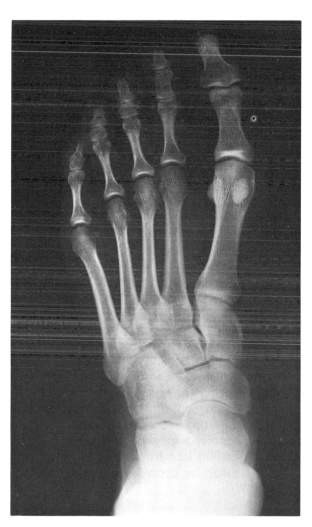

Fig. 376. A well-balanced dorsoplantar foot roentgenogram

plane in reference to the film-holder, the central ray should be directed perpendicular to a line that will bisect the surface–film-holder angle (Figs. 380-382).

Rule 3. When it is desired to visualize an articulation between two bones, the central ray should be directed through the articulation. Anatomic judgment governs the direction of the central ray.

POSTURE OF PATIENT

Weight-supporting Attitude (Figs. 383 and 384)

The natural weight-supporting attitude gives more information concerning pathomechanical conditions which may be present in the foot than other postures the patient may assume. The integrity of the foot regulates the degree of structural change visualized when the foot structure is in the anatomic situation that exists under the stress and strain created by body weight. The excursion of the joints and the alignments of the bones are all significant in determining the degree of functional disability present in the foot.

Other advantages of the weight-supporting attitude:

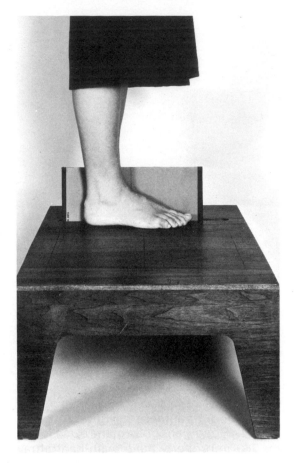

Fig. 383. Standing foot position.

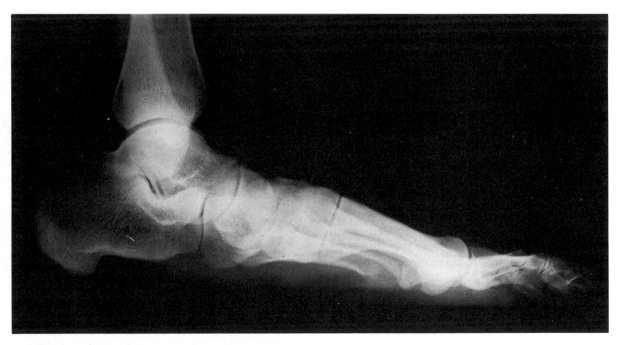

Fig. 384. Roentgenogram of standing foot (same case as in Fig. 386)

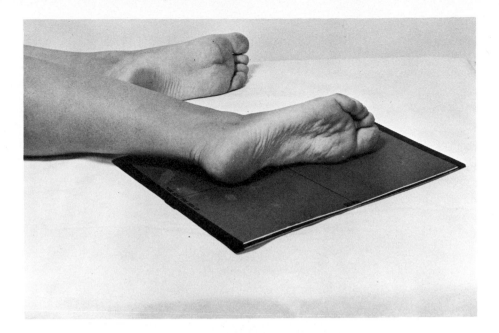

Fig. 385. Recumbent foot position

1. The foot is fundamentally aligned at a right angle to the leg, which contributes to standardization of projection.

2. Good foot immobilization is secured without the need of auxiliary devices.

3. The patient can more easily and quickly assume the various positions required for the examination.

Recumbent Attitude
(Figs. 385 and 386)

1. Uses:

a. Where traumatic lesions or pathologic conditions prevent weight support.

b. Where views of foot areas cannot be brought into profile in standard weight-supporting projections.

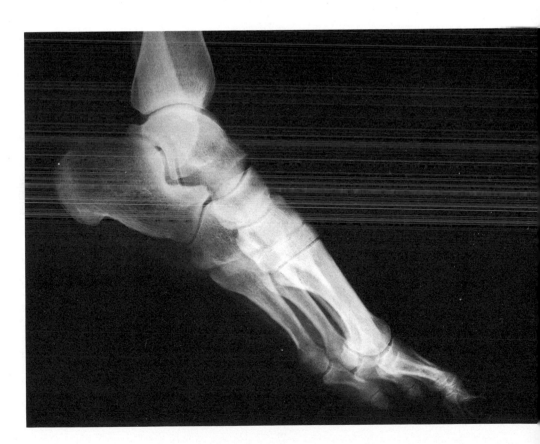

Fig. 386. Roentgenogram of recumbent foot

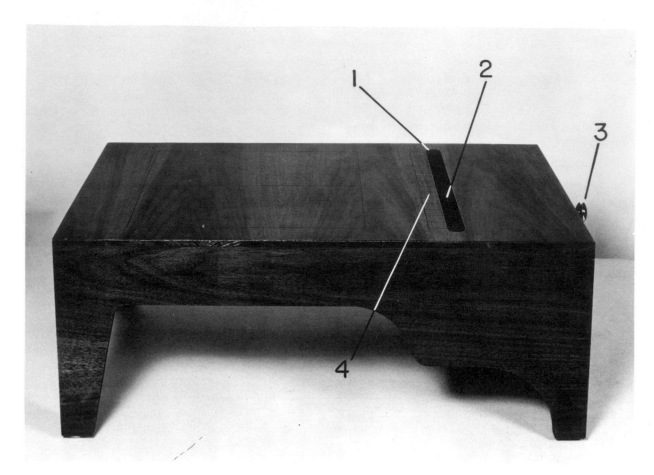

Fig. 387. Ortho-x-poser — foot X-ray examination stand. *Structural* features:

1. Radiation-proof well to protect film in lateral exposures. Provision for ray to undercut foot.
2. Cassette engaging bar holds film-holder in fixed vertical position.
3. Pull knob used to engage bar against film-holder.
4. Foot position scale in 1-inch gradations in front of film well insures duplication of film position for stereoscopy.
5. Guide lines are present on front of device to assist in positioning central ray.
6. Fixed depth of protection in well equal to one-half the 10-inch dimension of either 8 × 10 inch or 10 × 12 inch exposure holder.
7. Cassette holder for vertical or horizontal position.
8. Durable cabinet to withstand hard clinical use with patients of maximal weight. Easy to mount— 11 inches high.

2. Precautions in obtaining views in recumbent attitude:

a. Central ray must be directed to duplicate standard position requirements.

b. Relationship between foot and film should duplicate standard position requirements as closely as possible.

c. Unless sufficient weight can be applied to the foot by the patient to control motion, there will be an increased need for immobilization devices.

X-RAY EXAMINING STAND (ORTHO-X-POSER)

To fulfill the special needs of foot roentgenography — roentgenograms made in standard projections with the patient in the weight-supporting attitude — the author devised this apparatus and the technic used with it. The many features that were incorporated to achieve these purposes are listed in the legend for Figure 387.

To the advantages of recording the functional disability of the foot, standardization of projections, immobility of the foot, and efficiency of use are added the abilities to secure the lateral projection of weight-supporting foot with sufficient undercut to record the complete outline of the underlying soft tissues and to direct the central ray at an angle perpendicular to the foot and the film. Stereo-roentgenography of the foot in stance is also made possible.

ROENTGENOGRAPHIC PROJECTIONS

When the roentgen beam reaches its roentgenographic objective, its course is described in anatomic terms with the surface of entry named first and of exit last. These anatomic descriptions are used to designate roentgenographic projections.

Each projection will permit visualization of only one anatomic plane. To gain a three-dimensional impression, two projections must be produced at right angles to each other. Further information can be obtained by taking projections from other angles, depending on the plane of the bone to be examined.

Standard Projections
(Figs. 388-405)

To produce a standard roentgenographic projection, there must be a fixed relationship between the foot, the film, and the central ray

that can be duplicated. These relationships have been chosen to give optimal visualization to the majority of the bones in the foot.

In any projection of the foot there will be some overlapping of the bones. If the projections are standard, the interpreter becomes familiar with the amount of overlapping present in the normal foot and can determine the significance of variations from the normal. In a similar manner, other variations in relationships between the structures gain significance from the use of standard projections, and this is particularly important in demonstrating the changes that take place at intervals during the course of treatment. The use of standard projections is basic to any research study of biomechanical conditions of the foot.

Special Projections (Figs. 406-420)

Although they cannot be easily duplicated because of the varied angles and positions of the foot, special views of the foot can be extremely useful and are often added to the standard projections to complete a diagnostic survey.

Functional Projections
(Figs. 421-423)

These views taken with the foot in the position in which it becomes symptomatic can give important information concerning causative factors.

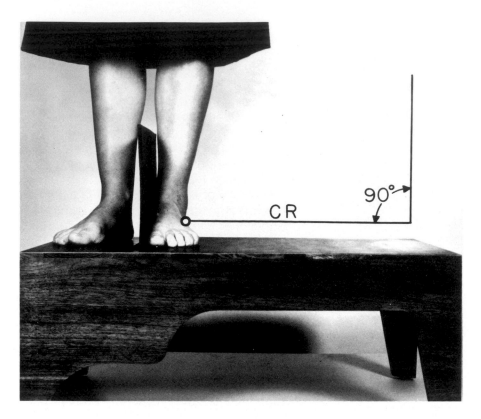

Fig. 388. Basic projection technic. Standard lateral foot projection.

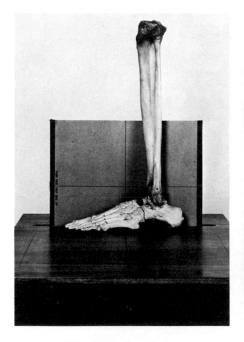

Fig. 389. Centering

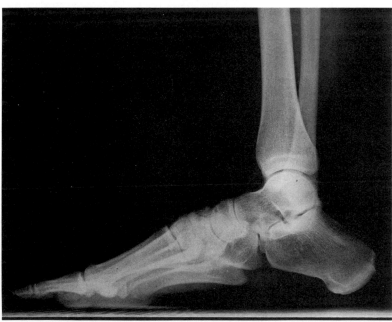

Fig. 390. Roentgenogram

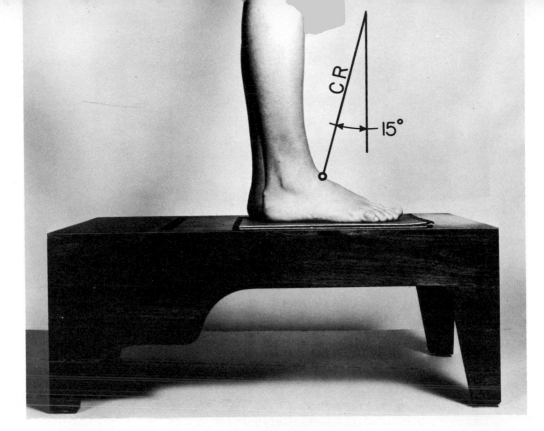

Fig. 391. Basic projection technic. Standard dorsoplantar foot projection

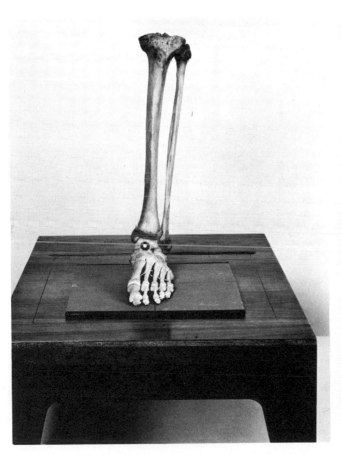

Fig. 392. Centering

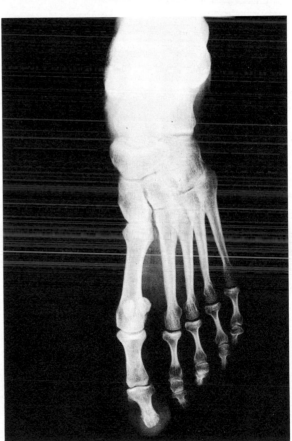

Fig. 393. Roentgenogram

FOOT ROENTGENOGRAPHIC TECHNIC/331

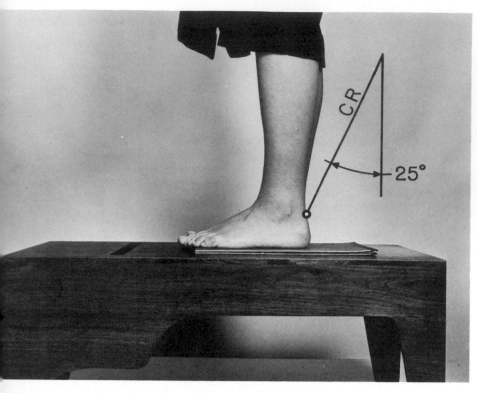

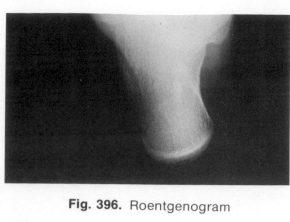

Fig. 396. Roentgenogram

Fig. 394. Basic projection technic.
Standard posteroplantar calcaneus projection

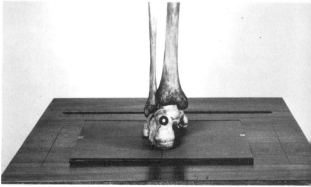

Fig. 395. Centering

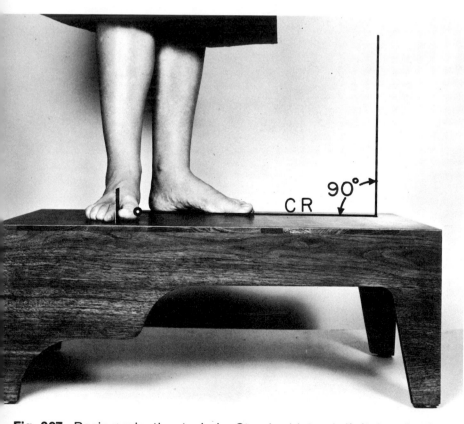

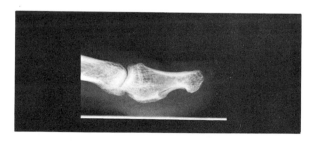

Fig. 399. Roentgenogram

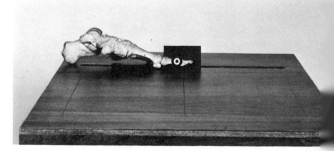

Fig. 397. Basic projection technic. Standard lateral digital projection

Fig. 398. Centering

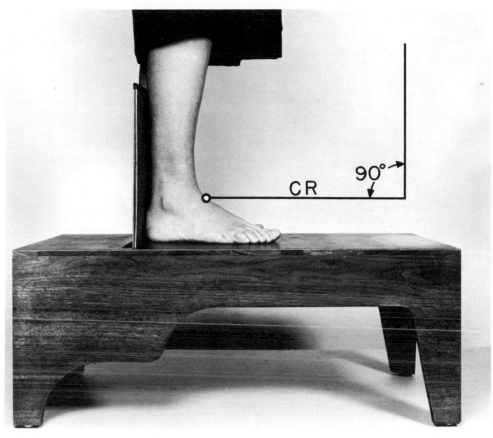

Fig. 400. Basic projection technic. Standard anteroposterior ankle projection

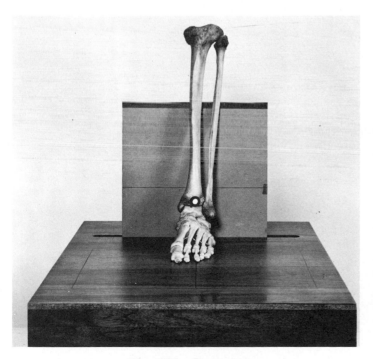

Fig. 401. Centering

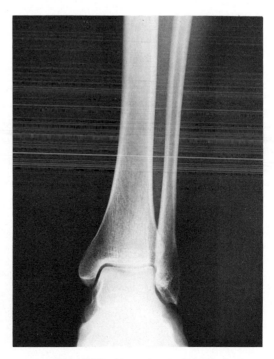

Fig. 402. Roentgenogram

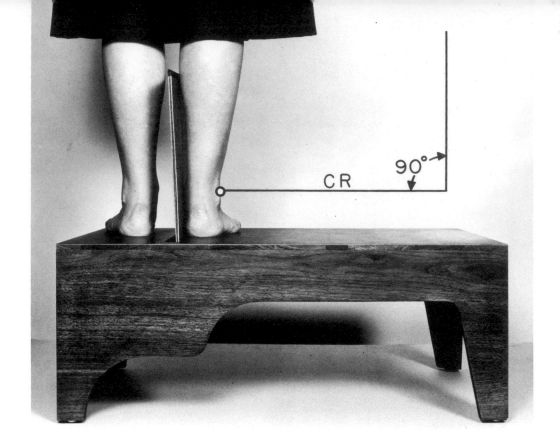

Fig. 403. Basic projection technic. Standard lateral ankle projection

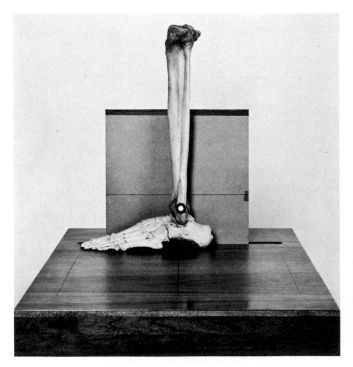

Fig. 404. Centering

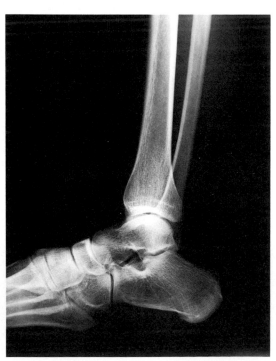

Fig. 405. Roentgenogram

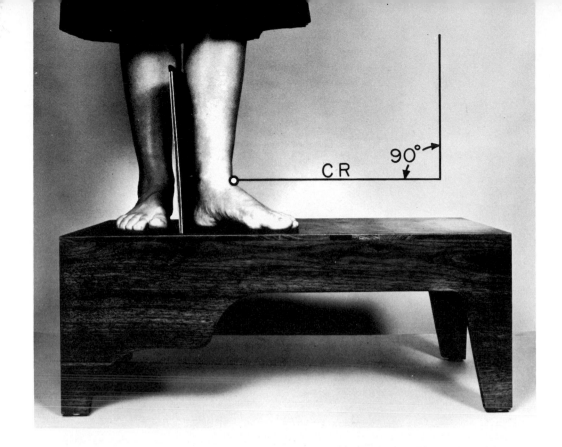

Fig. 406. Basic projection technic. Special oblique ankle projection

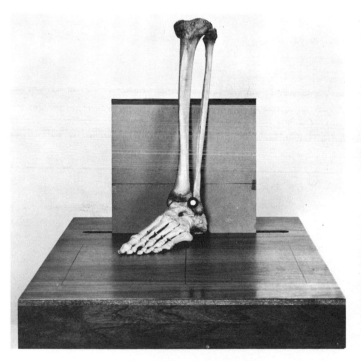

Fig. 407. Centering

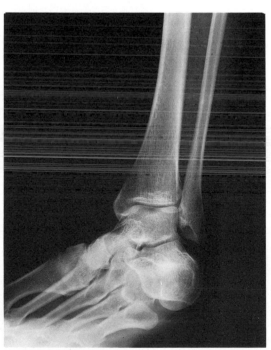

Fig. 408. Roentgenogram

FOOT ROENTGENOGRAPHIC TECHNIC/335

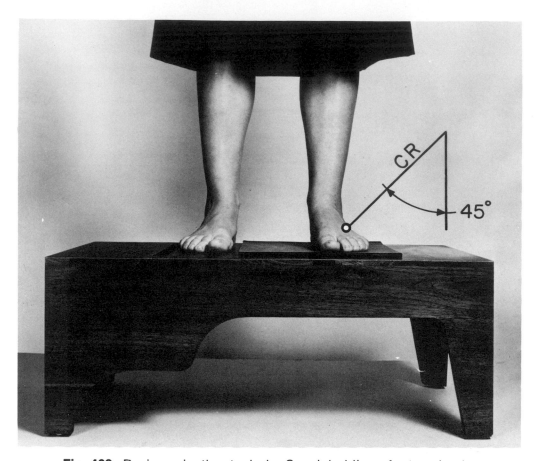

Fig. 409. Basic projection technic. Special oblique foot projection

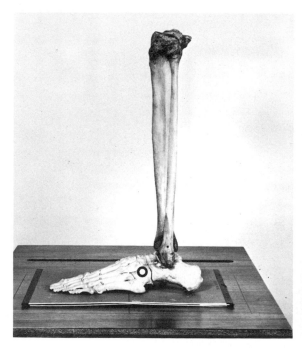

Fig. 410. Centering

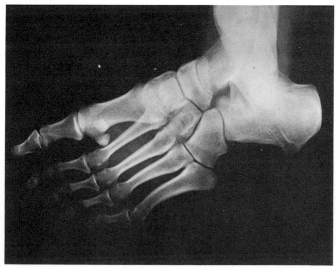

Fig. 411. Roentgenogram

336/FOOT ROENTGENOGRAPHIC TECHNIC

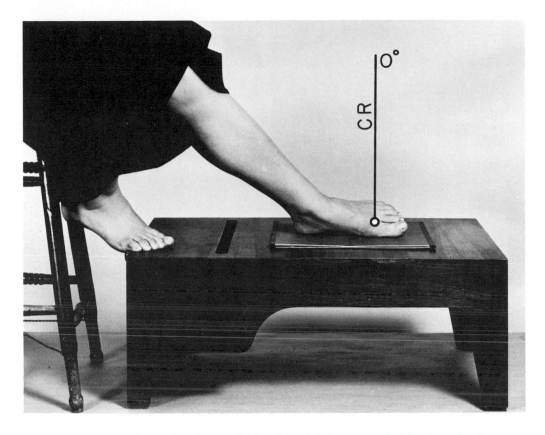

Fig. 412. Basic projection technic. Special dorsomedial foot projection

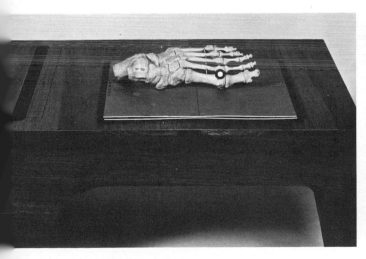

Fig. 413. Centering

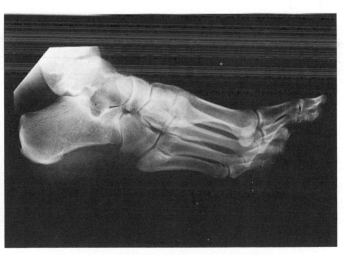

Fig. 414. Roentgenogram

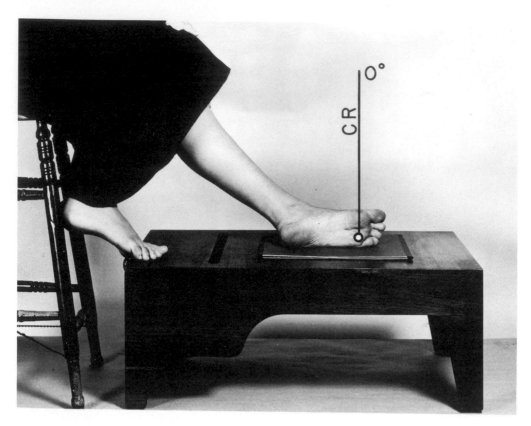

Fig. 415. Basic projection technic. Special plantolateral foot projection

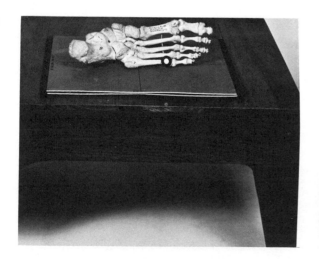

Fig. 416. Centering

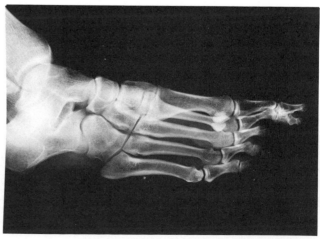

Fig. 417. Roentgenogram

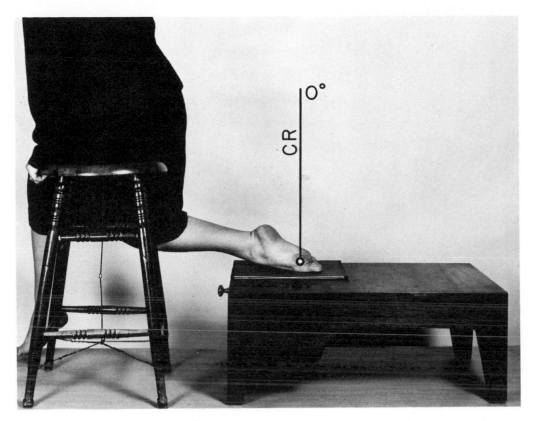

Fig. 418. Basic projection technic. Special plantomedial foot projection

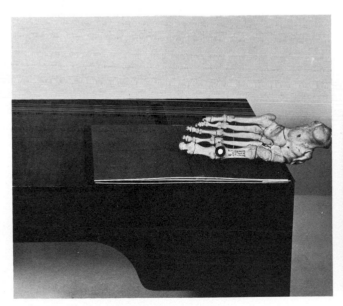

Fig. 419. Centering

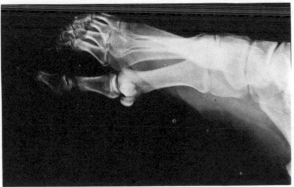

Fig. 420. Roentgenogram

FOOT ROENTGENOGRAPHIC TECHNIC/339

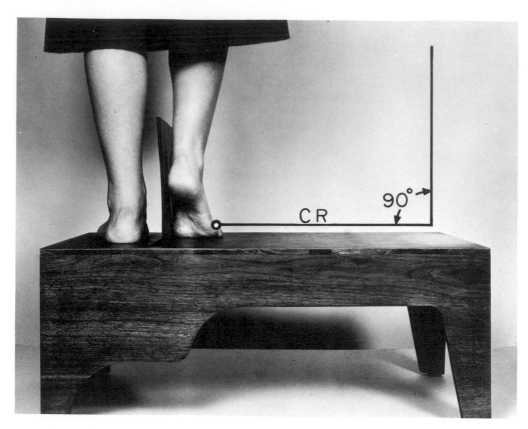

Fig. 421. Basic projection technic. Functional first metatarsophalangeal joint projection

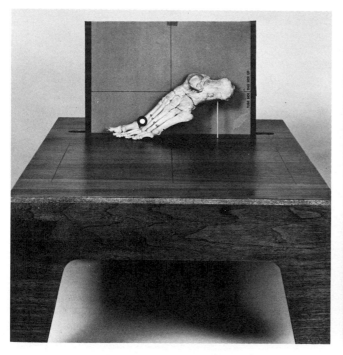

Fig. 422. Centering

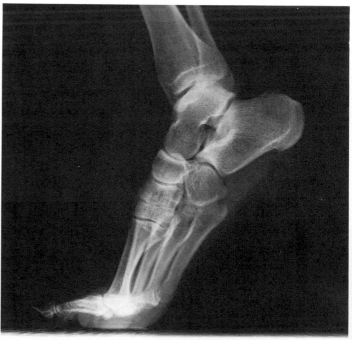

Fig. 423. Roentgenogram

340/FOOT ROENTGENOGRAPHIC TECHNIC

NEWLY ADOPTED SPECIAL PROJECTIONS

This group of projections have special significance in the diagnosis of the biomechanical status of the foot. All of the technics have evolved in recent years. Balsa wood blocks of appropriate sizes are used to gain the special profiles desired in several of the projections.

Details concerning posing the patient, using various height balsa blocks, directing the central ray, and the centering point involved are given for each of the new projections.

The special axial anteroposterior ankle and hindfoot projection (frontal plane) presents information similar to that from the Lewis posteroanterior projection.

The special oblique sinus tarsi, subtalar, and calcaneocuboid projection is somewhat similar to the oblique ankle projection; however, this newly adopted view includes additional foot joints and presents information concerning this bony alignment previously unattainable in conventional stance lateral views.

Special Axial Sesamoid and Metatarsophalangeal Area Projection (Figs. 424-427)

This method and device developed by Downey and Dorothy (1969) produce a roentgenogram of the sesamoid bones in a frontal plane axial view that is easily achieved and consistently accurate due to the standardized technique involved. The metatarsophalangeal area is also in good plantar profile (Fig. 427).

The device consists of balsa wood wedges used to raise the heel and toes so that the plantar aspect of the hallucal sesamoids and metatarsophalangeal area may be roentgenographed in profile with the patient standing. The balsa wood blocks are mounted on a hardwood base with a heel wedge adjustable to foot length. The dimensions of the device are: base board, 4½" × 14" × 1"; heel wedge, 4⅝" × 6" × 1½"; toe lift, 4½" × 1½" × 1", curved to accommodate the metatarsal parabola and varus rotation of the fifth ray (Fig. 426). The slope of the heel wedge is approximately 12° and of the toe lift 32°. Two devices are needed so that the patient may be posed with both heels elevated uniformly to avoid unequal balance and stress to the foot structure.

In practice, a device is used for each foot, with the foot under examination on a device perpendicular to the vertical film-holder with the toes just touching it. The indifferent foot is posed on a device positioned at the patient's predetermined angle of gait. The central ray is directed at 90° from one-half inch above the platform level in a heel-to-toe direction. The entire positioning procedure is repeated for the other foot. The film may be protected so that views of both feet are side by side on one film.

Commercial copies of the device made of plastic are on the market. It is a moot question whether roentgenologic detail is better when balsa wood or plastic is interposed during exposure.

Special Axial Calcaneal Plantar Profile Projection (Figs. 428-430)

The object of this technic is to produce a frontal plane axial view of the plantar profile of the calcaneus in stance so that any varus or valgus position may be appraised. The relative levels of the contours of the internal and external tuberosities of the calcaneus are the key to the evaluation (Fig. 428).

A set of balsa wood blocks is all that is needed to position the foot for this axial view of the calcaneus. Each block is 4½" × 2" × 1½". Each foot should be roentgenographed separately so that the one under examination may be aligned perpendicular to the vertical film-holder and the indifferent foot posed at the patient's predetermined angle of stance. The heel touches the film-holder. After positioning the patient in this manner, a 1" or 1½"-high balsa wood block is placed under the forefoot of the indifferent foot and the foot to be exposed. The central ray is then directed at 90° from one-half inch above the Ortho-x-poser in a toe-to-heel direction. The procedure is repeated for the other foot. Two views may be placed on one film by properly protecting half of the film during each exposure.

Special Axial First and Second Metatatarsocuneiform Segments Projection (Figs. 431-433)

The object of this technic is to produce a frontal plane axial view of the forefoot with special reference to the articulation between the first and second metatarsocuneiform segments to assess possible hypermobility. Adduction of the first metatarsal and its varus or valgus position may be visualized. Depending on the framework of the foot under study, the alignment of the lesser metatarsals and the metatarsocuboid articulation may be visualized.

A set of balsa wood blocks, 4½″ × 2″ × 2″, is needed to raise the heel for this technic. An auxiliary set of blocks, 2½″ in height, may be useful for exceptionally long feet. Each foot should be roentgenographed separately so that the one under examination may be aligned perpendicular to the film-holder and the indifferent foot posed at the patient's predetermined angle of stance. The heel touches the film-holder. After positioning the patient in this manner, a 2″-high balsa wood block is placed under the heel of the indifferent foot and the foot to be exposed, and the central ray is directed at 90° from 2″ above the Ortho-x-poser in a toe-to-heel direction. The procedure is repeated for the other foot. Two views may be placed on one film by proper protection of half of the film during each exposure.

Special Anteroposterior Ankle and Hindfoot Projection (Figs. 434-436)

The object of this technic is to demonstrate the tibiofibular relationship to the talus and the subtalar position of the calcaneus. The body of the talus is profiled in the frontal plane. The neck and head of the talus are obscured by tarsal bones. The calcaneus is normally directly beneath the talus.

A set of balsa wood blocks, 4½″ × 1½″ × 2″, is needed to raise the heel for this technic. Each foot should be roentgenographed separately so that the one under examination may be aligned perpendicular to the film-holder and the indifferent foot posed at the patient's predetermined angle of stance. The heel touches the film-holder. After positioning the patient in this manner, a 1½″-high balsa wood block is placed under the heel of the indifferent foot and the one to be exposed, and the central ray is directed at 90° from 1″ above the Ortho-x-poser in a toe-to-heel direction. The procedure is repeated for the other foot. Two

views may be placed on one film by proper protection of half of the film during each exposure.

Special Oblique Sinus Tarsi, Subtalar, and Calcaneocuboid Projection (Figs. 437-439)

The object of this technic is to demonstrate the integrity of the sinus tarsi, to visualize all subtalar articulations, and to appraise the position of the cuboid as it articulates with the calcaneus and the external cuneiform.

The foot under examination is posed at a 30° angle from the vertical film-holder with the hindfoot touching the film-holder. The central ray is directed perpendicular to the film-holder at 90° from one-half inch above the Ortho-x-poser at a centering point at the calcaneocuboid joint level.

INDIVIDUAL BONE PROJECTIONS

If the plane of a particular bone varies markedly from the plane of the majority of bones in a standard projection or if its image is obscured by the overlapping of the images of other bones, it is sometimes possible to bring it into position for a plane profile view by careful manipulation of the plane of the foot and the angle of the central ray.

ROENTGENOGRAPHY OF SELECTED FOOT CONDITIONS

A roentgenologic study of a foot condition requires enough roentgenographic views of the area to provide complete diagnostic information. A number of factors affect the selection of projections and the arrangement of the views.

Composing A Roentgenographic Examination

1. Exposures from at least two divergent planes are necessary to gain a three-dimensional impression.

2. Lateral and dorsoplantar views are basic.

3. Add views needed to give special information about the specific condition under examination.

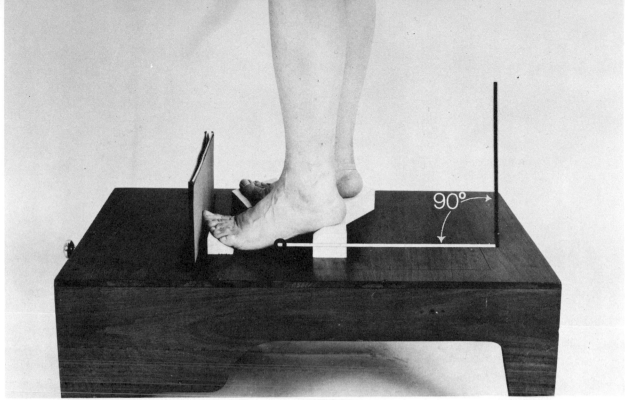

Fig. 424. Basic projection technic. Special axial sesamoid and metatarsophalangeal area projection (Downing and Dorothy technic)

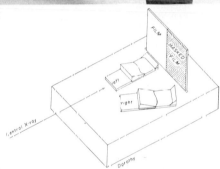

Fig. 426. Downing and Dorothy device. (Courtesy of Journal of American Podiatry Association and W.L. Dorothy, D.P.M.)

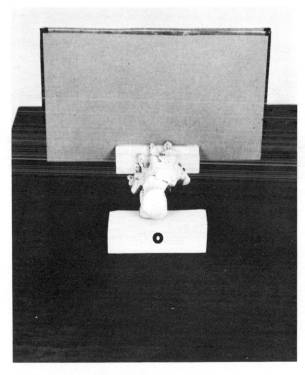

Fig. 425. Centering

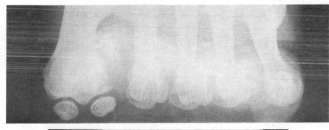

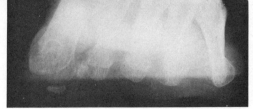

Fig. 427. Roentgenogram. *Above,* balsa wood wedge only; *below,* 1-inch firm foam plus wedge.

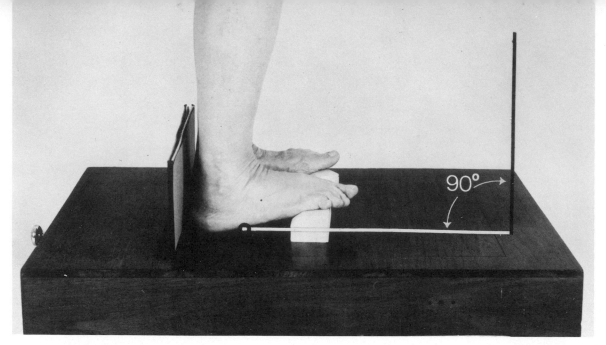

Fig. 428. Basic projection technic. Special axial calcaneal plantar profile projection

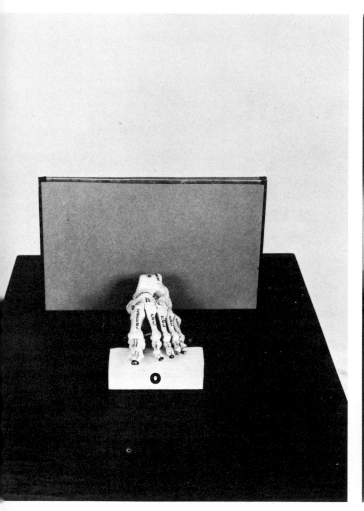

Fig. 429. Centering

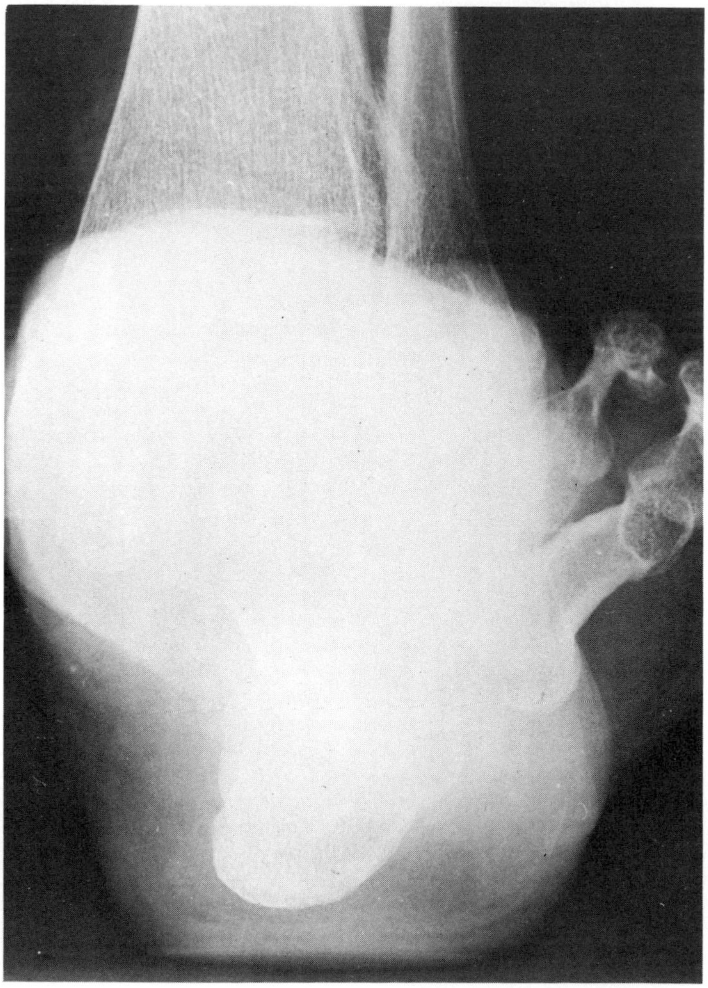

Fig. 430. Roentgenogram

344/FOOT ROENTGENOGRAPHIC TECHNIC

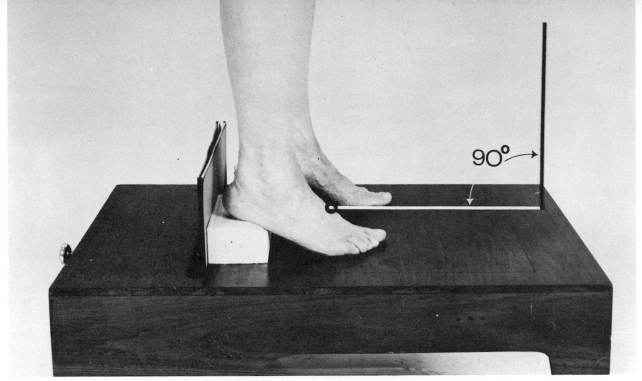

Fig. 431. Basic projection technic. Special axial first and second metatarsocuneiform segments projection

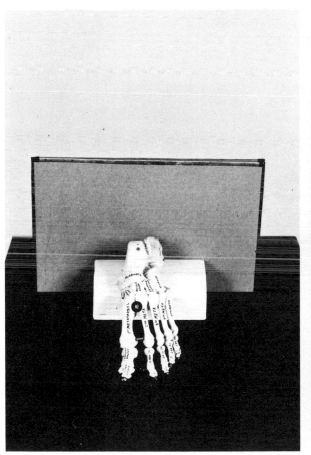

Fig. 432. Centering

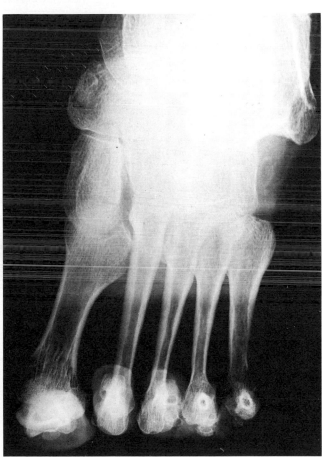

Fig. 433. Roentgenogram

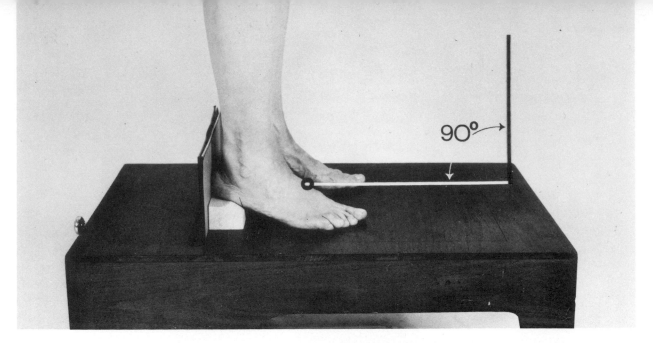

Fig. 434. Basic projection technic. Special anteroposterior ankle and hindfoot projection

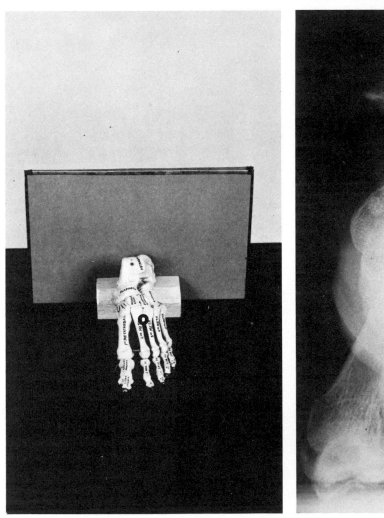

Fig. 435. Centering

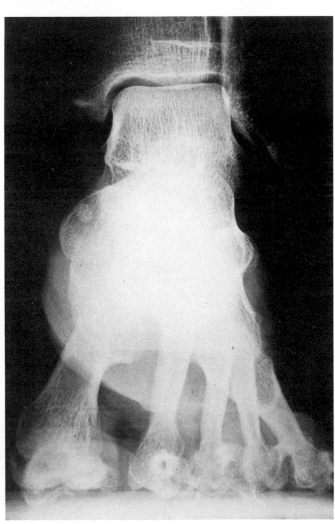

Fig. 436. Roentgenogram

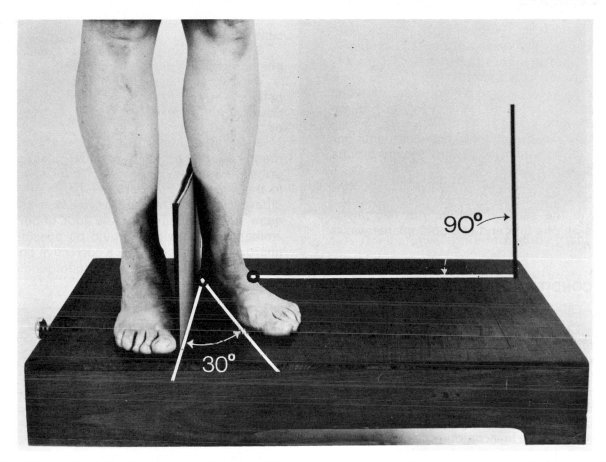

Fig. 437. Basic projection technic. Special oblique sinus tarsi, subtalar, and calcaneocuboid projection

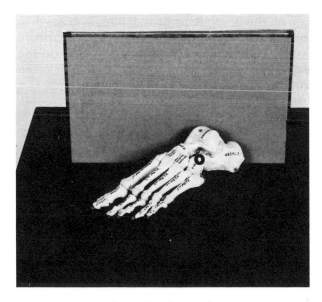

Fig. 438. Centering

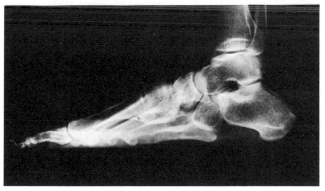

Fig. 439. Roentgenogram

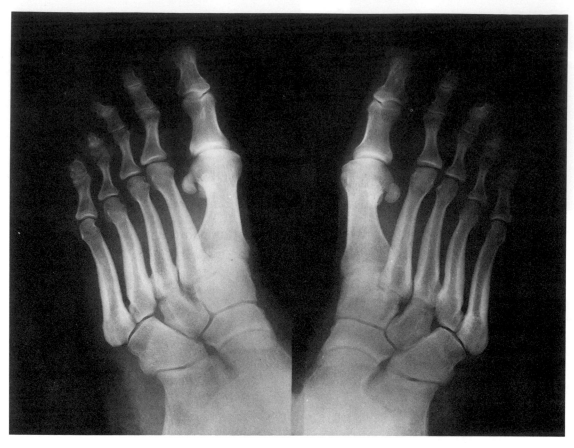

Fig. 446. Supplementary examination in pathoanatomic conditions: all nonspecific foot conditions (comparative)

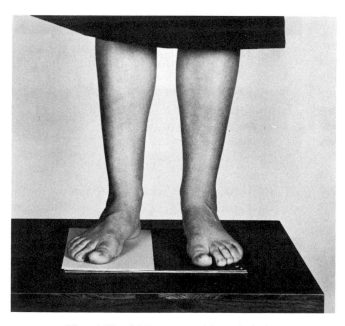

Fig. 447. Oblique position, left foot

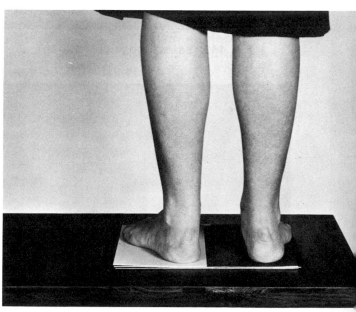

Fig. 448. Oblique position, right foot

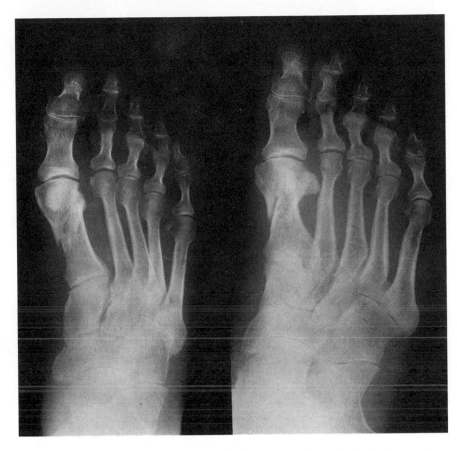

Fig. 449. Fracture of metatarsal or phalanx, metatarsalgia, hallux valgus, hammer toe, orthodigital conditions

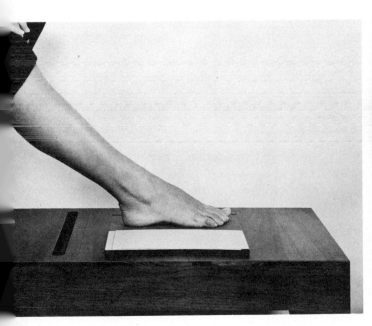

Fig. 450. Dorsoplantar position

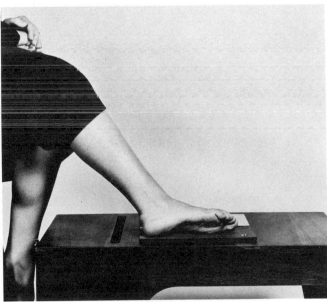

Fig. 451. Dorsomedial position

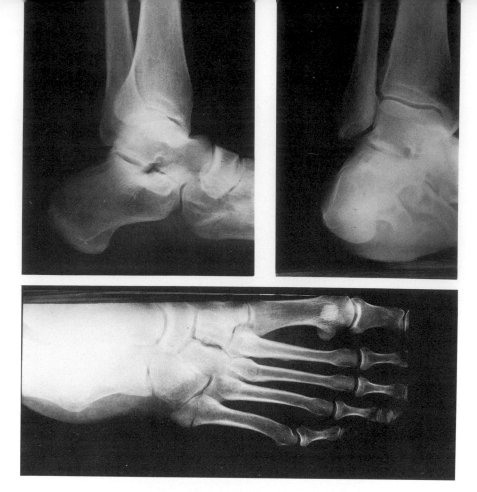

Fig. 452. Ankle area and base of fifth metatarsal

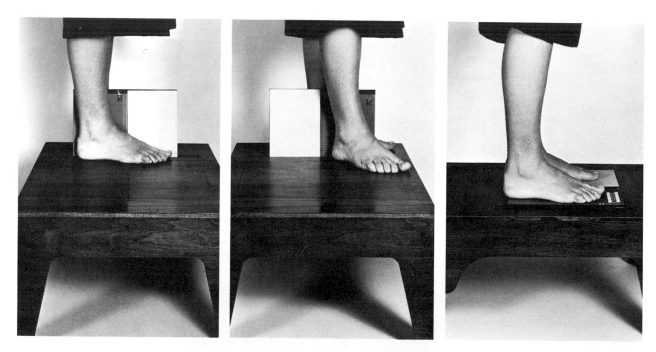

Fig. 453 *(left).* Lateral ankle position
Fig. 454 *(center).* Oblique ankle position
Fig. 455 *(right).* Dorsoplantar foot position

352/FOOT ROENTGENOGRAPHIC TECHNIC

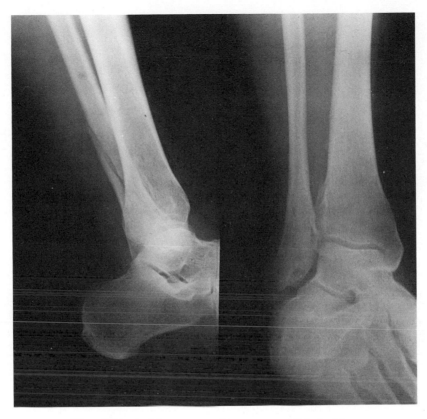

Fig. 456. Ankle area and lower one-third of leg

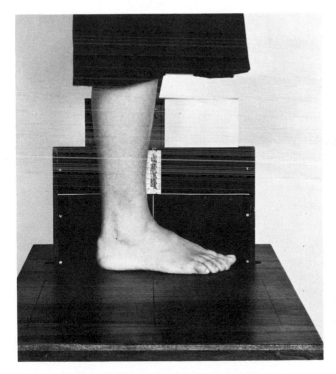

Fig. 457. Lateral ankle position

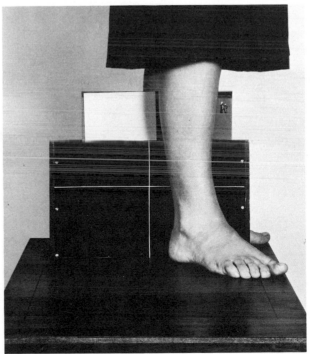

Fig. 458. Oblique ankle position

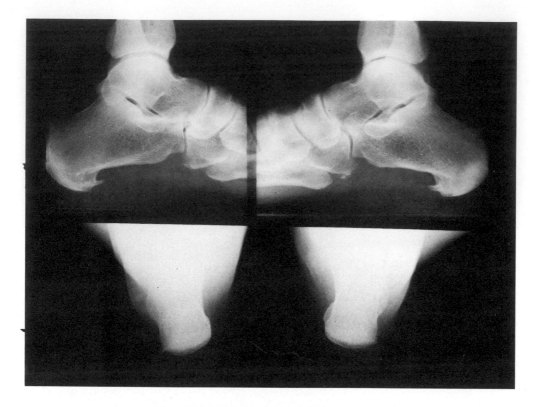

Fig. 459. Heel study (comparative)

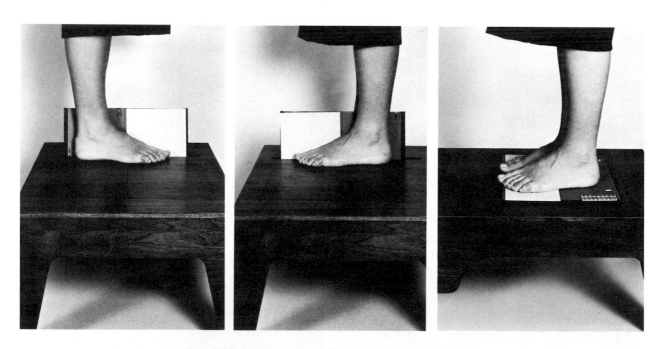

Fig. 460 *(left).* Lateral foot position, right heel
Fig. 461 *(center).* Lateral foot position, left heel
Fig. 462 *(right).* Posteroplantar calcaneus position

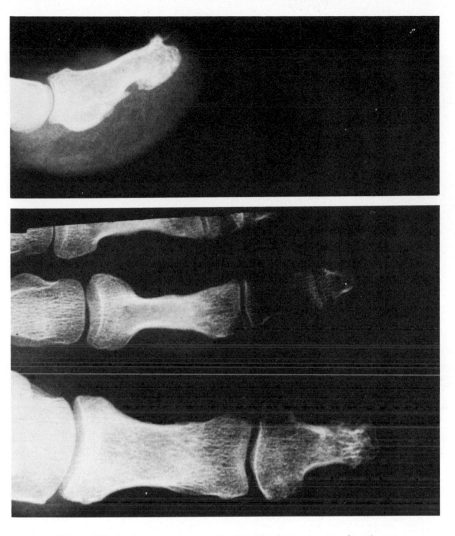

Fig. 463. Subungual exostosis, single toe examination

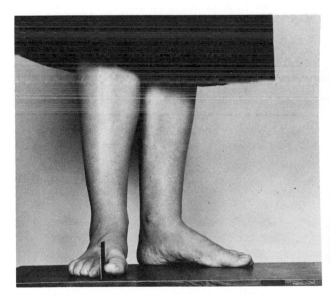

Fig. 464. Lateral digital position

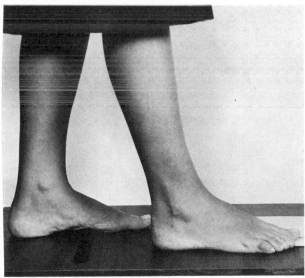

Fig. 465. Dorsoplantar position

FOOT ROENTGENOGRAPHIC TECHNIC/355

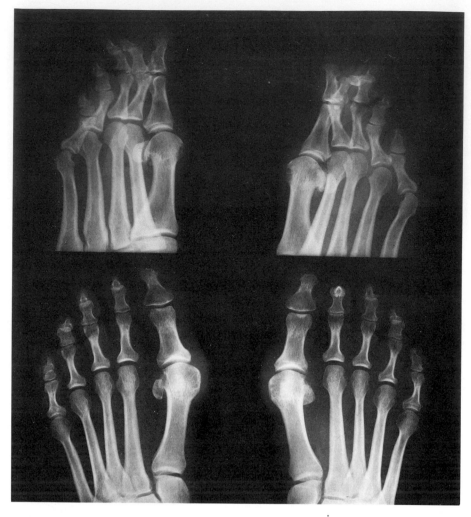

Fig. 466. Hallux valgus, metatarsalgia, hammer toe, fracture of metatarsal or phalanx, orthodigital conditions

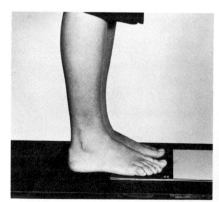 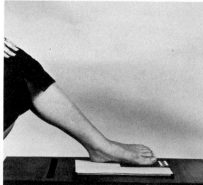 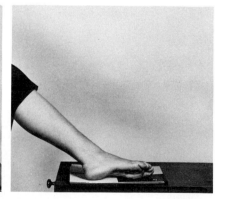

Fig. 467 *(left).* Dorsoplantar position
Fig. 468 *(center).* Dorsomedial position, left foot
Fig. 469 *(right).* Dorsomedial position, right foot

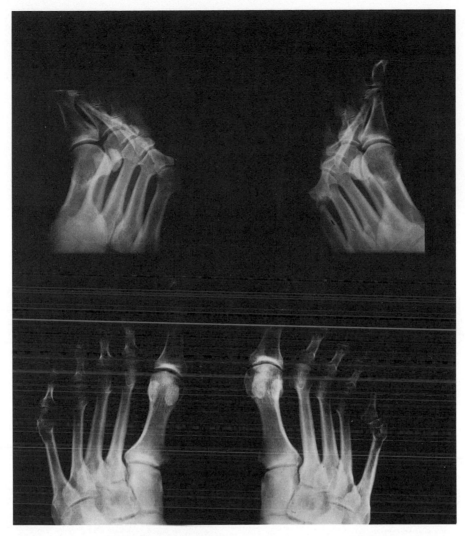

Fig. 470. Quinti digiti adductus (comparative)

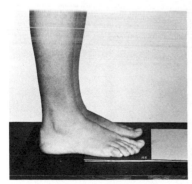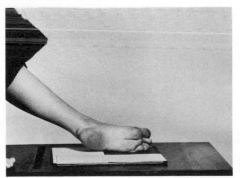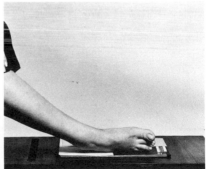

Fig. 471 *(left).* Dorsoplantar position
Fig. 472 *(center).* Plantolateral position, left foot
Fig. 473 *(right).* Plantolateral position, right foot

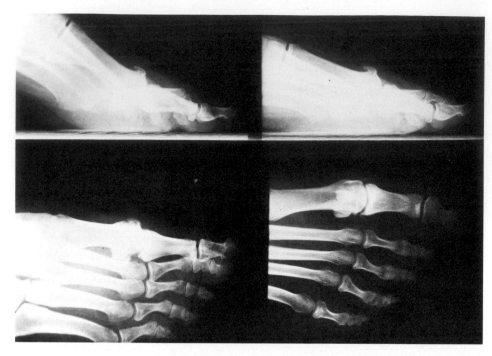

Fig. 474. Hallux limitus

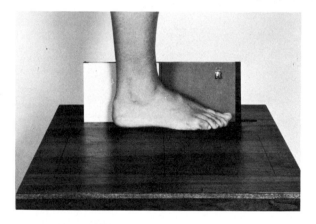

Fig. 475. Lateral foot position

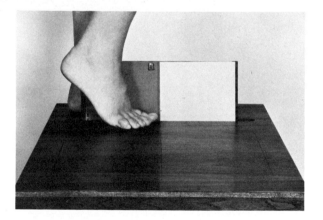

Fig. 476. Function foot position

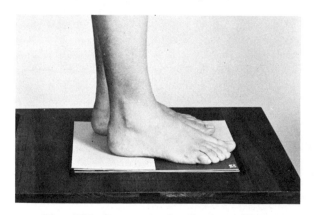

Fig. 477. Dorsoplantar foot position

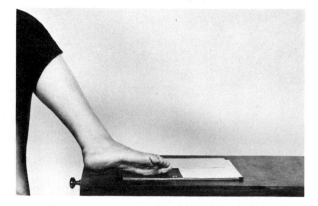

Fig. 478. Dorsomedial foot position

358/FOOT ROENTGENOGRAPHIC TECHNIC

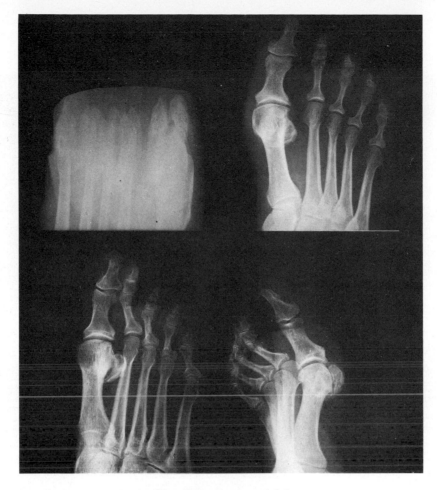

Fig 479. Sesamoiditis

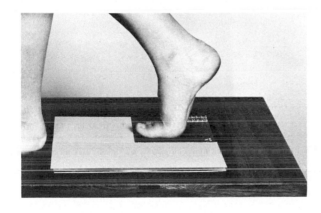

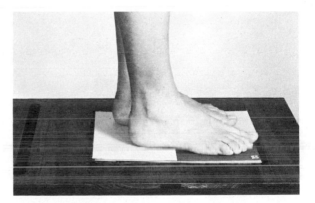

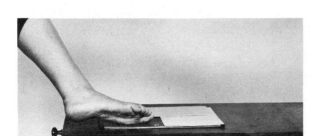

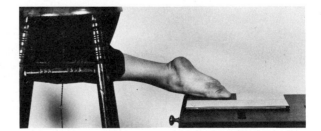

Fig. 482. Dorsomedial position
    Fig. 483. Plantomedial position

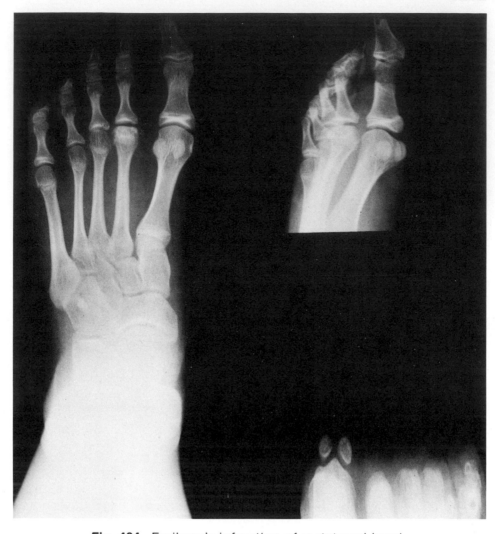

Fig. 484. Freiberg's infraction of metatarsal head

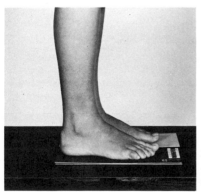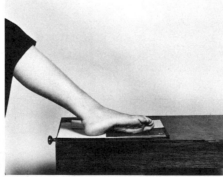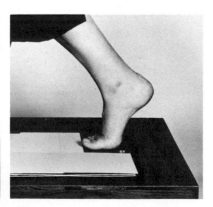

Fig. 485 *(left).* Dorsoplantar foot position
Fig. 486 *(center).* Dorsomedial foot position
Fig. 487 *(right).* Axial sesamoid position

25 SPECIAL ROENTGENOGRAPHIC PROCEDURES

Additional roentgenographic information may be obtained in certain cases through the use of special technics. The following methods will be explained: composite full-foot roentgenographic technic, stereoroentgenography of the weight-supporting foot, planigraphy, macroradiography, fine bone detail technic, use of filter for uniform exposure of the forefoot, special soft-tissue roentgenographic technic (angle block positioning), special projections of the subtalar joint, simultaneous foot-imprint roentgenograms, Polaroid roentgenography, positive X-ray paper, and Hammonds' postural tri-plane scanogram roentgenography.

COMPOSITE FULL-FOOT ROENTGENOGRAPHIC TECHNIC
(Figs. 488-492)

In the conventional dorsoplantar roentgenogram, the complete outline of the foot is lacking because the thickness of the leg and ankle causes an opacity that results in a panel of unexposed film in the hindfoot area. Although this view is an acceptable standard for diagnostic study, it lacks a complete outline of the foot with the posterior view of the calcaneus portrayed. This composite roentgenogram has special use in determining a foot axis reference line drawn from the center of the calcaneus to a point between the second and third metatarsal heads. It is also of value as a guide in appliance construction since measurements may be taken from the soft-tissue outline of the heel to anatomic areas for placement of corrections.

The composite roentgenogram with complete foot outline is accomplished by making two exposures: a dorsoplantar projection and then a superimposed posteroplantar projection on the same film. The patient stands immobile until both exposures have been made.

During each exposure, the tube is brought close to the body and the leg structures act as radiopaque shields. The most accurate rendition is accomplished by exposing each foot separately. Care must be taken to center the ray along the long axis of the foot from both front and hind positions. Careless centering may result both in overlapping density across the forefoot and double images.

Overlapping density may also occur when extremely thin leg structures do not afford an adequate protection for the forefoot. The same may occur in extremely wide forefoot or hallux abductus valgus. An acceptable composite roentgenogram of both feet may be made at the same time by posing the feet parallel and close together. The central ray must follow a central axis in both dorsoplantar and posteroplantar projections.

The full-foot view is accurate with respect to foot size at the point where the roentgen ray meets the skin-film contact. In any lateral view of the entire foot, there is always an overall magnification of foot size because the divergent rays from one projection extend the foot at each end.

STEREOROENTGENOGRAPHY OF THE WEIGHT-SUPPORTING FOOT

In the process of viewing conventional foot roentgenograms, the examiner is confronted by the fact that he is dealing with an image depicting bones that does not convey a three-dimensional effect such as would be observed in viewing a foot skeleton. Rather, it is necessary to organize in one's mind a three-dimensional concept by combining the impressions gained from two roentgenograms taken from two divergent projections, usually dorsoplantar and lateral views.

Instantaneous visualization of the three di-

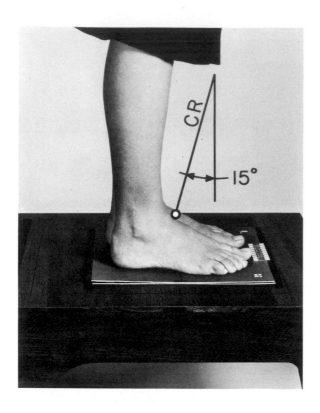

Fig. 488. Dorsoplantar foot projection

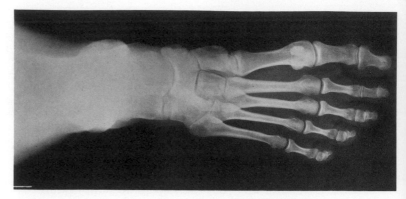

Fig. 490. Dorsoplantar foot roentgenogram. Note the incompletely exposed portion of film in the heel region.

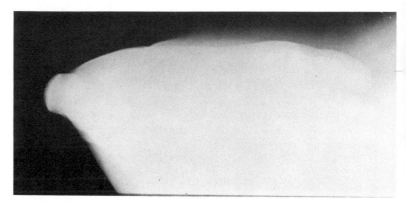

Fig. 491. Posteroplantar calcaneus roentgenogram. Note the incompletely exposed portion of film in the anterior region of the foot.

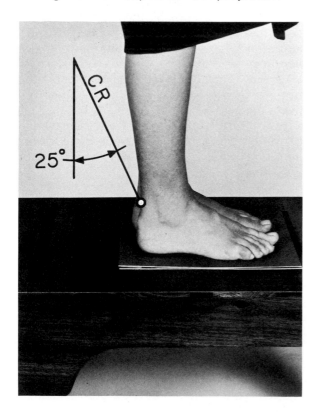

Fig. 489. Posteroplantar calcaneus projection

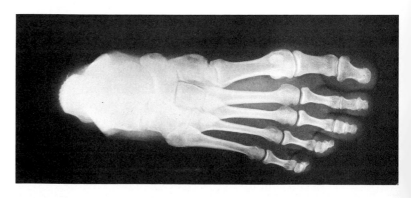

Fig. 492. Composite dorsoplantar and posteroplantar roentgenograms of the same foot projected on one film. Patient immobile as tube is moved and two projections are superimposed. Make the dorsoplantar exposure first, then the posteroplantar.

mensions of the foot bones may be achieved by stereoroentgenography. Stereoroentgenography of the weight-supporting foot not only produces three-dimensional visualization of the individual bones, but it also shows their anatomic spatial relationships. Thus, fault syndromes and alignment changes may be appraised with the foot appearing as a standing skeletal framework.

In normal binocular vision, everyone utilizes stereopsis to gain three-dimensional images. The left eye views an object from a slightly left-sided angle, while the right eye views the same object from a slightly right-sided angle. Each eye receives a two-dimensional image upon the receptive area of the retina, known as the fovea, which in turn transmits the image to the brain. The brain then fuses the two images together by superimposing each view to produce a single three-dimensional impression from the two views.

The roentgenographic system of stereoscopy will be explained. Two roentgenographic images of the foot must be produced. The first is made by projecting the central ray slightly from the left side, the second roentgenogram slightly from the right side. In each case, the central ray is moved left or right from the normal centering position. These roentgenographic views correspond to those that would be observed by each eye. (Each roentgenographic view corresponds to that which would be observed by a single eye.) A stereoscope is utilized to view the roentgenograms. In principle, the stereoscope is an optical device that isolates the eyes, thus allowing each eye to view the appropriate roentgenogram and transmit an image to the brain on an individual basis. There the images are superimposed to give the concept of depth.

STEREOROENTGENOGRAPHIC TECHNIC FOR WEIGHT-SUPPORTING FOOT (Figs. 493)

1. It is imperative to use the Ortho-x-poser or similar device to obtain accurately standardized views.

2. Pose the patient for standard lateral view of the foot.

3. Note position of film-holder on film-well scale so that the second film-holder of the stereo pair may be placed in exactly the same ref-

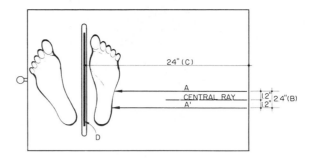

Fig. 493. Stereoroentgenographic technic. *A,* Exposure of right view of stereoscopic pair. *A',* Exposure for left view of stereoscopic pair. *B,* Total tube shift — 2.4 inches, divided equally from normal centering point. *C,* Film-anode distance — 24 inches. *D,* Film placement precisely the same for both views of the stereoscopic pair.

erence to the foot.

4. Affix stereo marker for the left view of the stereo pair.

5. Align the central ray to proper direction for focus. Mark centering point.

6. Total tube shift should be one tenth of tube-anode distance (24-inch tube-anode distance = 2.4 inch total tube shift).

7. Shift tube 1.2 inches to the left of normal centering point.

8. Expose left stereo view.

9. Without patient moving, second film is placed in duplicate position.

10. Affix stereo marker for right view of stereo pair.

11. Shift tube 1.2 inches to the right of normal centering point.

12. Expose right stereo view.

This completes the pair of stereoroentgenograms for one foot. The same procedure is repeated for the other foot.

VIEWING STEREOROENTGENOGRAMS (Fig. 494)

1. View one foot at a time by matching the left and right stereo views for that foot and viewing them by the stereoscope. The films require some adjustment to obtain perfect register.

2. In stereoscopic viewing, the visual acuity of the observer is a factor. In instances of poor

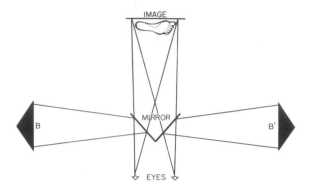

Fig. 494. Stereoscopic viewing (Wheatstone principle). *B,* Roentgenogram illuminated for left eye. *B',* Roentgenogram illuminated for right eye.

accommodation to convergence, it is difficult to break fusion and create the stereoscopic impression.

PLANIGRAPHY (Figs. 495-497)

There are instances when it is highly desirable to demonstrate a section of the foot that is obscured by superimposed images in the conventional roentgenogram. Exploration of the talocalcaneal relationships at the subtalar joint is an example of where lateral views at various metatarsal levels would be of great value. A planigram, in which a sectional view may be performed at any desired level, is the answer to these problems.

The principle of planigraphy consists of making the roentgenogram with the tube moving in an arc in one direction while the film moves in the opposite direction. The part remains immobile. Both tube and film are connected to the movable arm, and the axis upon which it turns is the key to the depth of the section being roentgenographed. At this level, the stationary axis chosen is the section; consequently, a detailed roentgenogram is produced at this level, whereas all other parts are blurred as a result of the motion of the tube and film.

Planigraphic attachments are added to standard roentgenographic tables and equipment. Unfortunately, planigrams are made in the recumbent attitude. There is at present no commercially feasible attachment for the Ortho-x-poser to do planigrams of the weight-supporting foot.

MACRORADIOGRAPHY

Direct magnification of roentgenographic images may be obtained by special technic and equipment. A localizing "spot film" apparatus, which is commonly used in institutional roentgenography, is utilized in connection with a tube of 0.3-mm focal spot. With the tube located 20 inches below the table, the part positioned on the table, and the film located 25 inches above the table, the magnification will be approximately twice.

FINE BONE DETAIL TECHNIC

Weiss (1972) has described a technic for demonstrating fine detail in bones of the hands that is applicable to bones of the foot provided the technical requirements may be met. A rotating anode tube with a 1-mm focus, single-phase-four-valve generator X-ray unit is needed. Kodak industrial AA film without screen is used. Exposure factors are: film-focus distance — 75 cm; 36-37 kVp; 250 ma; and 2.1 sec exposure time. All additional filtration is removed. Film development is by hand, using D19 Kodak developer, 5 min at 25° C. Viewing is assisted by using a modified helio contraster (D'Oude Delft), as for miniature chest films, which gives a magnification of 5-7 linear (25-49 square).

Obviously this technic will only be applied under very special circumstances, such as for a pathology that requires very critical demonstration, for example, the early changes seen in early rheumatoid arthritis, as described by Norgaard (1965).

USE OF FILTER FOR UNIFORM EXPOSURE OF TOES AND TARSUS

A dorsoplantar roentgenogram of the forefoot is commonly overexposed in the toe area if the tarsal area has been properly penetrated. This is particularly true if sufficient exposure is made to insure visualization of the medial aspect of the calcaneus where it articulates with the cuboid. One of the reference points used in charting the midline of the hindfoot is made at this point; the other is at the center of the heel.

Numerous types of wedge-shaped filters have been devised to be placed at the orifice of the X-ray tube, in the cone regulating the

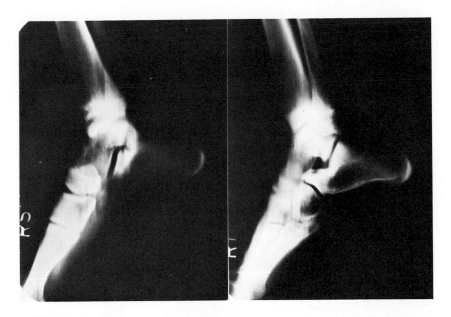

Fig. 495. Planigram, recumbent lateral foot position. *Left,* 5-cm level, medial foot segment. Note anterior subtalar articulation. *Right,* 3-cm level, lateral foot segment. Note posterior subtalar articulation.

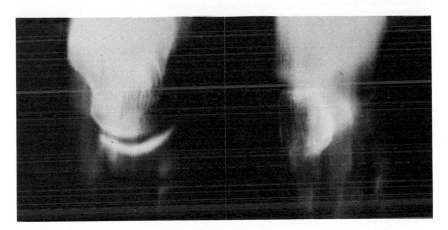

Fig. 496. Planigram, recumbent dorsoplantar (midtarsal) foot position. *Left,* 8-cm level, medial foot segment and talonavicular articulation. *Right,* 3-cm level, lateral foot segment and calcaneocuboid articulation.

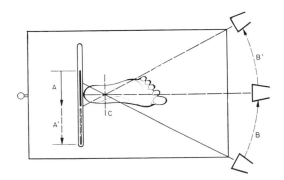

Fig. 497. Principle of planigraph. *A-A',* Film moves in one direction. *B-B',* Tube moves in opposite direction. *C,* Film-tube axis remains immobile. This plane is roentgenographed; other parts are blurred by the motion.

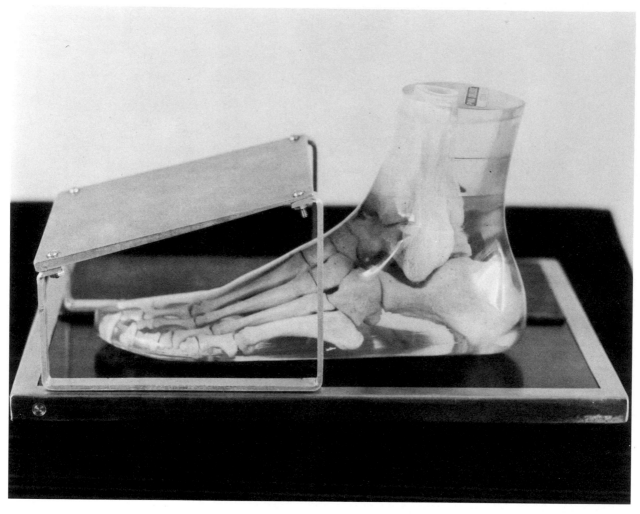

Fig. 498. Foot X-ray filter in place for dorsoplantar view of phantom foot model

beam, or on the plate that carries the filter into the tube housing in front of the useful beam. In each case, there have been problems associated with their use. Since the filter is only needed for the dorsoplantar projection, it needs to be removed for other projections. The off-and-on procedure is time consuming, and the chance of failing to remove the filter and spoiling an exposure is a possibility. Directing the central ray in such a manner as to obtain the most effective value from the filter can also create a problem.

A simple bridgelike device containing a wedge-shaped filter of aluminum (Fig. 498) that can be placed over the foot for each dorso-plantar exposure has been developed by the author. This is easy to manage and provides an improvement in the uniform exposure from toes to tarsus. One size is provided. The thin end is placed at the midtarsal level for the feet of children and small women and moved out so that the thick part of the wedge is over the toe area in large feet. Exposure factors are selected to satisfy exposure of the thickness of the tarsus. The balanced roentgenogram more than compensates for a slight sacrifice in contrast (Fig. 499). An interesting transverse line is exposed across the talus and calcaneus from the end of the wedge that provides a reference line that may be used for charting purposes.

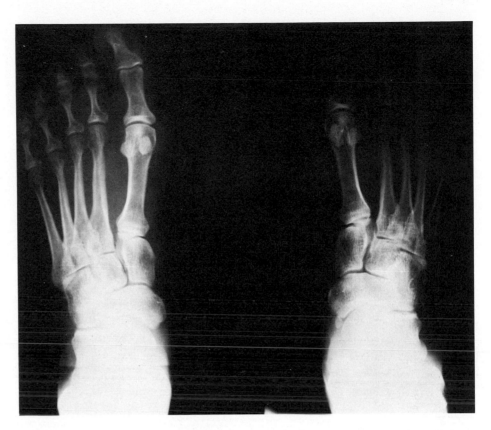

Fig. 499. Comparison of uniformly exposed dorsoplantar view using wedge-shaped filter with conventionally exposed dorsoplantar view. Same exposure factors.

SOFT-TISSUE ROENTGENOGRAPHIC TECHNIC

There are many soft-tissue changes of a physiologic and pathologic nature occurring in foot conditions that warrant roentgenographic examination (Chapter 2). Swellings, soft-tissue tumors, heterotopic calcifications, and early bone callus are demonstrable on the roentgenogram. Many radiopaque contrast media may also be used to show the extent of sinus tracts, cavities, cysts, and the patency of veins and arteries. Location of foreign bodies in soft tissue requires roentgenograms whose density demonstrates soft tissue as well as bone.

The inherent long-scale gradation of density obtained by using special roentgenographic film, such as the Lo-dose mammography film (Du Pont), nonscreen, or industrial type, in conjunction with lower kilovoltage values will produce maximal contrast of the elements within the soft-tissue density.

ANGLE BLOCK POSITIONING

There are occasions when non-weight-supporting oblique view of the foot are desirable, such as in the examination of traumatic conditions or in a comprehensive examination of the tarsus and subtalar joint when specific pathology is suspected, or if the patient cannot sustain body weight. In these instances, angle blocks made of radiolucent plastic foam materials provide a means of helping to steady the foot in the desired position. The standard shape for this type of block is a wedge with a 45° angle at the apex. Several blocks with varying apical angles are useful. An angle block of this kind is also useful if the X-ray equipment has an overhead tube that must be used in a vertical position and the foot has to be placed at an angle for special views. Angle blocks are helpful in immobilizing the foot under many circumstances.

It should be emphasized that anatomical

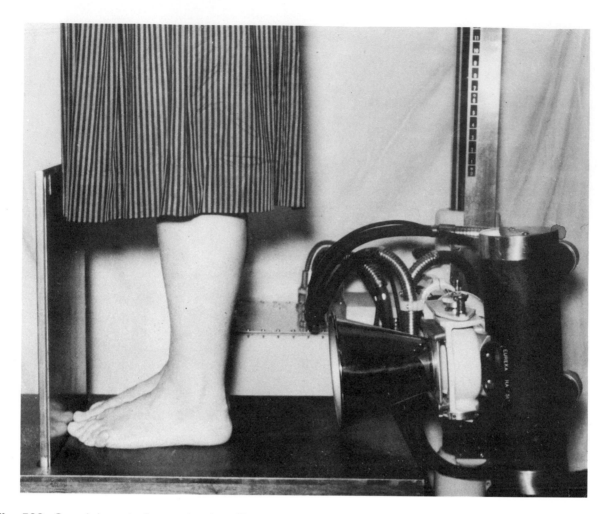

Fig. 500. Special posterior projection.(Reproduced with permission from *Atlas of Foot Roentgenology,* Milton R. Lewis, Chicago, 1964)

judgment should be exercised in choosing the angle of the foot and the direction of the projected central ray to insure that the bones involved will be shown in profile. The central ray should be parallel to the articulation. It should also be observed that due to the geometric laws of image production the part in contact with the film-holder will show greater detail and more accurate size than the part raised on an angle block.

A device consisting of a wooden base having slots that establish angles of 10°, 20°, and 30° with transparent plates held in an apex at the desired angle has been developed by Gabriel and Burger (1967) for fixed positions of the foot and ankle. Roentgenograms exposed in this manner may be accurately reproduced for serial studies.

SPECIAL PROJECTIONS OF SUB-TALAR JOINT

Both the calcaneus and talus are subject to positional changes in three directions. Forward and plantar displacements of the talus can be determined from the lateral view, but a dorso-plantar view is required to demonstrate the medial rotation. Likewise, the position of the calcaneus can be altered by several directional changes, including eversion on its long axis. The subtalar joint is often the key to understanding the altered position of its components. This joint area, including the sustentaculum tali, requires special projections to demonstrate the relative positions of the calcaneus and talus.

Lewis (1963) poses the patient with toes to-

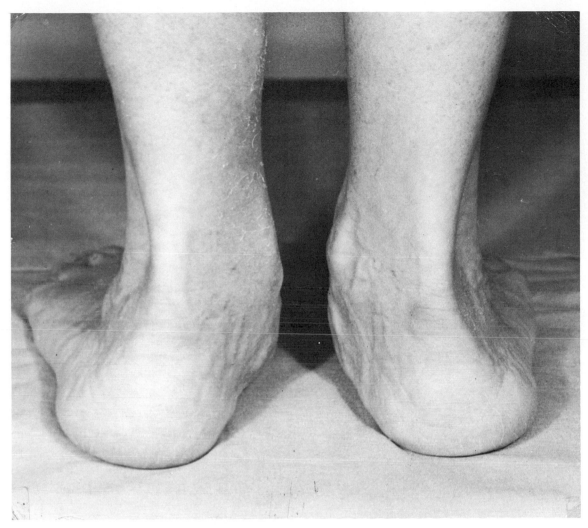

Fig. 501. Subtalar pathology, more in left foot. (Reproduced with permission from *Atlas of Foot Roentgenology*, Milton R. Lewis, Chicago, 1964)

ward the film and the roentgen-ray beam directed from a posteroanterior projection to produce a roentgenogram demonstrating the relationship of the calcaneus to the talus. In addition to showing the plane of the subtalar joint and the position of the sustentaculum tali, the position of the calcaneus is related to the fibula. A slight heel elevation (12/8 inches) is recommended to bring the calcaneus into complete profile, and exposure factors of 60 kVp, 50 mas, and 36 inches are suggested (Figs. 500-503).

Kleiger and Mankin (1961) have demonstrated the posterior aspect of the subtalar joint by means of a posterotangential view similar to the posteroplantar view described in Chapter 24, except that the angle is increased to 45°. This has an elongating effect on the appearance of the calcaneus but does show a profile of the sustentaculum tali that is informative in regard to gross alterations. This view is most effective in the study of the child's foot.

Feist and Mankin (1962) utilize a 45° angle wedge to demonstrate the tarsus and subtalar joint. The medial border of the foot is placed in contact with the 45° wedge so that the lateral border of the foot is elevated and the medial border of the foot touches the film-holder. The central ray is projected vertically to a point just distal to the lateral malleolus. This view shows the anterior subtalar joint and the cuboid and navicular. The middle and posterior

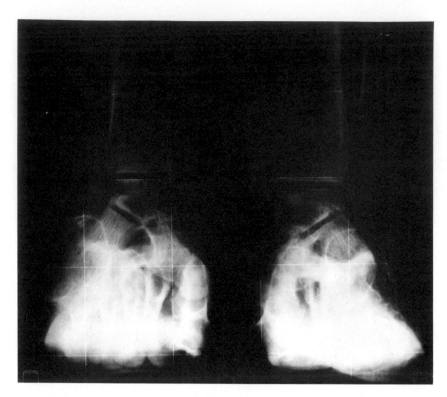

Fig. 502. Severe pronation. Calcaneus appears below the fibula. Talocalcaneal articulation is markedly oblique. Greater change in left foot. (Reproduced with permission from *Atlas of Foot Roentgenology,* Milton R. Lewis, Chicago, 1964.)

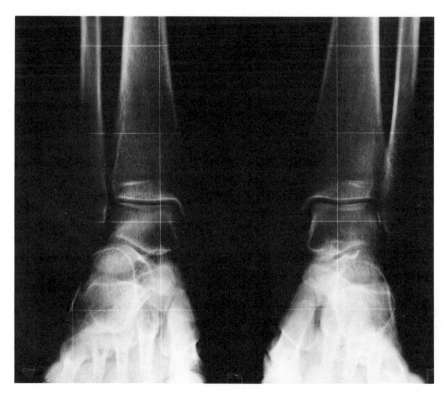

Fig. 503. Normal foot. Calcaneus directly beneath talus. (Reproduced with permission from *Atlas of Foot Roentgenology,* Milton R. Lewis, Chicago, 1964.)

articulations of the subtalar joint are demonstrated by a superoinferior oblique lateral projection with the patient lying on the affected side and the dorsum of the foot touching the film-holder as the heel is slightly raised and the foot extended. The central ray is directed to the ankle joint at a 5° anterior tilt and a 23° angle distally.

Isherwood (1961) demonstrated the three subtalar articulations in a slightly different profile by individual recumbent positions:

    1. Anterior subtalar articulation

      a. Oblique lateral projection.

      b. 45° angle block holds foot in oblique position

      c. Medial-plantar surface of foot on film-holder

      d. Centray ray perpendicular to 1 inch distal to the lateral malleolus.

    2. Middle subtalar articulation

      a. Medial oblique axial projection

      b. 30° angle block supports foot with toes up

      c. Medial surface of foot on wedge while heel is on film-holder

      d. Patient holds foot inverted and dorsiflexed by a bandage sling around forefoot

      e. Central ray angle 10° dorsally to 1 inch distal to lateral malleolus

    3. Posterior subtalar articulation

      a. Lateral oblique axial projection

      b. 30° angle block supports foot with toes up

      c. Lateral border of foot on wedge with heel on film-holder

      d. Patient holds foot dorsiflexed by a bandage sling around forefoot

      e. Central ray at 10° angle to 1 inch distal to medial malleolus

SIMULTANEOUS FOOT-IMPRINT ROENTGENOGRAPHY
(Figs. 504 and 505)

A weight-distribution imprint made while the foot completes a step provides a gross indication of the forces that are transmitted as the patient's weight meets the resistive surface reactions and propulsive action of gait. It is sometimes desirable to record this imprint in accurate register on a roentgenogram of the foot. Although in an earlier chapter we have discussed the independent imprint made on transparent paper that may be used as an overlay on a roentgenogram of the foot, it does not convey the accuracy of an imprint registered directly on the film simultaneously with its roentgenographic exposure. When roentgeno graphic paper is used instead of film and a composite full-foot roentgenogram is made, it may be used in charting for appliances.

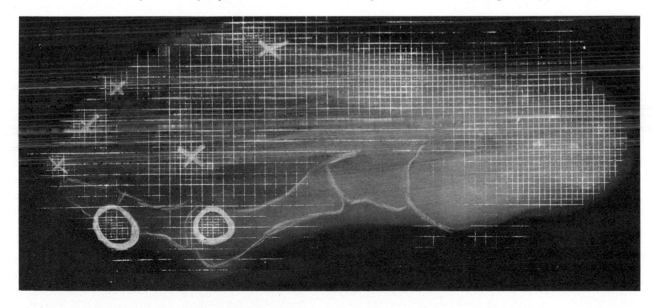

Fig. 504. Orthodynamic roentgenogram (X-ray paper), hallux valgus foot type. Excess imprint to medial sesamoid and interphalangeal joint area of great toe.

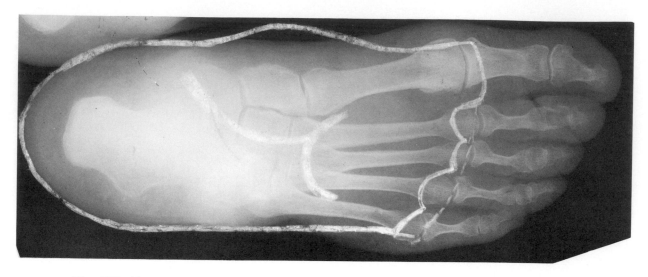

Fig. 505. Roentgenographic chart for parabola compensator (R. Sansone mold)

METHOD

A flexible plastic film-holder (nonevacuated, vacuum-pack type), 10 × 12 inches, is loaded with an inked imprint mat. A sheet of roentgenographic paper with the emulsion side facing the mat is loaded in the film-holder, taking care that its natural bowing helps to hold it away from the ink. The loaded holder is carefully handled and placed on the floor in front of the roentgen unit. The patient is instructed to stand a pace away from the holder and with a natural step place his foot in the center of the holder. Then he brings the other foot alongside and stands still in this position for the exposures. The dorsoplantar view is taken first; then the tube is moved in back of the patient and the superoplantar view is made. The patient is then instructed to step forward off the exposure holder. Repeat for the other foot.

POLAROID ROENTGENOGRAPHY

Polaroid film that provides a 4 × 5-inch roentgenographic print in 15 seconds processing time has been applied to foot roentgenography. The image is a photographic positive with background white and tissue elements and bone dark. Polaroid film has special applications. Detection and location of a foreign body by surface wire plotting and checks of instrument position during removal has been demonstrated by Block (1972) (Fig. 506). Roentgeno-graphic identification and location of a calcaneal exostosis by injected needles and immediate postoperative results have been demonstrated by Kaplan and Stone (1971). Toe bones and their irregularities and malalignments related to helomata are demonstrable. Position of fragments, splinting reduction, and healing progress of phalangeal fractures may be shown. Pathoanatomy and bone outlines in the tarsus are possible, although limited to the 4 × 5 inch size of the polaroid film. Bone pathology or fracture should be confirmed by X-ray film.

Perhaps the first thing to be considered in using Polaroid roentgenography is to establish the same safety precautions as those used under normal film roentgenography governing radiation exposure to doctor, patient, and personnel. The warning applies particularly to its use during surgical procedures when a portable or auxiliary X-ray machine is used in the surgery. It is suggested that a special collimating cone be used that reduces the useful beam to an area not more than one inch greater than the film size used. The X-ray beam should not be directed at anyone in the operating stage. The Polaroid film cassette should be wrapped in a sterile cloth for the procedure. Under no circumstances should the tube-film distance be less than 24 inches. Technics for a 6-inch distance are unwarranted and extremely hazardous. A short exposure technic with intensifying

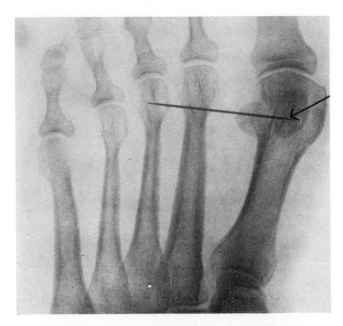

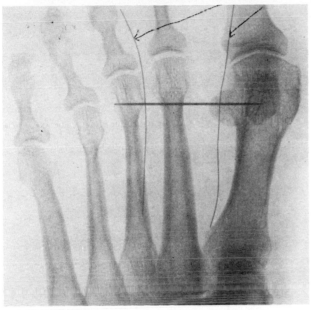

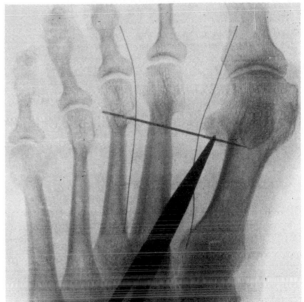

Fig. 506. Polaroid roentgenogram showing *1,* needle in foot, *2,* locating wires, *3,* hemostat grasping needle for removal. (Courtesy of I.H. Block, D.P.M. J. Florida Podiat. Ass.)

screens must be used. Sterility should be maintained by draping the X-ray unit.

There are two types of Polaroid film applicable to foot roentgenography. Type 52 film is of medium contrast, fine grain, and an excellent tonal range. It will yield relatively finer detail than Type 57 film, which is a faster film used to minimize exposure factors. A rule of thumb is to use Type 52 for forefoot and digital work and Type 57 for the tarsus.

Both film types should be used in a cassette provided with a detail intensifying screen. This reduces exposure factors needed to a minimum. Polaroid film should not be X-ray exposed in the processor (holder). This device constitutes the "darkroom" into which the exposed film is placed for development. Full instructions come with the equipment.

Polaroid roentgenography is a two-step procedure: exposure in the cassette with intensifying screen and development in the film processor holder.

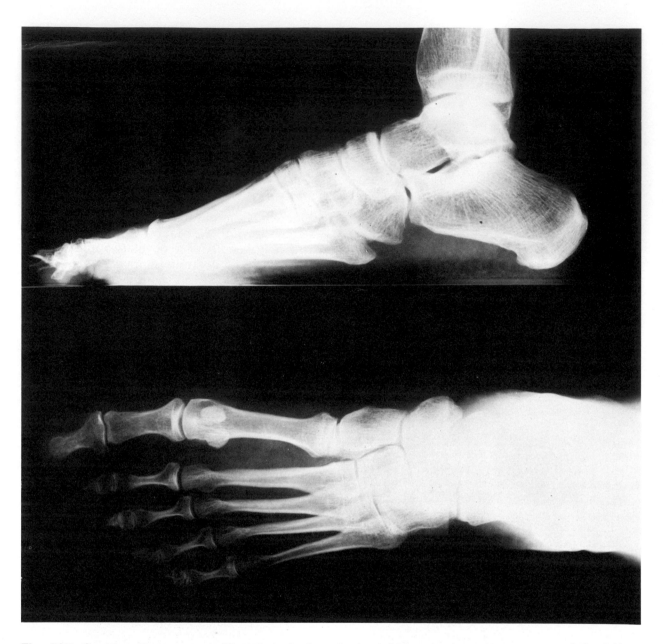

Fig. 507. Positive X-ray paper (Kodak Industrex Instant 600 paper) roentgenogram. A foot X-ray filter was used in the dorsoplantar view.

SUGGESTED TECHNIC GUIDELINES:

Forefoot and toes: Film Type 52, 60 kVp, 10 ma, 30″, 1/4 sec.

Tarsus: Film Type 57, 60 kVp, 10 ma, 30″, 1/8 sec.

As in using any technic guideline, a set of trial exposures should be made and appropriate corrections in technic instituted. Time is the preferable factor to vary. Overexposed films will be too light; reduce exposure to correct. Underexposed films will be too dark; increase exposure to correct. Overdevelopment increases contrast. Underdevelopment produces images that may be faint and muddy.

POSITIVE X-RAY PAPER ROENT-GENOGRAM

A type of photosensitized paper (Kodak Industrex Instant 600 paper[1]) provides a roentgenogram (Fig. 507) of good detail, contrast, and density. The areas of increased density appear white, grading to black for areas of decreased density to yield an appearance similar to that of a film roentgenogram. The high contrast and fine resolution of Kodak Industrex Instant 600 paper is of superior quality.

If the paper is loaded in a cassette with a single Cronex Hi-Plus intensifying screen, the exposure factors should match those used for exposing a nonscreen film in a cardboard holder. Use of a Cronex Lightning Plus intensifying screen will reduce mAs approximately 30 percent.

The Kodak Industrex Instant 600 paper is processed in 10 seconds by feeding it through a Kodak Industrex instant processor model P-1, Kodak Ektamatic processor, or a stabilization photographic paper processor, using Hi-Speed processing solutions. The paper roentgenogram is immediately readable, though damp. It dries quickly and flat if laid on a smooth surface. The image will be stable for weeks without further treatment; however, to insure a permanent image, the paper should be placed in a fixing solution, washed and dried.

Although not very practical, if a stabilization processor is not available, the paper may be manually processed in trays by developing by sight 30 to 60 seconds in Kodak Liquid X-ray Developer, agitating continuously, rinsing in Kodak Stop Bath SB-1, fixing 2 to 4 minutes in Kodak Rapid Fixer while agitating continuously, and washing for 30 minutes.

The positive paper roentgenogram has many interesting applications.

1. Diagnosis of bony factors involved with hyperkeratosis.
2. Instant reading for control during surgical procedures.
3. Foreign-body detection.
4. Foreign-body orientation for surgical removal. Instant reading for positioning instruments for delivery of foreign body.
5. Instant reading before and after reduction of fractures.
6. Biomechanical foot studies.
7. Charting for anatomical orientation.
8. Pattern for foot appliances.
9. Medical illustrations; for example, exhibits and publication reproduction.
10. A direct-reading "X-ray picture" for case presentation with no need for a view box.
11. If properly processed, may be filed in a case folder for easy access.
12. A duplicate roentgenogram that may be sent to a consultant.

SIMULTANEOUS PAPER AND FILM ROENTGENOGRAMS

The simultaneous exposure of X-ray paper and X-ray film will provide a conventional roentgenogram and an X-ray paper duplicate. To obtain this combination:

1. Prepare a cassette with a Cronex Hi-Plus intensifying screen on the tube side and a Cronex fast detail screen on the back side.
2. Load by facing the X-ray paper against the Hi-Plus screen and the Kodak Blue Brand Medical film[2] against the single fast detail screen.
3. Interspace black paper or a previously totally exposed film as an opaque buffer between the paper and film to prevent extraneous light from filtering through the back of the paper during exposure and fogging the film.
4. Expose by using factors for the X-ray paper; the X-ray film will receive a balanced exposure simultaneously.
5. Process film in usual manner and X-ray paper with a stabilization processor.
6. Warning: do not use a cassette prepared for the special film-paper procedure for any other purpose, since the mismatched screens will produce an unsatisfactory roentgenogram.

Essentially, the X-ray film-paper combination achieves the instant reading of the paper and a permanent legal record on film. Numerous applications of the two media will be apparent.

The foot is ideally suited for X-ray paper roentgenograms because of its size and osse-

---

1. Kodak Industrex Instant 600 paper is supplied in useful sizes of 14 × 17, 4½ × 17, and 8 × 10 inches in boxes of 100 sheets. One 14 × 17 sheet may be cut to make one 10 × 12, two 5 × 7, and two 4 × 6 sheets. Special orders for the 10 × 12 inch paper in minimum quantities of 1,500 sq ft are available to distributors.

2. Kodak Blue Brand Medical X-ray film is an Eastman Kodak company product.

ous nature. Positive X-ray paper roentgeno-grams are recommended for the special applications noted. It should not be used for general roentgenography.

SUGGESTED TECHNIC GUIDELINES
(AVERAGE WOMAN'S FOOT):

Cronex Hi-Plus Screen[1]
    Lateral view: 25″, 55 kVp, 10 mA, 2½ sec.
    Dorsoplantar view: 25″, 55 kVp, 10 mA, 2 sec.
Cronex Lightning Plus Screen[1]
    Lateral view: 25″, 55 kVp, 10 mA, 1¾ sec.
    Dorsoplantar view: 25″, 55 kVp, 10 mA, 1½ sec.

Note: When making a simultaneous exposure of positive X-ray paper and Kodak Blue Brand Medical X-ray film[2] or Cronex 2 X-ray film, using a cassette prepared with a Cronex Hi-Plus front screen and Cronex Fast Detail back screen. Use the exposure factors above to match Cronex Hi-Plus Screen technic.

Although the conventional cassette may be used to hold the X-ray paper and intensifying screen, a plastic vacuum-packed cassette (E-Z-EM Vacupac[3]) has a theoretical advantage of improved detail sharpness by improving screen-paper contact. A vacuum pump is attached to the special cassette loaded with X-ray paper and intensifying screen to evacuate air from the cassette before exposure. The reusable cassette and method of use were developed for use with Du Pont's Lo-dose mammography film[1] and screen which may also be used for soft-tissue roentgenograms of the foot.

HAMMONDS' POSTURAL TRI-PLANE SCANOGRAM ROENTGENOGRAPHY

Significant information is to be gained by a proper roentgenographic tri-plane scanogram

---

1. Cronex intensifying screens and Lo-dose mammography film are Du Pont photo products.

2. Kodak Blue Brand medical X-ray film is an Eastman Kodak Company product.

3. The Vacupac cassette may be obtained from the E-Z-EM Company, Inc., 111 Swalm Street, Westbury, N.Y. 11590. Mityvac, a hand-held and hand-operated vacuum pump, may be obtained from Neward Die & Manufacturing Co., Inc., 2066 West 11th Street, Upland, California 91786.

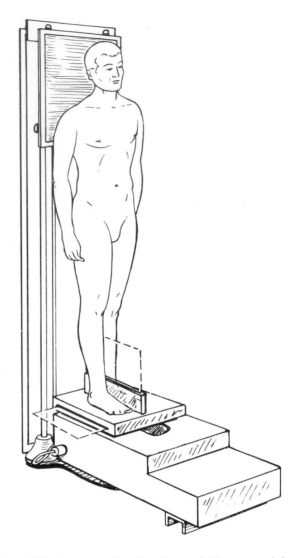

Fig. 508. Schematic drawing of Hammonds' Posture-Poser (courtesy of C.M. Hammonds, D.P.M.)

survey of the spine, pelvis, knees, ankles, and feet to determine the presence of superstructural abnormality or accommodation in patients who have a postural malalignment, according to Hammonds (1959). He claims that postural malalignment cannot be isolated to any one part but involves the entire postural complex.

Hammonds has developed a device (U.S. Pat. 3,524,057, 1970) that produces comparative tri-plane scanograms of the spine, pelvis, knees, ankles, and feet at various levels and planes of exposure with the patient posed in the static stance attitude with the feet in natural angle

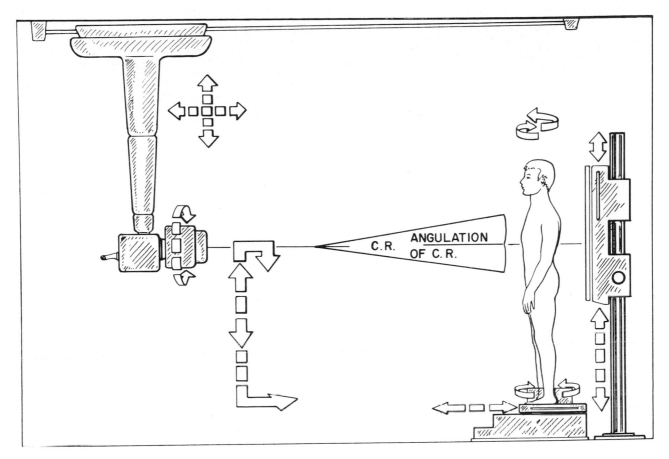

Fig. 509. Schematic diagram of adjustments needed to perform tri-plane scanograms in conjunction with Hammonds' Posture-Poser (courtesy of C.M. Hammonds, D.P.M.)

and width of stance. The device consists of a stance platform, a vertical film cassette for lateral foot view, a film well beneath the platform to hold the film cassette for dorsoplantar and oblique views, and a vertical cassette holder using a Bucky diaphragm that is adjustable from foot to head (Fig. 508). The stance platform is automatically adjustable to rotation and fore-and-aft positions by a controlled power source. X-ray equipment with a capability of doing heavy-body roentgenography is needed. The tube head should adjust for lateral, oblique, and vertical views from head to foot (Fig. 509).

A standardized technique is used that may be duplicated. Of most importance is that once the patient is properly positioned on the device an entire series of views may be exposed while the patient retains the same position. This is accomplished by utilizing cassette holders that do not interfere with the patient's stance and by rotation of the stance platform in front of the vertical film cassette holder that is adjustable to any desired level.

With the assurance that all roentgenographic views reflect the natural skeletal alignment of the patient, the scanograms are charted and coordinated through a system of anatomical reference lines and measurable angles by which the biomechanics of the feet are related to the pelvis and spine (Chapter 26). A comparison is made of the left side with the right side of the composite chart by a plus or minus measurement of the angles shown. The clinical significance of these contralateral relationships indicate the alignment of each foot and the position of each component in the postural complex. Each angle reflects specific alignment problems (Chapter 26).

BIBLIOGRAPHY

Armstrong, R.H.: Foot Opacities — Non-osseous, J. Amer. Podiat. Ass. 53:431, 1963.

Barnes, R.B., and McLachlan, D., Jr.: Roentgenographic Techniques: Soft Tissue Surface Detail, Foreign Body Localization, Amer. J. Roentgen. 50:366, 1943.

Batson, O.V., and Carpentier, V.E.: Stereoscopic Depth Perception, Amer. J. Roentgen. 51:202, 1944.

Becker, M.L.: Personal communication, Chicago, Ill.

Becker, R.R.: Shoes are Medicine, J. Natl. Ass. Chiropodists 4(4):29, 1950.

Beckman, H.: Personal assistance in developing forefoot filter, 1973.

Block, I.H.: Polaroid Radiography in Podiatry, J. Florida Podiat. Ass. 27:10, 1972.

Block, I.H.: Wedge-shaped Filters for Radiography of the Foot, J. Amer. Podiat. Ass. 58:182, 1968.

Campbell, C.J., Roach, J.F., and Jabbur, M.: Xeroroentgenography, J. Bone Joint Surg. 41-A:271, 1959.

Carvahal-Forrero, J., and Thompson, M.R.: Roentgenography of Soft Tissues by Monochromatic Roentgen Radiation and Color Forming Developers, Amer. J. Roentgen. 50:248, 1943.

Cullinan, J.E.: *Illustrated Guide to X-ray Techniques.* Philadelphia: J.B. Lippincott, 1972.

Downey, M.A., and Dorothy, W.L.: A Radiographic Technique to Demonstrate the Plantar Aspect of the Forefoot in Stance, J. Amer. Podiat. Ass. 59:140, 1969.

Feist, J.H., and Mankin, H.J.: The Tarsus — Base Relationships and Motions in the Adult and Definition of Optimal Recumbent Oblique Projection, Radiology 79:250, 1962.

Ferguson, A.B.: *Roentgen Diagnosis of the Extremities.* New York: Paul B. Hoeber, Inc., 1939.

Field Emission Corporation: Personal communication re: Polaroid Land Film Holder No. 545 and Flexitron Model 1320 X-ray Cassette. McMinnville, Oregon, 1972.

Gabriel, G.R., and Burger, E.S.: Angulation Plates for Fixed Angle Radiography, J. Amer. Podiat. Ass. 57:1, 1967.

Gamble, F.O.: A Radiographic Pattern for Foot Appliance Construction, Clin. J. Chirop. Podiat. & Pedic. Surg. 11:1, 1940.

Gamble, F.O.: A Special Approach to Foot Radiography, Radiog. Clin. Photog. 19:78, 1943.

Gass, C.C., and Hatchett, C.S.: A Simple Inexpensive Set of Prisms for Viewing Stereoscopic Roentgenograms, Amer. J. Roentgen. 61:715, 1952.

Geissberger, H.: Wedge-shaped Filters for Improved Radiography of the Thoracic Vertebrae and the Foot: Med. Radiog. Photog. 42:6, 1966.

Gill, G.G.: A Simple Roentgenographic Method for the Measurement of Bone Length: Modification of Millwei's Method of Slit Scanography, J. Bone Joint Surg. 26-A: 767, 1944.

Hammonds, C.M.: Personal communication. Chief of Podiatry, Veterans Administration Hospital, Ft. Miley, San Francisco, California.

Hammonds, C.M.: Concept of Dynamic Relationships of the Whole Human Mechanism in Bipedal Position, Podiatry Record (Sept.-Oct.), 1959.

Hammonds, C.M.: Hammonds' Posture-Poser, U.S. Pat. 3,524,057, 1970.

Hammonds, C.M.: Personal interview. Chief of Podiatry, Veterans Administration Hospital, Ft. Miley, San Francisco, California, 1970.

Harris, R.I., and Beath, T.: *Army Foot Survey.* Ottawa: National Research Council of Canada, 1947.

Havey, H.J.: The Use of Radiopaque Substances in Foot Radiography, Chiropody Record 35:2 (Feb.), 1952.

Hickey, P.M.: Teleroentgenography as an Aid in Orthopedic Measurements, Amer. J. Roentgen. 11:232, 1924.

Isaid, J.H., Ostru, B.J., and Cullinan, J.E.: Magnification Roentgenography, Med. Radiog. Photog. 38:92, 1962.

Isherwood, I.: A Radiological Approach to the Subtalar Joint Surg. 43-B:566, 1961.

Jones, C.L.: The Damaging Effects of a Disaligned Musculoskeletal System, J. Amer. Podiat. Ass. 61:369, 1971.

Jones, L.: *The Postural Complex.* Springfield, Ill.: Charles C Thomas, 1955.

Johnson, M.L.: Personal communication. Technical Sales Representative, Radiography Markets, Eastman Kodak Company, Phoenix, Arizona, 1974.

Kaplan, E.G., and Stone, J.A.: A New View on Calcaneal Spur Surgery, J. Foot Surg. 1:8, 1971.

Kieffer, J.: The General Principles of Body-section Radiography, Radiog. Clin. Photog. 19(1):2, 1943.

Kleiger, B., and Mankin, H.J.: A Roentgenographic Study of the Calcaneus by Means of the Posterior Tangential View, J. Bone Joint Surg. 43-A:961, 1961.

Klein, E., Klein, M., Klein, H., and Newman, A.T.: An Investigation into Some Practical Aspects of Roentgen-ray Stereoptics, Amer. J. Roentgen. 49:682, 1943.

Lawrence, D.J.: Written communication concerning Kodak Industrex instant 600 paper: Acting Director, Medical Trade Relations, Radiography Markets Division, Eastman Kodak Company, Rochester, N.Y., May 8, 1974.

Lewis, M.R.: An X-ray Technique to Visualize the Subtalar Joint, J. Amer. Podiat. Ass. 53:128, 1963.

Lewis, M.R.: *Atlas of Foot Roentgenology.* Chicago: M.R. Lewis, 1964.

Merrill, V.: *Atlas of Roentgenographic Positions,* ed. 3, Vol. 1. St. Louis, C.V. Mosby Co., 1967.

Meshan, I.: *Analysis of Roentgen Signs in General Roentgenology.* Philadelphia: W.B. Saunders Co., 1973.

Millwie, R.H.: Slit Scanography, Radiology 28:483, 1937.

Moore, H.D.: New Method of Venography, Brit. J. Surg. 57:78, 1949.

Nelson, D.H.: Forced Inversion of Ankles, J. Bone Joint Surg. 42-B:793, 1960.

Norgaard, F.: Earliest Roentgenological Changes in Polyarthritis of the Rheumatoid Type: Rheumatoid Arthritis, J. Radiology 82:325, 1965.

Sedlin, E.D.: A Device for Stress Inversion of Eversion Roentgenograms of the Ankle, J. Bone Joint Surg. 42-A: 1184, 1960.

Thompson, E.: Electrical Engineering, March 11, 1896.

Tisa, V.N.: Forefoot Exposer, J. Amer. Podiat. Ass. 62:146, 1972.

Walton, G.J.: Personal communication. X-ray Technical Representative, Photo Products Department, E.I. Du Pont de Nemours & Co. (Inc.), Tucson, Arizona, 1974.

Weiss, A.: A Technique for Demonstrating Fine Detail in Bones of the Hands, Clin. Radiol. 23:185, 1972.

26 CHARTING IN FOOT ROENTGENOLOGY

Charting the foot roentgenogram for clinical purposes is the recording on the roentgenogram of the diagnostic features that will add a graphic description to the usual written exposition of findings and diagnostic conclusions.

In an academic context, charting the foot roentgenogram consists of determining reference points, lines, and angles that may be compared or measured so that numerical values, indexes, and ratios may be provided as criteria for assessing relative positions of the foot bones to assist in the classification of foot abnormalities.

As a practical matter, charting is a very valuable schooling exercise for the tyro. It has merit when discretely used in making a case presentation to the patient. The value of charted criteria in research and for statistical surveys is recognized. The charted roentgenogram is needed when it is an integral part of a diagnostic correlation with biomechanical measurements.

The student of foot roentgenology will find it useful to chart roentgenograms routinely until confident that he is knowledgeable enough to limit his charting to critical diagnostic features. The experienced practitioner studies the overall pathology and pathoanatomy and quickly analyzes the specific areas that contribute to a comprehensive roentgen diagnosis. However, it is most interesting that charting may provide some startling reappraisals of criteria that have been accepted as irrefutable diagnostic evidence.

It is recommended that either an X-ray paper duplicate exposed simultaneously with the film or a transparent overlay on the roentgenogram be used upon which markings may be recorded.

There are many pitfalls in producing, marking, and measuring a foot roentgenogram for charting purposes. Likewise, the use of a charted foot roentgenogram for diagnostic purposes has many limitations. Small, subtle changes may be overlooked if too much attention is given to gross configurations of the diagram. The human foot is so variable in the size and shape of its framework that it is difficult to assign a range of numerical values to chartable criteria of normalcy. However, a chart that points out the signs and direction of alignment change serves a useful purpose. Quantitative analysis of numerical criteria is best applied to a comparison between the feet of an individual rather than to a statistical norm. Statistical values are interesting, and each case may be measured to compare its values with the means and modes of the particular categories. But the fundamental issue is the ability to make a clinical value judgment concerning the pathoanatomy demonstrated by the charted foot roentgenogram.

Several methods of charting proposed by various investigators will be presented, and the purpose of each method will be individually discussed. In the orientation and critique of the principles of charting, certain deficiencies will be indicated.

In the section of this book on the diagnosis of foot pathoanatomy, diagrams have been provided to show the relative anatomic bone positions of a normal foot, functional foot faults, orthodigital problems, and abnormal foot types. The comprehensive descriptions of the bone shapes and positions that have been offered explain normal and abnormal anatomy in a concrete manner, and the charting and measurements have been limited to the clinically important items, such as calcaneal inclination, talo-longitudinal axis angle, first and second intermetatarsal angle, hallux abductus angle, and the parabola angle of the metatarsophalangeal joints. The other roentgen signs and indicators used include midtarsal joint cyma, congruent or closed sinus tarsi, pseudo-sinus tarsi, gaping joints, overlapping bones, tightly bound bones, loosely bound bones, and abnormal bone shapes. This chapter elaborates on charting.

At the end of this chapter, an entirely different category of charts related to the clinical application of foot roentgenograms will be presented: (1) a check list for a systematic survey of a foot roentgenogram for diagnostic entities; (2) a case presentation chart that coordinates diagnosis, prognosis, and the treatment program; and (3) a master chart for comparison of traditional, roentgenological, and biomechanical terms, descriptions, and sequelae of foot deformities.

In addition, a new system will be offered that charts medial and lateral longitudinal segments of the foot to show pathoanatomical directional shifts. Appropriate angles will be shown for contralateral comparison of left and right feet.

A highly critical attitude is taken of charting in general because indiscriminate, arbitrary, and inconsistent reference lines have been applied in some methods that create unrealistic anatomic relationships. A framework of reference should reflect acceptable anatomic alignment patterns. If charted criteria consisting of numerical indexes and ratios have validity, there is, of course, no objection to their use in elaboration on pathoanatomic positions. As will be pointed out, there are special uses of charting that are clinically and statistically significant. On the other hand, charting is not a diagnostic panacea nor a substitute for a basic and comprehensive knowledge of the bone images that is basic to the roentgenological interpretation of the pathoanatomy of the foot. As so aptly stated by Catterall (1968): "The study of radiographs is a practical art." He decries the fact that when a ruler is produced, lines tend to get drawn, angles appear, measurements are expressed as ratios, and pseudo-mathematical calculations emerge with an aura of inviolable scientific law, when, in fact, they can be no more than useful approximations. We agree.

ORIENTATION

Methods of reducing the sources of errors in

charting will be discussed and the value of determinations from charting will be placed in proper perspective in the following discussions.

AVOID INCOMPATIBLE COMPARISONS

Values from charted roentgenograms are often compared to criteria established by other investigators. It therefore becomes imperative that any roentgenogram used for comparative information must be made by the same precise technique as the one used for the roentgenograms from which the criteria were developed. Even if comparable techniques are used in producing the roentgenogram, the reference points, lines, and angles must be marked and measured in precisely the same manner as those for the roentgenogram used to obtain the comparative criteria. It is invalid for diagnostic purposes to select at random a roentgenogram for charting, unless these conditions can be satisfied.

INSURE STANDARDIZED TECHNIC

Since investigators generally follow a standardized technic in producing the roentgenograms used for charting, the strict acceptability of roentgenograms for charting purposes depends on precise standardization of positioning technic, as has been advocated throughout this text. The size, shape, and relative positions of foot bones on the roentgenogram are determined by the geometries of X-ray image formation; consequently, chartable roentgenograms must be made by following the rules for accurate image production.

In an extensive study of the validity of standardized production of foot roentgenograms and their measurement, Venning and Hardy (1951) ascertained that under precise conditions of standardization and measurement, the statistical sources of error were minimal. Our experience in producing standardized foot roentgenograms has been one of high fidelity in duplicating roentgenograms. This has been demonstrated by comparing roentgenograms of the feet of the same patient taken over a span of 20 years. A simple test to prove bone position fidelity is to place one film over the other on a viewbox and check the matching of bone images. The only differences that should be seen are those due to pathoanatomical changes that have taken place in the interval.

The natural weight-supporting attitude is the most feasible one for establishing standardization of roentgenograms used for charting to demonstrate the biomechanical status of the foot.

It is interesting to note that the roentgenograms in the extensive survey of 7,167 feet by Harris and Beath (1947) were not taken in a completely natural standing position. The patient was posed on a platform inclined 15 degrees with the feet placed parallel instead of at the natural angle of stance. This plantarflexed position of the foot precludes natural weight distribution and pull of the tendo achillis so very important to the determination of joint excursions and bone alignment in the foot under stress. The natural alignment of the angle of stance is lost if the feet are posed parallel or if the central ray is projected between the two feet when both feet are roentgenographed together in the dorsoplantar view. This latter procedure also creates sideway geometric distortions (Fig. 510). However, since these procedures have been standardized, it may be argued that the statistics obtained from the study are valid, and this is technically true under the specific limitations discussed.

In some surveys involving children too young to cooperate in the proper stance (Davis and Hatt, 1955; Templeton, McAllister, and Zim, 1965; Ritchie and Keim, 1968), simulation of the weight supporting position has been attempted by pressing a board against the bottom of the foot while the child is in a supine position. The resulting roentgenograms used for charting present only gross alignment profiles. The same is true of roentgenograms made with the foot in a relaxed position. The technic and frame devised by LeNoir (1966) to produce standardized roentgenograms of infants' feet produces standardized roentgenograms, and his method of charting and interpretation give acceptable judgments.

ASSESS POSSIBLE GEOMETRIC INACCURACIES

Although the foot roentgenogram may have been made using a standardized technic, the general foot shape and individual bone shapes have multiangular planes that are difficult to resolve into accurate-size images in a single-plane roentgen view. Some indexes of charting involve angular relationships of the foot bones that rely on angles formed by lines bisecting geometrically distorted shapes of individual bones. It is difficult or often impossible to apply accurately a true angular value to relative bone positions in a single-plane roentgen view. Trigonometric formulae would be needed to calculate values for the polyhedral angles present in the foot.

The transverse-plane intermetatarsal angle between the first and second metatarsal bones is a commonly used index for the adduction of the first metatarsal in cases of hallux abductus valgus, but this angle is subject to geometric aberration in both the high and low foot structure. According to Turvey (1952), the higher the metatarsal inclination, the greater the intermetatarsal angle, if both feet are roentgenographed at the same time with the central ray centered between the two feet, because the intermetatarsal angle is reduced due to distortion by sideway divergence of the central ray. If each foot is roentgenographed separately with the central ray centered over the base of the second metatarsal, maximal reliability may be presumed for the alignment of all metatarsals and the rest of the foot (Fig. 510).

Inversion of the entire foot is another factor that alters the intermetatarsal angle by adducting the metatarsals, yet subluxation in the transverse metatarsal articulations can cancel some of the adduction. Abduction or adduction of either the first or second metatarsal would also influence the intermetatarsal angle. It is thus obvious that the position of any line or angle of reference within the foot structure is dependent on the alignment of adjacent bones and of the entire foot. Consequently, the entire foot should be critically evaluated before the significance of any one charted value is assessed.

Attention is drawn to a possible gross misconception obtained from the dorsoplantar view concerning the direction taken by a line bisecting the roentgen image of the head of the talus because the relationships between the talus and calcaneus are different in the normal foot than in the pronated or supinated foot. In pronation, the talus adducts, extends distally, and plantarflexes, with a severely everted cal-

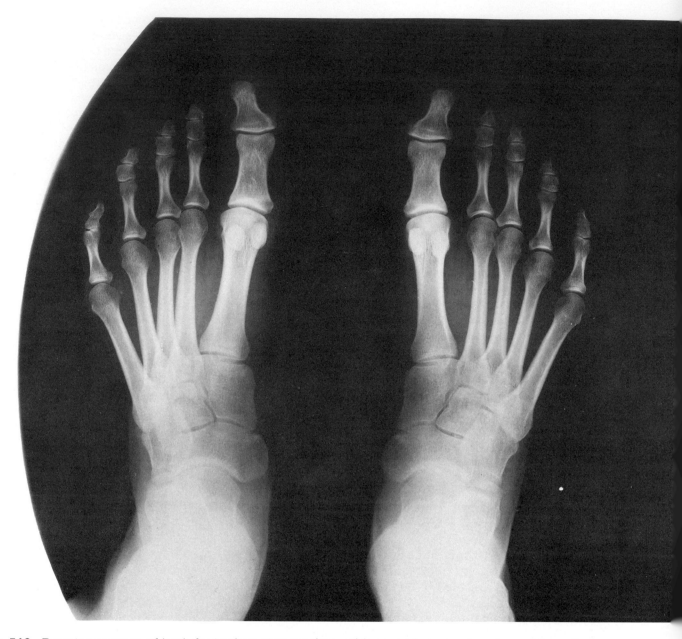

Fig. 510. Roentgenogram of both feet taken at same time, with central ray centered over base of second metatarsal, right foot. Note overlapping metatarsal bases of left foot caused by geometric distortion due to divergence of X-ray beam. (Left side is cone cut.)

caneus and subtalar joint. Therefore, the narrowest dimension of the head of the talus is presented in the roentgenogram, and the apparent curve and size of the talar head are less than those of the normal foot. In supination, the talus abducts, moves proximally, and dorsiflexes, with a severely inverted calcaneus and subtalar joint. This foot presents the broadest dimension of its talar head in profile, and the

apparent curve and size of the head are greater than in the normal foot. Selection of reference points at the apparent extremes of each side of the head of the talus for the construction of a bisecting line creates a line of reference that drastically belies the common concept that the talocalcaneal angle of which it is one side is greater in pronation and lesser in supination.

An angle formed by a line extended from the

bisector of the head of the talus with the calcaneus to the longitudinal axis of the foot or of the first metatarsal will be materially decreased in extreme eversion of the talus and increased in extreme inversion of the talus (Figs. 511A, B, C). In extreme cases, an arbitrary compensation of ± 10° is suggested to allow for variance. In average moderate eversion or inversion of the talus, a profile of the head is preserved that provides acceptable relationships between the talus, calcaneus, longitudinal foot axis, and first metatarsal (Figs. 511D, E. F). In moderate cases, a ± 5° compensation is suggested. The amount of talar head exposed is subject to the same variations of measurement and a 10% latitude should be made to compensate for the extreme range and 5% for the moderate range of eversion or inversion.

Measurements of talar tilt under stress have been made by Rubin and Witten (1960) on frontal plane roentgenograms of 150 normal subjects. They found talar tilts of 3° to 23° in 56 percent of the subjects. They also found a similar range of talar tilt in 72 percent of 18 subjects with severe flexible flatfoot. An unstable sprained ankle was found to have a talar tilt of 31°. Such a range of talar tilt indicates the possible malposition that may occur in pronated or supinated feet and the variable range for talocalcaneal angles that may be demonstrated.

Not only is the positional change a misleading factor, but an abnormal shape of the neck and head of the talus should be equally suspect. A clue to the evasive inclination of ontogonic origin of the neck and head of the talus in the frontal plane would be a narrow profile if the inclination is large and a broad profile if the inclination is small.

These dramatic examples of the gross variance possible for the talocalcaneal angle are an indictment of the sacrosanctity of the use of the angle as an infallible criterion for diagnosis. The total status of the foot should be correlated. Of most importance, a value judgment should be made regarding position by considering the amount of overlap or gap between the head of the talus and the distal end of the calcaneus.

IDENTIFY ABNORMAL BONE SHAPES THAT CAUSE CHARTING FAULTS

A major source of error in arriving at definitive biomechanical evaluations of charted roentgenograms is the variable shape of the talus (Chapter 13, Figs. 254-256). The shape of the head and neck of the talus may vary in three aspects: (1) inclination of the head in the frontal plane, (2) inclination of the neck and head in the transverse plane, and (3) declination of the neck and head in the sagittal plane. The talus may also present either a long or short neck or head which can greatly alter charting values. In the conventional roentgenographic views of the foot usually used for charting, it is impossible to assess the total implications of the geometries of these variations. If the investigator recognizes the abnormality in the shape of the talus and discounts the resulting discrepancy in angular measurements, some useful information may be obtained by charting.

Variations in the shape of the calcaneus can be a source of error in charting. An excessively long or short anterior part of the calcaneus will influence charting interpretation. An excessive laterosuperior margin of the calcaneus can distort any measurement of overlap of the talus and calcaneus visualized in the sagittal plane on the lateral view. The distal end of the calcaneus, as visualized in the transverse plane, can have two distinctly different shapes: the distal-medial margin either ends abruptly or it slopes gradually in a curve to unite with the sustentaculum tali. If the latter, the location of a specific point to represent the distal-medial margin of the calcaneus is practically impossible (see Fig. 514).

PROVIDE SUFFICIENT ROENTGEN VIEWS

Both the lateral sagittal-plane roentgenogram and the dorsoplantar transverse-plane roentgenogram should be charted for comprehensive analysis of relative bone positions. In addition to providing a key to the possible source of error in values assigned to a polyhedral angle, determinations can be made from biplane views that help to assess the type, level, and degree of foot deformity. A single plane view is an isolated, inconclusive observation.

greatest chance for errors is in locating the marker so that it will record the true center of the posterior aspect of the calcaneus. Clinical judgment must be exercised in locating this point. A line bisecting the posterior aspect of the heel may be marked on the skin prior to taking the patient to the X-ray stage to assist in placing the marker. However, even with great care, the relative proportions of tendon tissue, fibrous tissue, fat tissue, and skin may distort the true center of the calcaneus. Within these limitations, this procedure is acceptable and recommended.

3. After the patient has been positioned as for (2), the center of the posterior margin of the heel may be marked directly on the film by punching a hole through the paper film-holder and the film. A stylus is convenient. The same limitations as in (2) apply and the procedure is tedious and only reasonably reliable. The pin-hole through the paper film-holder should be covered with a piece of tape to prevent the entrance of light. This procedure is acceptable but not recommended, and technic (2) is preferred.

4. The full-foot technic (Figs. 488-492), in which the superoplantar heel view is superimposed on the dorsoplantar view, with the patient maintaining the standardized stance position for both views, provides as accurate a profile of the posterior calcaneus as can be obtained. The center point can be accurately located on the film. The only disadvantage to this procedure is the occasional overlap of bony structures in the hindfoot that may obscure the center point in the distal area. This can be avoided by using a relatively brief exposure for the superoplantar view, just enough exposure to demonstrate the posterior calcaneal profile. In comparison with the other technics discussed, this technic is highly acceptable and recommended.

CENTER OF DISTAL ASPECT OF THE HINDFOOT. The true center of the distal aspect of the hindfoot (rearfoot) should be equidistant from the medial extreme margin of the talus and the lateral extreme margin of the calcaneus at the level of the distal margin of the calcaneus. Regardless of pronation of supination of the foot, this center point will represent the midpoint of the hindfoot. Other reference points are used for hindfoot axes.

Comparison of the roentgenogram of a dis-

sected specimen severed at the crural joint with the talus in place (Fig. 512) with one with the talus removed to expose the true position of the longitudinal axis of the calcaneus and the elements of the subtalar joint (Fig. 513) will illustrate the relative proportions of the widths of the talus and of the distal part of the calcaneus and will show the very important shape and volume of the sustentaculum tali and the relative position of midline reference points. A roentgenogram of a viable foot (Fig. 514) shows the difficulty of selecting a precise reference point for the distal dorsomedial end of the calcaneus, it may be appreciated by observing the lack of an anatomic landmark on the slope of the calcaneus to the sustentaculum tali. A reference point can be defined at the distal calcaneocuboid joint.

CENTER OF THE FOREFOOT AT THE DISTAL METATARSAL LEVEL. The true center of the forefoot related to the width of the forefoot at the first to fifth metatarsal parabola can be marked from the following geometric construction (Fig. 512).

1. Extend a line from the center of the posterior aspect of the calcaneus through and beyond the center of the first metatarsophalangeal joint.

2. Extend a line from the center of the posterior aspect of the calcaneus through and beyond the point at the center of the fifth metatarsophalangeal joint.

3. Using the compass as a divider, measure the distance from the center of the heel to the first metatarsophalangeal joint and draw an arc on a line extended through the fifth metatarsophalangeal joint.

4. In the same manner, measure the distance from the center of the heel to the fifth metatarsophalangeal joint and draw an arc on the line from the center of the calcaneus to the first metatarsophalangeal joint.

5. Draw a line from the center point at the head of the fifth metatarsophalangeal joint to the point marked by the arc on the line from the center of the heel to the center of the first metatarsophalangeal joint.

6. Draw a second line from the center point of the head of the first metatarsophalangeal to the point marked by the second arc.

7. The point of intersection of these transverse lines is the center point of the forefoot.

The position of this precisely located center

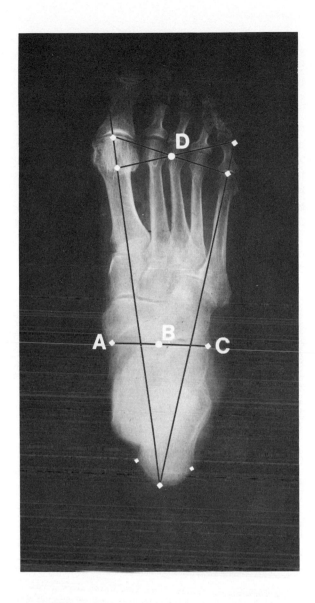

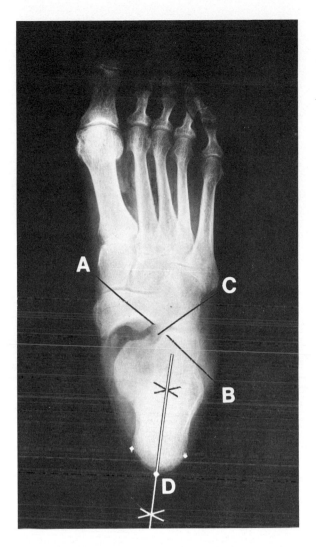

Fig. 512. Roentgenogram of dissected foot specimen removed from leg, illustrating:

B, Geometric center of distal aspect of hindfoot at calcaneocuboid joint level (*A-B* and *B-C* are equidistant).

D, Geometric center of forefoot at intersection of lines drawn from center of posterior calcaneus to equidistant arcs measured on first and fifth metatarsal coordinates.

Note that hindfoot center and forefoot center do not coincide on a longitudinal axis from center of posterior calcaneus to center of forefoot (Dissection, courtesy of G. Elmer Harford, D.P.M.; roentgenogram, courtesy of Leon E. Kehr, D.P.M.; specimen, courtesy of Pennsylvania College of Podiatric Medicine.)

Fig. 513. Roentgenogram of dissected foot specimen (same foot as in Fig. 512) with talus removed to expose size and shape of sustentaculum tali, subtalar joint features, and with selected reference points marked and defined.

A, Dorsal medial anterior aspect of calcaneus reference point.

B, Plantar medial anterior aspect of calcaneus reference point. Note that the dorsal medial image is less dense than the image of the superimposed density of the plantar medial margin.

C, Medial calcaneocuboid joint reference point.

D, A line perpendicular to a bisector of the posterior aspect of the calcaneus bisects the body of the calcaneus exclusive of the sustentaculum tali. The axis of the calcaneus is not parallel to the midline of the foot.

point will be influenced by the amount of adduction of the first metatarsal and abduction of the fifth metatarsal, or converse changes in position. Further changes in the position of this center point occur with altered alignment of the lesser tarsals, metatarsals, or the total forefoot. Under such restrictions, it is obvious that this center point may be used as a valid reference point only for an individual foot. There may be special charting or statistical uses for this reference point for which its validity would be acceptable and recommended within the limitations specified.

Reference Lines

GENERAL PURPOSES FOR REFERENCE LINES

1. Bisection of longitudinal bones.
2. Transection of small or irregular bones.
3. Transection of groups of bones.
4. Geometric diagramming.
5. Formation of angles.

LOCATION OF REFERENCE LINES

1. Line drawn to unite two reference points (bisection of metatarsal bone).
2. Line drawn perpendicular to established reference line for geometric reference (line perpendicular to the bisection of the talar head).
3. Line drawn parallel to established reference line or cortical margin of bone or joint for geometric reference (line parallel to lateral margin of calcaneus).
4. Line extrinsic to the foot exposed on the roentgenogram (line indicating plane of stance for lateral view).
5. Margin of film.

SPECIAL REFERENCE LINES

BASE LINE. A base line is one whose location is constant and not influenced by variations in bone shape, bone alignment, or irregular articulations. This primary line of reference is used to relate bone positions. A base line may be located on the roentgenogram in several ways: it may be exposed on the film, drawn on the film, or it may be the margin of the film itself.

A base line for the sagittal plane on a lateral view of the foot is automatically achieved when the horizontal weight-supporting surface is exposed beneath the foot in stance. This reference line is unquestionably recommended.

A base line for the transverse plane on a dorsoplantar view of the foot is not easily achieved. A longitudinal midline of the foot would seem to be an ideal base line; however, there are sources of error that cause the use of this line to be questioned, such as variations in bone shape and alignment that may influence the constancy of the line. The transverse plane of the foot is best determined on a segmental basis with reference lines and angles that indicate directional alignment changes.

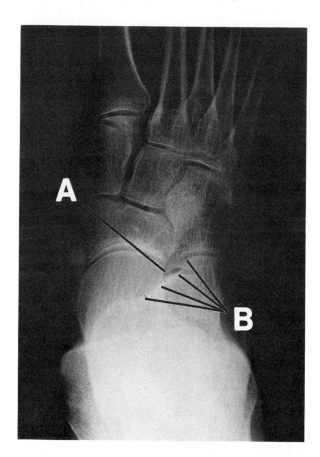

Fig. 514. Viable foot roentgenogram showing anterior margin of calcaneus sloping into the sustentaculum tali. It is possible to locate a reference point *A* at the medial calcaneocuboid joint, whereas it is practically impossible to define a specific point of reference for the distal dorsomedial margin of the calcaneus *B* on the oblique slope.

MIDLINES AND LONGITUDINAL AXES.
Lines applied to the dorsoplantar view are frequently indiscriminately referred to as midlines of the foot, when in truth they represent a selected longitudinal axis of the foot. A midline is a line connecting the center points that divide the foot or a part of the foot into halves. A selected longitudinal axis may be drawn to connect reference points that does not necessarily create an equally divided foot or part of a foot. A longitudinal axis may be drawn connecting selected reference points and have validity as a line of reference under specified circumstances. A true midline has a similar reference value with the added value of designating an absolute central location.

Axes drawn on the roentgenogram for charting purposes may differ from the theoretical axes that represent the line of reference for directional motion of the foot (Fig. 223). Theoretical axes are obtained from experimental data, whereas charted lines are specifically applied as positional references to orient topography of the foot structure.

BISECTOR OF A BONE. Judgment is necessary to insure the validity of the center points used to bisect an irregularly shaped bone. For example, the use of the center point of the head and the base of the metatarsal is a source of error because of the unequal flare of the base. Also, a rotated metatarsal shaft may present a distorted width on the roentgenogram. A line which best fits several center points located equidistantly along the shaft is the most accurate bisector. Bisectors of bones represent fairly reliable indicators of bone position.

A TABLE OF SELECTED REFERENCE LINES. Midlines, longitudinal axes, cortical margin lines, and bisectors, as used by various investigators, are placed in perspective by a table that indicates their locations, purposes, values, and limitations (Table 11). To illustrate the various axes chosen for the hindfoot and the total foot, a roentgenogram of a foot (Fig. 515) is marked with lines to represent them. This figure shows that each line serves only a specific purpose as related to the method of charting for which it was designed.

Reference Angles

In charting a foot roentgenogram, the angular relationship between two designated refer-

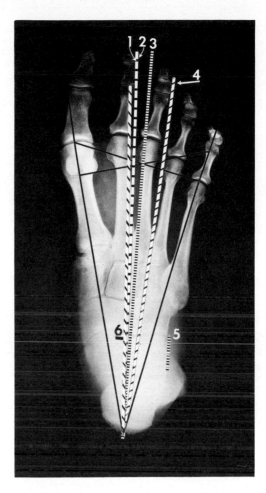

Fig. 515. Composite of midline and longitudinal foot axes

1, Center of posterior aspect of calcaneus through a point at distal calcaneocuboid joint to digits.

2, Center of posterior aspect of calcaneus through a point between heads of second and third metatarsals. (Note, in this foot *1* and *2* coincide).

3, Center of posterior aspect of calcaneus through junction of transecting lines drawn from equidistant arcs measured on first and fifth metatarsal coordinates. (Foot midline)

4, Center of posterior aspect of calcaneus through a point on the distal dorsomedial margin of calcaneus to digits.

5, A line drawn parallel to cortical margin at distal lateral third of calcaneus.

6. Center of posterior aspect of calcaneus through a point equidistant between medial margin of talus and lateral margin of calcaneus to digits. (Hindfoot midline)

TABLE 11. SELECTED REFERENCE LINES, DORSOPLANTAR VIEW, TRANSVERSE PLANE

Reference Line	Location	Purpose	Values & Limitations
Midline of Hindfoot	center posterior aspect of calcaneus to a point equidistant between medial margin of talus and lateral margin of calcaneus, distal level	accurate midline of hindfoot; related to second metatarsal forefoot axis by Harris and Beath	although geometrically accurate, mobility of talus may move the line medially or laterally from calcaneus; this midline does equate hindfoot position relative to other foot segments
Longitudinal Axis of Hindfoot #1	center of posterior aspect of calcaneus to a point on the distal dorsomedial margin of calcaneus	stable long axis of hindfoot; extendible as a base line for all other segments; used in Root and Sgarlato charting methods	not a true midline because distal calcaneus is only 2/5 wide at this level; hard to define a precise point on the dorsomedial margin; stable line related to a calcaneal axis but may be related to other segments
Longitudinal Axis of Hindfoot #2	center of posterior aspect of calcaneus to a point at distal medial calcaneocuboid joint	stable long axis of hindfoot; extendible as a base line for all other segments; Gamble charting method, usable in Root and Sgarlato charting methods	not a true midline due to variable width of calcaneus and talus at this level, but oriented to a more precise distal point than (1); a stable calcaneal axis that may be related to other segments
Midline of Midfoot (lesser tarsus)	perpendicular to the center of a transection: equidistant points: talonavicular and first cuneiform-first metatarsal and calcaneocuboid-cuboid-fifth metatarsal	used to approximate lesser tarsus abduction or adduction and forefoot-related abduction and adduction; used in Root and Sgarlato charting methods	many variables involved, such as shape of talus and first cuneiform; influenced by subtalar and midtarsal joint alignment; only gross approximations allowed
Longitudinal Axis of Midfoot (medial segment)	center of distal talar head to meet bisector of second metatarsal at cuneiform joint	used to indicate alignment of medial midfoot segment; Gamble charting method	a directional indicator; it ranges from the unstable talus to the stable second metatarsocuneiform joint
Longitudinal Axis of Total Forefoot	perpendicular to the center of a transection; lateral calcaneocuboid joint through distal center of head of talus to medial navicular	used to indicate the effect of distal talar position on position of forefoot relative to hindfoot; Gamble text	a fairly reliable index of total forefoot abduction or adduction; influenced by change in talocalcaneal angle
Midline of Foot	center posterior aspect of calcaneus to junction of lines from calcaneus to arcs measured on first and fifth metatarsal coordinates	geometrically accurate midline of foot for comparison of bony alignment between feet of same individual	although geometrically accurate for a given foot, it is not a constant reference line; influenced by adduction and abduction of first and fifth metatarsals, all metatarsals, or forefoot
Longitudinal Axis of Total Foot #1	extension of longitudinal axis of hindfoot #1 through forefoot	an axis related to the calcaneus used as a base of reference for other segments in Root and Sgarlato charting methods	a stable axis when accurately located; distal dorsomedial point can be difficult to locate; not a true midline
Longitudinal Axis of Total Foot #2	extension of longitudinal axis of hindfoot #2 through forefoot	same as longitudinal axis of total foot #1	distal reference point accurate; a stable axis but not a true midline
Longitudinal Axis of Balance (Morton, 1935)	center of posterior aspect of calcaneus through a point between heads of second and third metatarsals	establishes a long foot axis related to a point independent of forefoot width and first or fifth metatarsal alignment for contralateral comparison: Gamble text diagram	although not a true midline, does coincide in a normal foot with the geometric midline and may be used as a reference for talar deviation (normal $15° \pm 5°$)
Longitudinal Bisector of a Long Bone #1	joins center points at each end of bone or joint surfaces	establishes a central long axis for a long bone	does not bisect bone equally if either end of bone or joint flares unequally
Longitudinal Bisector of a Long Bone #2	best-fit line for center points equidistant along shaft of bone	establishes a central long axis for a long bone	distortion of width of metatarsal shaft caused by rotation may produce error in presented width
Cortical Margin Axis of a Bone	line drawn from cortical margins at each end of bone	establishes a cortical axis along margin of a bone	valid for bones of normal shape; distorted axes produced by irregular bone shapes

ence lines constitute a reference angle, expressed in degrees. While for some purposes "greater" and "lesser" are all that is needed to express a comparison, there are instances when the numerical value of an angle is highly significant. For example, the degrees measured for the angle of inclination of the calcaneus are used to indicate increments in the height of the foot framework. In other cases, the numerical value is significant in a contralateral foot comparison.

GENERAL PURPOSES OF REFERENCE ANGLES

1. Demonstration of normal angular relationships of the foot structure.
2. Expression of degree of malalignment.
3. Orientation of foot segments by angular relationships.
4. Computation of ratios of altered anatomy.
5. Assessment of amount and kind of surgical intervention needed.

TYPES OF REFERENCE ANGLES

1. Angle between bisectors of two bones.
2. Angle between a base line and a bisector of a bone.
3. Angle between a base line and the cortical margin axis of a bone.
4. Angle between a reference line and a bisector of a group of bones.

Various investigators use different angles to express their methods of charting. They will be described and illustrated as each method is presented.

METHODS OF CHARTING

Many methods of charting have been proposed by investigators, and each method serves the special purpose of its originator. It is the practitioner's prerogative to adopt a method that is compatible with the clinical evaluation that he employs or the method that presents the most logical and informative clinical demonstrations. Interpretation of a chart should be dynamic to be meaningful, according to Hammonds (1974). The ultimate concept of charting is to be able to predict function from designated positional relationships of the foot bones. In a static sense, a charted foot roentgenogram shows the abnormal alignment status of foot deformities.

Most investigators have limited numerical measurements to the relatively few angles of importance, and where numerical values are given, a liberal range has been assigned for any consideration of normalcy. Most investigators point out that charted measurements should apply to the individual patient and be evaluated with clinical findings in arriving at a diagnosis.

Unfortunately, since different investigators use different reference lines and angles upon which to base their reference criteria, there is a lack of standardization of reference criteria. In spite of the vagaries of individual charting methods, if pursued consistently, the criteria will set up a pattern that supports the method and may be used within its special framework of reference.

Perhaps the greatest possible chance for misconception in the interpretation of the data of charting has been consideration of numerical values and representations of normal angular ranges that have been determined from non-standardized recumbent roentgenologic studies. In the past decade, most studies have been performed using weight-supporting roentgenograms, resulting in more reliability.

Very few studies meet the requirements that would qualify them as statistically valid. A statistically normal profile implies that the numerical values have been calculated to obtain the means, standard deviations, and boundaries of normalcy from data supplied by some specific survey (Feinstein, 1967). The scopes of many surveys lack a sample population of adequate size and demographic features, such as age, sex, race, and occupation, to relate to the general population and uncommon variables to be encountered.

Charted foot roentgenograms and their interpretations are, in the final analysis, at best only a guide to the relative positions of foot bones to be used as a diagnostic tool correlated with other features of a comprehensive clinical examination.

Charting can enhance or limit roentgenological interpretation. The danger prevails that the subtle bone changes are lost in engrossment with the lineal and angular features of a chart. Certainly, the chart should not be more difficult to interpret than the usual roentgen features. In no way should a charted roentgenogram become merely a plotted geometrically contrived configuration. It needs to be an easily understood graphic diagram of the relative anatomic positions of the individual bones and their segmental relationships within the total foot.

An investigator usually coordinates his charting method with a plan of interpretation. The following are some of the schemes:

1. Comparison of measurements with standards of normalcy.

2. Comparison with contralateral foot and postural complex.

3. Direct clinical interpretation of specific measurements.

4. Relating of criteria to statistical data concerning specific problems.

5. Relating of charted criteria to the diagnosis of faults, abnormal foot types and deformities.

6. Interpretations designed to classify deformities.

7. Interpretation of segmental alignments.

8. Interpretation of plotted angular configurations for planning of surgical procedure.

If the practitioner is familiar with the different types of charting, he will be better able to interpret the various methods that may confront him.

SPECIAL STUDIES BASED ON ROENTGENOLOGICAL CHARTING

Roentgenological charting has been applied in the investigation of a number of diagnostic projects. A brief review of several studies will be given and a comparative table of related angles and rocntgen signs will be presented. Special emphasis will be given to pediatric surveys. This group is primarily concerned with congenital deformities and the charting is done on roentgenograms of infants and children.

Charting Pediatric Foot Roentgenograms

Davis and Hatt (1955) offer a technic for obtaining standard views of the infant foot by securing the foot in its natural position. From roentgenograms made in this manner they develop diagrammatic criteria to describe the normal foot, talipes equinovarus, "rocker deformity" (overcorrected clubfoot), flatfoot, metatarsus varus, and pes cavus. Their method uses a combination of angles and direction lines to define the positional deformities. The study did not report the number of cases and the numerical values are therefore not statistically significant. However, the criteria they offer have been used as a basis for subsequent studies and serve a very useful purpose.

Templeton, McAlister and Zim (1965) report a study similar to that of Davis and Hatt, using 160 simulated weight-bearing dorsoplantar and lateral roentgenograms of normal children, ages 12 days to 12 years, from which they established normal criteria on an age-dependent basis. Their method related to angular relationships rather than to directions of selected lines. To promote standardization of terminology they propose valgus, varus, equinus, calcaneus deformity, abduction and adduction as the best terms to describe congenital abnormalities of the feet. They point out that the normal range of angles presented should be used as a guide, with the final diagnosis depending on physical examination and subjective roentgenologic evaluation.

LeNoir (1966) presents the most comprehensive analysis of congenital idiopathic talipes in the literature. His roentgenological descriptions relate to segmental deviations shown as signs and angles on standardized roentgenograms made with a frame of his invention holding the infant foot. LeNoir's work is exhaustive and his report should be studied in detail. An overview of this study is given in Chapter 20 and illustrations of extreme forms of talipes are diagrammatically shown. LeNoir unequivocally recommends an X-ray diagnosis in clubfoot as an initial necessity for management of the problem.

Ritchie and Keim (1968) present a classification and X-ray analysis of major foot deformities in which he uses roentgenograms made in a simulated weight-bearing position for infants and in a natural stance for older children. These authors use established reference lines and angles to describe the deformities they analyze. They make clear that the measurements they offer are not statistically valid and should be used only as guides to interpretation. Consideration of angles should be related to the foot as a whole, with comparison of feet included if one is normal, otherwise available normal standards should be used. A total clinical evaluation is essential because of the many compensatory changes possible.

COMPARATIVE TABLE OF RELATED ANGLES AND ROENTGEN SIGNS

The criteria presented in Table 12 are illustrated in the composite drawings of Figure 516. All investigators are in agreement that the relationship between the talus and calcaneus is the most important criterion since it is influenced by abnormal movement of the talus and midtarsal joint. Altered axial relationships of the talus to the first metatarsal and of the calcaneus to the fourth metatarsal indicate subsidiary abnormal forefoot movements. The wide range of numerical values given for the talocalcaneal angle may be attributed to the fact that the data include infants and children with subsequent ontogenic variables. It is interesting to note that there is a lack of consistency regarding the location of reference lines for the longitudinal position of the calcaneus and fifth metatarsal. For example, in some studies a bisecting line is used, and in other studies the cortical margin is used. Investigators make each line serve a special purpose.

The Harris and Beath Canadian Army Foot Survey

Harris and Beath (1947) examined the feet of 3,619 recruits to determine the incidence and nature of certain foot abnormalities and deformities with special reference to their functional limitation of the individual in military service. A most comprehensive clinical examination and a standardized foot X-ray examination were performed. The weight-supporting foot X-ray technic was used exclusively. Roentgenograms of all subjects were carefully charted and measured, and the data compiled for some 32 anthropometric features were extensively explored statistically. The statistical significance of many features was minimal, but other features were shown to be important for identification of significant abnormalities. However, the isolated observation of a statistically significant measurement cannot be relied upon to provide a diagnosis of foot disability without clinical correlation because too many compensatory effects can alter an as-

sumed situation. Harris and Beath used other clinical aids in diagnosis. Among these was a pressure-sensitive mat of their design for recording on inked paper the fine degrees of impress from the weight-loaded foot.

Much of the survey related to a study of the hypermobile flatfoot with short tendo achilles and atavistic short first metatarsal (HFF-STA). Analysis of the statistical data for HFF-STA yielded the following information concerning eight specific measurements.

1. Angle between axis of talus and axis of calcaneus. Variation in values insufficient to identify HFF-STA.

2. Forward projection of head of talus in front of calcaneus. In general, greatest for HFF-STA and least for clawfoot.

3. Slope of sustentaculum tali. Greatest in severe HFF-STA and least in severe pes cavus.

4. Length of spring ligament. Longest in HFF-STA and shortest in pes cavus.

5. Distance of sustentaculum tali behind anterior end of calcaneus. Greatest in HFF-STA and least in normal feet and pes cavus. Significant and important. Tonguelike shape of sustentaculum tali of practical importance.

6. Proportion of diameter of talar head overlying calcaneus in dorsoplantar view. Least overlap in HFF-STA and greatest in pes cavus.

7. Proportion of diameter of talar head overlying calcaneus in lateral view. Greatest in HFF-STA and least in pes cavus.

8. Length of calcaneus. Differences of little value in identifying HFF-STA.

Harris and Beath conclude that roentgenograms are of great value in anthropometric studies.

1. Standardized measurements are directly comparable.

2. Relationship of bony structure to clinical foot types and function may be studied.

3. Diagnosis of specific foot types from measurements is of limited value in individual cases.

4. Overlapping of statistical range of measurements from type to type makes it impossible to define precisely the limits of normal.

The Harris and Beath survey was a tremendous undertaking and has provided insight into HFF-STA and other concepts that have been followed by many other investigators. The statistical study points out the importance of examining every diagnostic roentgen feature and

TABLE 12. MAJOR PEDIATRIC FOOT DEFORMITIES AND ABNORMALITIES

(A composite of roentgenological criteria from the studies of Davis and Hatt, Templeton, McAlister and Zim, and Ritchie and Keim. Subjects for these studies range in ages from 12 days to 12 years.)

Sagittal Plane, Lateral View	Midtalar-Midcalcaneal Angle	Midtalar-First Metatarsal Angle	Inferior Cortex of Calcaneus-Fifth Metatarsal	Midtibial-Midcalcaneal Angle
Normal Foot	an acute angle (15°-50°)	no angle; lines coincide after age 5	obtuse angle (150°-175°), apex upward	10°-30° less than a right angle
Talipes Equinovarus	reduced or lines are parallel	obtuse angle; apex upward	obtuse angle (+ 175°), apex downward	obtuse angle
Overcorrected Clubfoot (rockerbottom)	reduced or lines are parallel	reverse angle, apex downward	reverse angle, apex downward	obtuse angle
Pes Planovalgus (flatfoot) (talipes equinovalgus has ankle equinus and vertical talus)	increased angle	obtuse angle, apex downward	obtuse angle, apex upward	in talipes equinovalgus, ankle equinus
Metatarsus Varus (adductus) (pes adductus has varus heel)	may increase; increased with varus	first metatarsal higher than fifth		
Pes Cavus	increased angle	increased angle, apex upward	increased angle, apex upward	

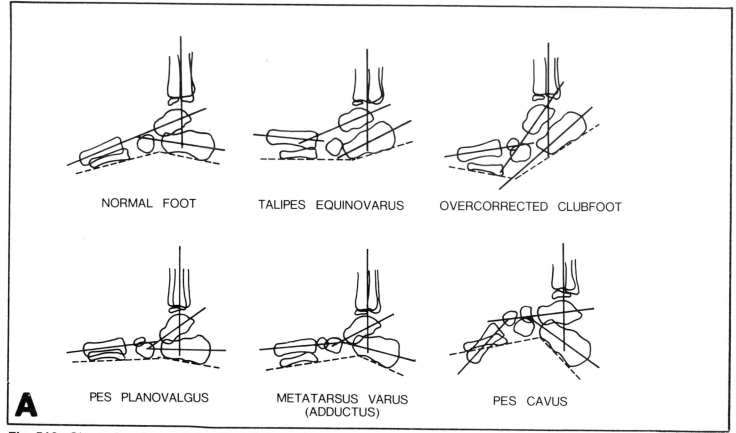

Fig. 516. Charted major pediatric foot deformities and abnormalities. A composite of roentgenological criteria from the studies of Davis and Hatt; Templeton, McAlister and Zim; and Ritchie and Keim (see Table 12 for interpretations).

A. *Sagittal plane, lateral view:* criteria charted — midtalar-midcalcaneal angle, midtalar-first metatarsal angle, inferior cortex of calcaneus-fifth metatarsal, midtibial-midcalcaneal angle.

Transverse Plane, Dorsoplantar View	Midtalar-Midcalcaneal Angle	Midtalar Line	Midcalcaneal Line	Metatarsal Shafts
Normal Foot	30°-50° in infants 15°-50° in children	coincides with first metatarsal head and midshaft	coincides with fourth metatarsal head and midshaft	parallel
Talipes Equinovarus	reduced or reversed	lateral to first metatarsal head; angle with shaft apex lateral	lateral to fourth metatarsal head and shaft	converge posteriorly; overlapping metatarsal bases
Overcorrected Clubfoot (rockerbottom)	reduced angle			forefoot may be normal or residual varus
Pes Planovalgus (flatfoot)	increased angle; 58° angle shown for age 2	medial to first metatarsal	placement varies	abducted forefoot
Metatarsus Varus (adductus) (pes adductus has varus heel)	varies; superimposed when hindfoot varus	forms angle with first metatarsal	passes lateral to normal position	converge posteriorly; overlapping bases; forefoot adduction
Pes Cavus	Normal findings unless associated with pes adductus or other abnormal components			

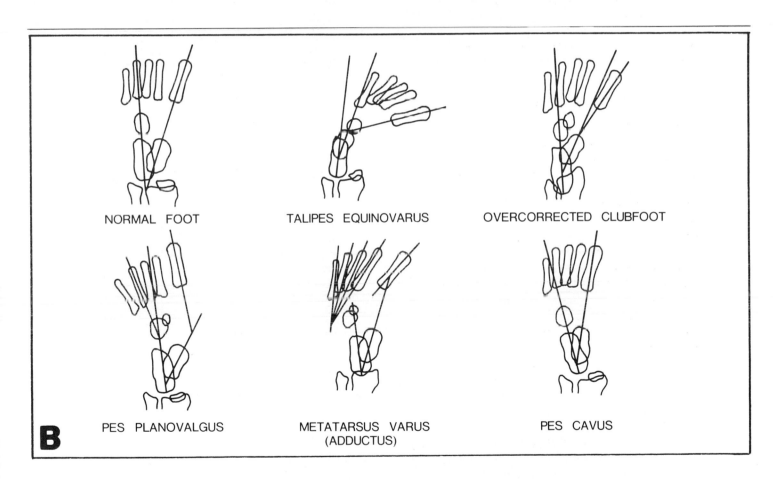

B. *Transverse plane, dorsoplantar view:* criteria charted — midtalar-midcalcaneal angle, midtalar line, midcalcaneal line, metatarsal shafts. (Drawings courtesy of A.K. Whitney, D.P.M.)

correlating all of them with clinical information in arriving at a diagnostic judgment. Demographically, the survey was limited to young men, ages 18 to 25, and this may have some bearing on statistical data for the general population.

SELECTED CHARTING METHODS

Charting methods of clinical value developed by several investigators will be presented. Each method imparts information keyed to an individual scheme of interpretation. All of these methods are designed to enhance a comprehensive clinical examination. The student or practitioner should strive to attain mastery of a basic plan of charting and interpretation. A comparison can be made of the different types of charting shown so that he will be familiar with the various methods. When confronted with various charting methods he will be better able to interpret them. Each investigator has the prerogative of assigning lines and angles to his concept of a framework of reference.

Tanenbaum Charting Method

A simplified method for determining talar rotation was originated by Tanenbaum (1952) to assist in diagnosing pes planus and pes cavus. A dorsoplantar view of a natural-stance roentgenogram of the foot is charted. The articular limits of the head of the talus are marked, and intersecting arcs are drawn from these points with a compass so that a common bisector of the head of the talus may be drawn through them. The base and head of the first metatarsal are bisected and a line drawn connecting these points represents a bisection of the first metatarsal. This line is extended to meet the talar-head bisector and forms an angle (Fig. 518).

Tanenbaum states that if the talar and first metatarsal lines do not cross, the foot is normal concerning talar rotation. If the first metatarsal bisector forms a distal angle with the talar bisector on the medial side, the talus is rotated medially and pes planus is present. If a distal angle is formed on the lateral side, the talus is rotated laterally and pes cavus is present.

A series of 25 patients with asymptomatic feet were examined and roentgenographed to determine a norm. One hundred patients with symptomatic feet were used to determine the range of abnormal rotation of the talus. Many patients exhibited different degrees of rotation

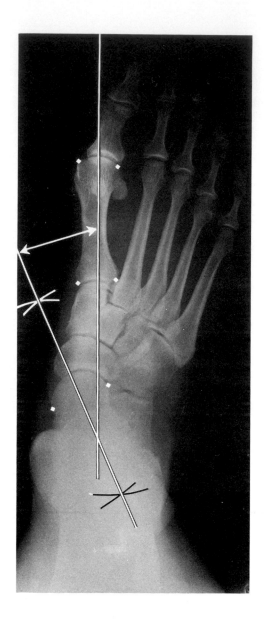

Fig. 518. Tanenbaum's charting method. The bisectors of the talar head and the first metatarsal form an angle. An angle medial to the metatarsal bisector indicates pes planus; an angle lateral to the metatarsal bisector indicates pes cavus. (Reference points and compass arcs show Tanenbaum's features for construction of bisectors.)

contralaterally. The roentgenographic assessment was related to the amount of orthotic wedging needed for correction. Although no reference line is applied to the calcaneus, Tanenbaum assumes that its position is responsible for talar rotation.

The conclusions drawn from this method of charting have limitations because of variations in the position of the first metatarsal, such as the adduction of the first metatarsal that may occur in the zigzag type of subluxed pes planus. It is better to include several charted anatomical relationships to insure comprehensive reliable diagnostic information.

Hammonds Charting Method

Hammonds uses an anthropometric measuring system of charting on scanograms made of the patient in natural standing position. This system is designed to indicate contralateral values of the angles and lines chosen to demonstrate the pathoanatomical status of the patient. A composite chart of scanograms of the pelvis and feet is illustrated (Fig. 517), and the lines of reference and the reference angles are described in Table 13.

Clinically, Hammonds associates the roentgen interpretation with a postural appraisal by observation of the patient in gait and stance and by palpation of bony landmarks. He indicates that his technic of roentgenographic and clinical examination is designed to relate the anatomy and functions of the foot to the following:

1. The primary center of gravity for the whole body and its vertical position as it is related to the foot.

2. The kinetic anatomical link theory (postural complex, Jones, 1955).

3. The effect of torque in the transverse plane rotation that is either created in the foot or dealt with by the foot if created by another link in the kinetic chain.

4. The relationship of foot function to balance and locomotion and to growth and deformity.

5. The effect of the balancing mechanisms of the eyes, ears, musculature, joints, and skin.

6. The evaluation of the use and mechanics of orthopedic braces.

7. The establishment and evaluation of corrective and supportive exercises for muscles that are affected.

8. The establishment of proper history by taking of signs and symptoms of disease, deformity, stress, injury, growth, and adaptation that occur extrinsic to the foot and record its relationship.

Stess (1972) confirms the applied value of tri-plane scanograms by relating the following clinical considerations:

1. Correlation of foot biomechanics to ankle, knees, hips, and shoulder girdle.

2. Appraisal of structural versus positional abnormalities and their effects on the feet and the postural complex.

3. Contralateral relationships of one extremity to the other.

4. Determination of limb length discrepancies in a closed kinetic chain.

5. Determination of actual limb length discrepancies or whether in fact the length discrepancy is due to abnormal pronator forces of one extremity.

6. Critical appraisal of the effects of orthotic control of the feet on the knees, pelvis, and shoulder girdle. Comparison of postural status with and without orthotic control. Comparison of the effect of the orthotic for one foot on the other foot.

7. Comprehensive interpretation of before and after scanogram surveys of a patient after use of an orthotic for a substantial interval.

Hammonds emphasizes that the composite chart (Fig. 517) is hypothetical and was prepared to illustrate the typical predictable guide to the interpretation of pathomechanics. In practice, charted scanograms should be related to a biomechanical examination of the patient which includes total postural complex and gait. Interpretation of charted roentgenograms should be dynamic and, in many instances, may predict certain postural and gait responses and other considerations. No precise contralateral pattern of alignment is to be assumed. If a charted angle does not coincide with a typical relationship, it is necessary to explore the pathomechanical situation to find the problem. Every angle has biomechanical significance.

TABLE 13. HAMMONDS' ANTHROPOMETRIC MEASURING SYSTEM CHARTED FROM ROENTGENOLOGICAL SCANOGRAMS

Angle	Sides of Angle
Frontal-Plane Reference Angles — Pelvis and Femora	
Iliac Wing List Angle (IWLA)	Line across top of iliac crests horizontal line to intersect highest point of first line
Center of Gravity Angle (CGA)	Extend bisector of head and neck of each femur to intersection. Relate to midline of pelvis with apex to show shift to right or left.
Pelvic Ring List Angle (PRLA)	Line from the right arcuate line of the lesser pelvic brim to the left arcuate line of the lesser pelvic brim to meet on each side the points touched by the bisectors from neck and head of femora. Horizontal line to intersect highest point of first line.
Intraacetabular Angle (IACA)	A line from superior outer margin of one acetabulum to same point on other acetabulum. Horizontal line to intersect highest point of first line.
Weight-bearing Angle (WBA)	A line perpendicular to the line across the iliac crest to the apex of the angle of inclination of the femur. The bisector of the head forms the measurable angle.
Femoral Inclination Angle (FIA)	Upper third of the bisector of the femur. Bisector of neck and head of femur.
Milch Triangle (inferior angle shown)	A line connecting superior outer margins of acetabula. From outer margin points draw a lines by the lateral margins of ischia. Draw a line perpendicular to the superior interacetabular line to meet the ischial line on both sides of pelvis. The inferior intersection is the measured angle.
Transverse Plane Reference Angles — Left and Right Feet	
Rear Calcaneus Angle (RCA)	A line drawn parallel to the lateral border of the calcaneus. The base line for both feet.
Rear Talus Angle (RTA)	Bisector of the talus. Base line for both feet.
Talus-Calcaneus Angle (TCA)	Bisector of the talus. A line parallel to the lateral border of the calcaneus.
Forefoot Angle (FFA) (dorsoplantar view)	Bisector of shaft of second metatarsal. Bisector of talus.
Chopart's Angle (CA) (mid-tarsal angle) (dorsoplantar view)	A line parallel to the anterior margin of the calcaneus. A line from the lateral margin of the calcaneocuboid joint to the distal center of the talus.
Sagittal-Plane Reference Angles — Left and Right Feet	
Tibia-Talus Angle (TTA)	Bisector of the tibia. Bisector of the talus.
Chopart's Angle (CA) (mid-tarsal angle)	A line parallel to the anterior margin of the calcaneus. A line from the inferior margin of the calcaneocuboid joint to the distal center of the talus.
Talus-Calcaneus Angle (TCA)	Bisector of head and neck of talus. Bisector of calcaneus.
Forefoot Angle (FFA) (lateral view)	A line from the base of the first metatarsal plantar contact center to the apex of the talus-calcaneus angle.

✛ and — RELATIONSHIP RIGHT TO LEFT - PELVIS, FEMUR, and FEET

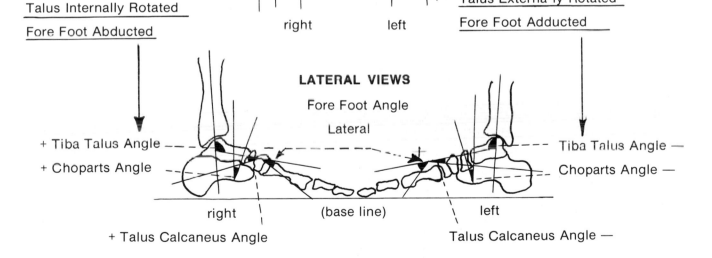

Right side   **AP VIEWS**   Left side

Apex IWLA Left (+)
Center of Gravity to the left
Apex PRL Left (+)
Apex IAA Left (+)
— WBA Left
+ Left FIA Angle
— Milch Triangle

+ WBA Right
— FIA Right
+ Milch Triangel

Leg and thigh internally rotated   Leg and thigh externally rotated

DP VIEWS
(base line)

Rear Calcaneus Angle —
Rear Talus Angle —
Talus Calcaneus Angle +
Fore Foot Angle +
Choparts Angle +

Rear Calcaneus Angle +
Rear Talus Angle +
Talus Calcaneus Angle —
Fore Foot Angle —
Choparts Angle —

Right Rear Foot Pronated
Talus Internally Rotated
Fore Foot Abducted

Left Rear Foot Supinated
Talus Externa-ly Rotated
Fore Foot Adducted

right   left

LATERAL VIEWS

Fore Foot Angle
Lateral

+ Tiba Talus Angle
+ Choparts Angle

Tiba Talus Angle —
Choparts Angle —

right   (base line)   left

+ Talus Calcaneus Angle   Talus Calcaneus Angle —

Fig. 517. Composite chart devised by Hammonds of anatomical orientation angles and their hypothetical biomechanical significance drawn from tracings of scanographic roentgenograms made with Hammonds' Posture-Poser, U.S. Pat. 3,524,057; courtesy of C.M. Hammonds, D.P.M.)

CHARTING IN FOOT ROENTGENOLOGY/399

Root Charting Method

The osseous relationships of the foot bones in the transverse plane have been the basis of a charting method devised by Root (1958) and adopted by Sgarlato (1971) and others relating the charted findings to the biomechanical status of the foot.

Root has chosen reference lines and angles that indicate four basic component relationships:

1. Forefoot angle, normally adductus, relates the rearfoot to the metatarsus.

2. Lesser tarsus angle, normally abductus, relates the lesser tarsus to the rearfoot.

3. Metatarsus angle, normally adductus, relates the lesser tarsus to the metatarsus.

4. Digital angle, normally abductus, relates the digits to the metatarsus.

Root has designated a line perpendicular to a chosen bisector of the entire lesser tarsus to represent the alignment of the lesser tarsus with the rearfoot and metatarsus. These component relationships convey an indirect demonstration of the effect of the movement of the talus on the lesser tarsus and forefoot through the movements of the subtalar and midtarsal joints. Other investigators use a bisector of the talar head in charting their framework and an entirely different set of lines and angles that demonstrate talar involvement directly. These examples are cited to illustrate why it is possible to have very different charting patterns according to individual concepts. The important issue is to analyze how each pattern conveys information concerning the structure under consideration.

Sgarlato has applied a very sophisticated relationship of the angle of gait to an elaboration of the Root charting method and biomechanical examination measurement of malleolar torsion. He describes the angle of gait for an individual as the amount of malleolar torsion plus or minus the relative adductus or abductus of the whole foot to the body of the talus. The position of the long axis of the calcaneus and the amount of abductus and metatarsus adductus are directly related to the given ratio.

The charted foot roentgenogram alignment that Root describes as metatarsus rectus compares with the normal foot described in this text (table 14).

TABLE 14. ROOT CHARTING METHOD

Transverse-Plane Reference Angle	Sides of Angle	Demonstration and Interpretation
Lesser Tarsus Angle (LTA)	longitudinal bisector of lesser tarsus (midfoot axis)	normally an abductus angle (lesser tarsus abductus, LTab)
	longitudinal rearfoot bisector (center of calcaneus to dorsomedial anterior point	
Metatarsus Angle (MA)	longitudinal bisector of second metatarsus (center of base to center of neck)	normally an adductus angle (metatarsus adductus, Mad)
	longitudinal bisector of lesser tarsus (midfoot axis)	
Forefoot Angle (FFA)	longitudinal bisector of second metatarsus (center of base to center of neck)	normally an adductus angle (forefoot adductus, FFad); influenced by positional change of midtarsal or subtalar joint
	longitudinal bisector of rearfoot (center of calcaneus to dorsomedial anterior point)	
Digital Angle (DA)	longitudinal bisector of digit (second toe, shaft of proximal phalanx)	normally an abductus angle (digital abductus, Dab); bisector of digit parallel to rearfoot longitudinal bisector
	longitudinal bisector of second metatarsus (center of base to center of neck)	

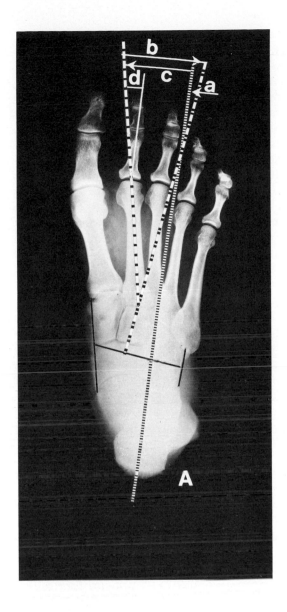

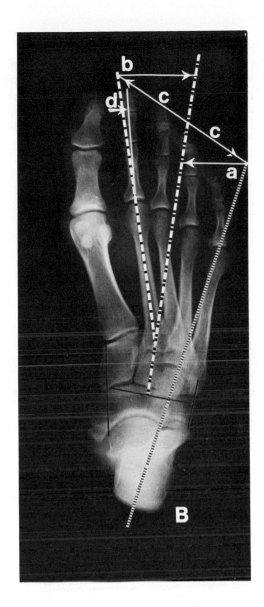

Fig. 519. Root's charting method. Comparative angular values of a relatively normal straight (rectus) foot (A) and an adductus foot type (B)

A. *Straight (rectus) foot*

a,	Lesser tarsus angle	8°
b,	Metatarsus angle	20°
c,	Forefoot angle	13°
d,	Digital angle	11°

B. *Adductus foot type*

a,	Lesser tarsus angle	11°
b,	Metatarsus angle	17°
c,	Forefoot angle	27°
d,	Digital angle	4°

The significant correlation is between the smaller lesser tarsus angle a and the larger forefoot angle c in roentgenogram B and the same angles in roentgenogram A that indicates that the foot in B may be interpreted as an adductus foot type and by comparison the foot in A is a rectus foot type.

Gamble Charting Method

In a paper entitled "The X-ray Analysis of Weakfoot" (Gamble, 1937), a diagrammatic approach to charting consisting of arrows to indicate pathoanatomic changes compared with the normal status of a weight-supporting foot on a roentgenogram was shown. After reviewing many charting methods, the simplicity of this basic graphic approach is recommended today. Certain angles and measurements were included in the original presentation, including calcaneal inclination and the "angle of pronation." Updated supplementary criteria are provided in the present method.

Roentgen signs, lines, and angles are applied to the foot roentgenogram to establish comparative and correlative charted information. Any pathoanatomic charting can be compared with normal and abnormal patterns shown in previous chapters of this book to assist in diagnosing pathoanatomic entities. Lines and angles are used to determine levels of deformity and to measure the degree of malalignment for comparative purposes.

The lateral view of the sagittal plane of the foot is most informative. Important clues concerning foot type and its abnormalities are simply and easily charted on this view.

The dorsoplantar view of the transverse plane of the foot is very deceptive. Both medial and lateral segments seem blended together. We prefer to divide the foot into functionally significant longitudinal segments with charting applied to hindfoot, midfoot, metatarsal, and toe components of these interrelated segments. Some investigators relate charting to transverse components primarily. It is difficult to perceive the arc shape that is formed from the cuboid up and around the three cuneiform bones in a dorsoplantar view; however, a flattening of this arc does occur in certain subluxations and independent charting of the segments helps to identify this changed alignment.

A far more complex interrelated framework is involved than is quickly perceived on the roentgenogram. It becomes important to realize that hindfoot varus and valgus and forefoot varus and valgus are either sustained or compensated by the medial forefoot segment or the lateral forefoot segment with corresponding transverse midfoot stability or subluxations. Charting should indicate their interrelationships as much as possible.

There are many implications that may be drawn from charting. From an objective standpoint, roentgen findings are static criteria. To be realistic, every diagnostic impression conceived by charting should be confirmed by clinical examination. It is common practice to view a foot roentgenogram and say, for example, that there is a hypermobile first metatarsal segment. In fact, hypermobility is not visible on a static film. It is a valid diagnostic assumption that hypermobility is present when a gaping joint is present. This is an extended roentgen interpretation based on clinical knowledge. As a general rule, a gaping joint or bones that spread apart suggest a weakened ligament integument, loosely bound articulations, subluxation, and hypermobility. According to Smith (1967), practitioners who attempt clinical correlation of the roentgenogram will become aware of errors to which others are oblivious.

Certain key alignments indicate important features of pathoanatomy. In many cases, directional arrows and roentgen signs make them apparent. If greater detailed analysis is desired, all angles may be charted and their numerical values determined and compared.

As a practical matter, the major chartable criteria will indicate what is happening to a foot. If both feet are charted and compared, the status of each foot may be appraised and it becomes apparent how each foot differs from the other. Sometimes one foot may show a normal pattern and provide the ideal control model to compare with the disordered foot. In other cases, completely opposite foot alignments occur, when one foot overcompensates the problem of the other foot.

RECORDING AND MEASURING CHARTABLE CRITERIA

Preservation of the diagnostic quality of the foot roentgenogram is essential for potential forensic purposes. Of immediate importance, markings cluttering a roentgenogram obstruct visualization of the trabecular structure of the bone and subtle changes of bone position as well as the features that are critical in diagnosing bone pathology that may be concurrent with the pathoanatomic pattern.

Several measures may be taken to avoid marring the roentgenogram. We recommend one of the following:

1. Make a duplicate X-ray paper roentgenogram simultaneously with the film roentgenogram. (See Chapter 25, "Special Procedures.") This roentgenogram made on X-ray paper may be drawn upon at will.

2. Use a transparent overlay on the roentgenogram and mark the charting on the overlay. A series of diagrams on tracing paper may be made to satisfy a critical analysis of the foot roentgenogram. Basically, one can be used for roentgen signs and another for lines and angles. Others may show angles related to the forefoot alone, a study of the interrelated angles associated with hallux abductus valgus, plotted angles for osteotomies, and so forth.

3. On a temporary basis, use pressure-sensitive tapes to form lines and angles directly on the film. Such tapes can be easily removed without leaving a mark on the film and come in various patterns and are easy to use.

4. As a last resort, use a china marking pencil to mark the film on a temporary basis. The marking may be removed with ether.

A protractor may be used to measure angles with an available apex on the film. Sometimes extended lines approach parallelism and the apex of the angle is beyond the film. A tractograph is needed to align with the lines to obtain the value of the angle.

A ruler is used for drawing straight lines and for making measurements. A compass is used to establish bisections of a curve, of small bone dimensions, and for other geometric plotting.

ROENTGEN SIGNS AND SPECIAL LINES

Roentgen signs are the indicators of bone position that make up patterns of alignment characteristic of the normal foot and pathoanatomic entities. Roentgen signs indicate intimate changes of bone position that affect individual joints. Charted roentgen signs represent the graphic demonstrations of the roentgen criteria that are used in arriving at a diagnostic roentgenologic impression.

Directional arrows — point in the direction of pathoanatomic change

Congruent lines — indicate a congruent articular margin

Noncongruent lines (zigzag line or lines on unequal levels) indicate a noncongruent articulation

Cyma line — a line uniting dissimilar curves

Broken cyma line — a break in the continuous curve of a cyma line

Circle — indicate a normal sinus tarsi or gaping joint

Circle enclosing an x — indicates an abnormal sinus tarsi or closed or overlapping joint spaces

Arrow — indicates a joint gap — points into gaping joint

x (single or in series) — indicates overlapping bones

Parentheses — indicate exposed articular margin; marked at each end

Plus angle — designates a large angle or greater angle

Minus angle — designates a small angle or lesser angle

REFERENCE LINES AND ANGLES

Reference lines and angles establish specific linear and angular criteria of the bony relationships within the foot and of other planes of reference, such as the weight-supporting surface upon which the patient stands. Reference lines and angles may be measured to provide diagnostic data, comparable criteria, and statistical information. This form of charting tends to lack the critical inspection of bone-to-bone achieved by assessing each bone in the foot in the process of charting roentgen signs, which is highly recommended.

The angular configuration of the foot that is considered normal is based on an alignment that is inherently structurally strong so that its components function in harmony without the need for unusual compensations.

Perhaps the greatest fallacy in charting is the unsubstantiated designation of the size of an angle. A large or small angle must relate to a standard of normalcy. An increased or decreased angle must relate to its previous size. A larger or smaller angle must compare with a standard of comparison: a previous roentgenogram showing a different angle, a comparison

TABLE 15. COMPOSITE CHART OF REFERENCE ANGLES (SAGITTAL PLANE — LATERAL VIEW), GAMBLE CHARTING METHOD

(Angle number refers to numbers shown on Fig. 520, lateral view. Terms for relative value: *plus* — large, larger or increased; *minus* — small, smaller, or decreased.)

No.	Angle	Sides of Angle	Demonstration: norms and correlation of major foot faults, positional abnormalities and deformities
1	Calcaneal Inclination	weight-supporting plane Cortical margin axis extended through plantar calcaneal tuberosity and plantar aspect of calcaneocuboid joint	*normal:* shows index of height of foot framework; 0°-10°, low; 10°-20°, medium; 20°-30°, high *minus:* HF-ST-midT fault; pronation; planus deformities, compensated talipes equinus, uncompensated subtalar valgus, compensated forefoot varus *plus:* supination; cavus deformities, uncompensated talipes equinus, subtalar varus, forefoot valgus, compensated forefoot valgus
2	Talar Declination[1] (for body of talus)	line parallel to weight-supporting plane line from posterior subtalar margin through a point at superior margin of sinus tarsi (level of talar body)	*normal:* both lines coincide, no true angle exists *plus:* body declines in HF-ST-midT fault; pronation; planus deformities usually, compensated talipes equinus, uncompensated subtalar valgus, compensated forefoot varus *minus:* may reverse with increased talar inclination in cavus and supination deformities
3	Talar Declination[1] (for head of talus)	line parallel to weight-supporting plane line perpendicular to bisector of head of talus; choose reference points at superior and inferior margins of talar head for bisector	*normal:* variable due to abnormal or ontogenically differing bone shapes; compare both feet *plus:* same as for (2) but a larger angle *minus:* same as (2), but angle is reduced not reversed

1. Angle between body of talus and head of talus represents inherent shape and ontogenic or abnormal declination of talus.

of angles in both feet, or a comparison with established angles for normal or abnormal foot types. Angles must be correlated in some manner to be meaningful. Atypical compensations of component foot segments can distort the classical patterns of angular relationships. Abnormal bone shapes also distort angular patterns and should always be given critical consideration.

Roentgen angles are described as follows:
1. Angles are measured in degrees from 0 to 180.
2. Acute angle — one less than a right angle (less than 90°).
3. Obtuse angle — one larger than a right angle (more than 90°).
4. An angle is described as large or small by comparison.

5. Plus angle — by comparison the larger angle.
6. Minus angle — by comparison the smaller angle.
7. An angle may be increased when made larger.
8. An angle may be decreased when made smaller.
9. Changes in the amount of an angle occur from alterations in bone positions.
10. The apex of an angle is the point where the angle originates and is used to designate its direction, i.e., apex upward, downward, medial, lateral, distal, or proximal.
11. The open end of an angle indicates where it spreads apart.
12. Basic angular configurations are used to make up the geometric pattern of alignments of the foot bones.

No.	Angle	Sides of Angle	Demonstration: norms and correlation of major foot faults, positional abnormalities and deformities
4	First Metatarsal Inclination	weight-supporting plane cortical margin axis of first metatarsal extended through plantar aspect of metatarsal head through plantar margin of first metatarsocuneiform joint	*normal:* related to height of foot framework; compare both feet *minus:* HF-ST-midT fault; pronation; planus deformities, compensated talipes equinus, uncompensated forefoot varus, metatarsus elevatus *plus:* supination; cavus deformities, uncompensated talipes equinus, subtalar varus and forefoot valgus; compensated forefoot valgus, plantarflexed first metatarsal
5	Talocalcaneal (sagittal plane)	bisector of talar head cortical margin axis of calcaneus	*normal:* compatible with normal open sinus tarsi; compare both feet *plus:* HF-ST-midT fault; pronation; planus deformities, compensated talipes equinus, uncompensated subtalar valgus, compensated forefoot varus *minus:* supination; cavus deformities, uncompensated talipes equinus, subtalar varus and forefoot valgus, compensated forefoot valgus
6	Midtarsal Joint	line parallel to calcaneocuboid joint line from plantar margin of calcaneocuboid joint through most distal point on head of talus	*normal:* compatible with a congruous midtarsal cyma line *plus:* distal displacement of talus in HF-ST-midT fault; abnormally long talar neck and head, pronation deformities *minus:* cavus, adductus and inverted foot deformities, abnormally short talar neck and head
	Naviculocuneiform (not charted on roentgenogram)	bisector of cuneiform bisector of navicular	*normal:* obtuse angle, apex down *minus:* second cuneiform shows as an inverted triangle, naviculocuneiform fault; may occur with plantarflexed talus in HF-ST-midT fault, pronation

USE OF THE CHARTED ROENTGENOGRAM FOR DIAGNOSIS

Tables 15 and 16 will explain the lines and angles chosen to demonstrate alignment of the foot structure. Norms for angles will be given and abnormal angles will be correlated with appropriate foot faults, foot abnormalities, and bone position abnormalities.

Charted roentgenograms are presented to illustrate the normal foot and several abnormal foot types (Figs. 520-529). Orthodigital abnormalities are not described in detail. (Refer to Chapter 16, "Orthodigital Problems.") Foot roentgenograms will be charted in which a center point is available at the posterior aspect of the calcaneus from which a line may be drawn to a point at the medial calcaneocuboid joint to establish a longitudinal axis of the hindfoot. This line may be extended to the forefoot to form a longitudinal axis of the foot. Other foot roentgenograms will be charted in which a center point for the posterior aspect of the calcaneus is absent and a line parallel with the laterodistal margin of the calcaneus is oriented through the medial calcaneocuboid joint to establish a longitudinal axis for the hindfoot and the entire foot.

TABLE 16. COMPOSITE CHART OF REFERENCE ANGLES (TRANSVERSE PLANE — DORSOPLANTAR VIEW), GAMBLE CHARTING METHOD

(Angle number refers to number shown on Fig. 520, dorsoplantar view. Terms for relative value: *plus* — large, larger or increased; *minus* — small, smaller, or decreased.)

No.	Angle	Sides of Angle	Demonstration: norms and correlation with positional abnormalities
1	Talus-Longitudinal Foot Axis	bisector of talar head	*normal:* 15° ± 5°; traditional indicator of adduction of talus from long axis of foot
		line from center of posterior calcaneus through point at medial calcaneocuboid joint to metatarsophalangeal area[1]	*plus:* adduction of talus; pronation *minus:* abduction of talus; supination
2	Talus-First Metatarsal[2]	bisector of talar head	*normal:* range ± 5°; lines normally coincide
		bisector of first metatarsal	*plus:* if talar bisector is medial, talar adduction; pronation *minus:* if talar bisector is lateral, talar abduction; supination
3	Talocalcaneal (longitudinal angle)	bisector of talar head	*normal:* 30° ± 5°
		bisector of distal part of calcaneus from point on lateral calcaneocuboid joint to medial calcaneocuboid joint margins; extend bisectors posteriorly to form apex	*plus:* adduction of talus; pronation *minus:* abduction of talus; supination
4	Midtarsal Joint (transverse talocalcaneal angle)	line from lateral calcaneocuboid joint parallel to this joint to medial border of foot	*normal:* 6° ± 2°
		line from lateral calcaneocuboid joint through point that bisects talar head	*plus:* distal displacement of talus (may be neutralized by excessive talar adduction); pronation; forefoot abduction *minus:* abduction of talus; supination; forefoot adduction
5	Talus-Medial Midfoot Axis	bisector of talar head	*normal:* none established; compare both feet; talus-medial segment alignment
		line from center of talar head to meet bisector of second metatarsal at cuneiform joint (*medial midfoot axis*)	*plus:* midfoot abduction *minus:* midfoot adduction
6	Medial Midfoot Axis-Second Metatarsal	medial midfoot axis (see 5) bisector of second metatarsal shaft	*normal:* none established; compare both feet; medial midfoot segment-second metatarsal alignment; correlate with long axis of foot *plus:* second metatarsal adduction *minus:* second metatarsal abduction

1. If no center point can be determined for posterior calcaneus, orient a line parallel to the laterodistal margin of calcaneus to pass through a point at medial calcaneocuboid joint to metatarsophalangeal area. This line is an acceptable longitudinal foot axis.

2. Influenced by metatarsal or forefoot abduction or adduction

No.	Angle	Sides of Angle	Demonstration: alignment of medial and lateral midfoot segments
7	Calcaneus-Lateral Midfoot Axis	bisector of distal part of calcaneus	*normal:* none established; compare both feet; calcaneus-midfoot lateral segment alignment; compare with talo-medial midfoot axis angle
		line from center of distal part of calcaneus to bisector of fourth metatarsal at cuboid joint *(lateral midfoot axis)*	*plus:* midfoot abduction
			minus: midfoot adduction
8	Lateral Midfoot Axis-Fourth Metatarsal	lateral midfoot axis (see 7)	*normal:* none established; compare both feet; correlate with fourth and fifth intermetatarsal angle (angle 12)
		bisector of fourth metatarsal shaft	*plus:* fourth metatarsal adduction
			minus: fourth metatarsal abduction
9	First-Second Intermetatarsal	bisector of first metatarsal shaft	relative adduction of first metatarsal
		bisector of second metatarsal shaft	compare both feet; correlate amount of angle with talus-first metatarsal angle to determine proportion of adduction or abduction; also check gap at base of metatarsals
10	Second Metatarsal-Longitudinal Foot Axis	bisector of second metatarsal shaft	index of second metatarsal-hindfoot alignment; second metatarsal is most stable of metatarsals
		longitudinal axis of foot extended from center of posterior calcaneus through point at medial calcaneo-cuboid joint	compare both feet
11	Third-Fourth Intermetatarsal	bisector of third metatarsal shaft	a key indicator of third metatarsal-cuneiform alignment
		bisector of fourth metatarsal shaft	apex normally at base of metatarsal; apex distal if third metatarsal is adducted
12	Fourth-Fifth Intermetatarsal	bisector of fourth metatarsal shaft	relative abduction of fifth metatarsal
		bisector of fifth metatarsal shaft	compare both feet
13	First Metatarsal-Proximal Phalanx of Hallus	bisector of first metatarsal shaft	indicator of hallux abductus or adductus
		bisector of proximal phalanx of hallux	correlate congruity of articulation
14	Metatarsal-Digital	bisector of a metatarsal shaft	relative alignment of metatarsal and toe
		bisector of proximal phalanx of a lesser digit	both lines normally coincide; correlate congruity of articulation
			apex medial—toe abducted; apex lateral—toe adducted

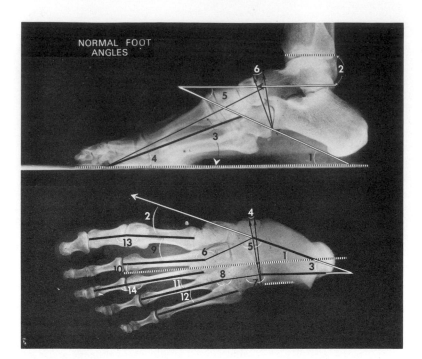

Sagittal-plane Angles
1, Calcaneal inclination
2, Talar (body) declination
3, Talar (head) declination
4, First metatarsal declination
5, Talocalcaneal
6, Midtarsal

Transverse-plane Angles
1, Talus-long foot axis
2, Talus-first metatarsal
3, Talocalcaneal
4, Midtarsal
5, Talus-median midfoot
6, Median midfoot-second metatarsal
7, Calcaneus-lateral midfoot
8, Lateral midfoot-fourth metatarsal
9, First-second intermetatarsal
10, Second metatarsal-longitudinal foot axis
11, Third-fourth intermetatarsal
12, Fourth-fifth intermetatarsal
13, First metatarsal-proximal phalanx, hallux
14, Metatarsal-digital

Fig. 520. Normal foot angles, medium foot height framework. A composite of demonstrable angles that indicate normal foot bone relationships. A standard for comparison with abnormalities. Consult Tables 15 and 16 for significance of angles. Numbers on charted roentgenogram are keyed with tables.

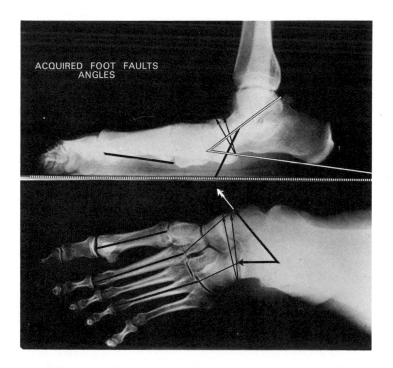

Sagittal-plane Angles

Calcaneal inclination—minus

Talar declination—plus

First metatarsal inclination—minus (reversed angle)

Talocalcaneal‖plus

Midtarsal—normal

Transverse-plane Angles

Talus-first metatarsal—plus

Talocalcaneal—plus
Midtarsal—normal
Talus-medial midfoot—plus
Medial midfoot-second metatarsal—plus
Calcaneus-lateral midfoot—plus

Lateral midfoot-fourth metatarsal—normal

Fig. 522. Acquired foot faults — extreme subluxations

Sagittal-plane Signs
1, Even posterior subtalar joint
2, Open sinus tarsi
3, Congruous midtarsal joint
4, Level sustentaculum tali
5, Plantar tuberosities defined
6, Peroneal groove defined
7, Parallelism of naviculocuneiform and cuneiform-first metatarsal joints

Transverse-plane Signs
1, Overlapping talocalcaneal joint
2, Congruous sinus tarsi
3, Closed first and second metatarsal segment joint
4, Closed fourth and fifth metatarsal segment joint
5, Parallelism of internal cuneiform and longitudinal foot axis

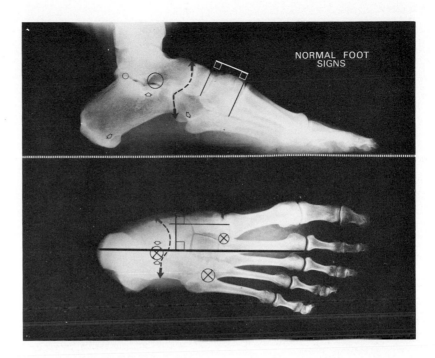

Fig. 521. Normal foot signs, medium foot height framework. A composite of roentgen signs and alignments that indicate normal foot bone positional relationships. A standard for comparison with abnormalities.

Sagittal-plane Signs
Arrows indicate malpositions

Pseudo-sinus posterior subtalar joint

Closed sinus tarsi
Broken midtarsal joint cyma

Transverse-plane Signs
Arrows indicate malposition

Gap at talocalcaneal joint

Broken midtarsal joint cyma
Gap at first and second metatarsal segment

Gap at second and third cuneiform joint

Gap at all intermetatarsal base joints

Gap at cuboid-fourth and fifth metatarsal bases

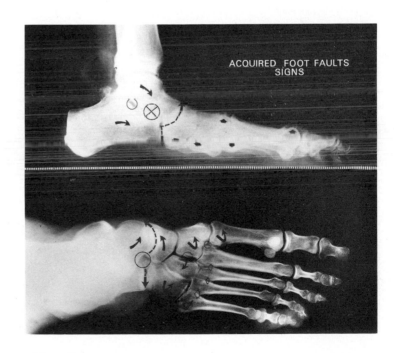

Fig. 523. Acquired foot faults — extreme subluxations

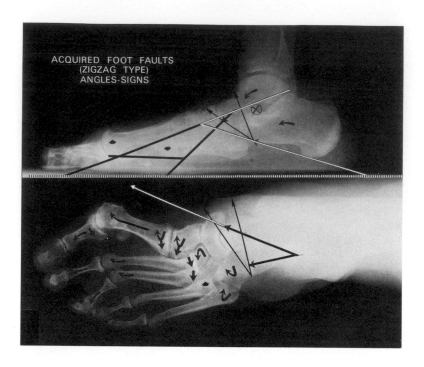

Sagittal-plane Angles
    Calcaneal inclination—minus
    Talar declination—plus
    First metatarsal inclination—
    (reversed)
    Talocalcaneal—plus
    Midtarsal—plus
Sagittal-plane Signs
    Arrows indicate malpositions
    Closed sinus tarsi
Transverse-plane Angles
    Talus-first metatarsal—normal
    (neutralized by adducted first meta-
    tarsal)
    Talocalcaneal—plus
    Midtarsal—plus
Transverse-plane Signs
    Arrows indicate malpositions

Fig. 524. Acquired foot faults — zigzag subluxation type (roentgenogram courtesy W.R. Walp, D.P.M.)

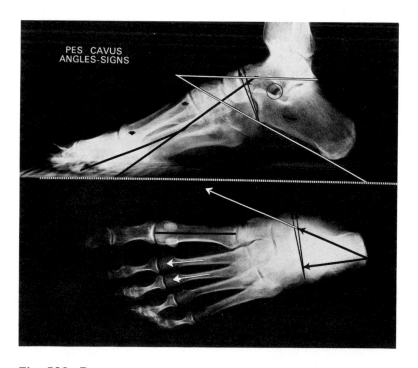

Sagittal-plane Angles
    Calcaneal inclination—plus
    Talar declination—minus
    First metatarsal inclination—
    plus
    Talocalcaneal—plus
    Midtarsal—minus
Sagittal-plane Signs
    Arrows indicate malpositions
    Open sinus tarsi
Transverse-plane Angles
    Talus-first metatarsal—plus
    Talocalcaneal—plus
Transverse-plane Signs
    Parallelism of metatarsal bones

Fig. 526. Pes cavus

410/CHARTING IN FOOT ROENTGENOLOGY

Sagittal-plane Angles
 Calcaneal inclination—minus
  —reversed
 Talar declination—plus
 First metatarsal inclination—minus
 Talocalcaneal—minus
 Midtarsal—plus
Sagittal-plane Signs
 Arrows indicate malpositions
 Closed sinus tarsi
Transverse-plane Angles
 Talus-first metatarsal—plus
 Talocalcaneal—plus
 Midtarsal—plus
Transverse-plane Signs
 Arrows indicate malpositions
 Gap at talocalcaneal joint
 Spreading transverse tarsal joints
 Gap at all intermetatarsal base joints
 Gap at tarsometatarsal joints

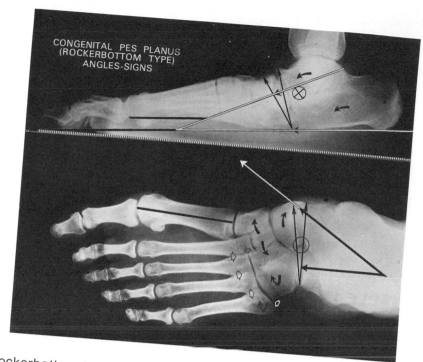

Fig. 525. Congenital pes planus — rockerbottom type

Sagittal-plane Angles
 Calcaneal inclination—plus
 Talar declination—minus
 First metatarsal inclination—plus
 Talocalcaneal—plus
 Midtarsal—plus
Sagittal-plane Signs
 Arrows indicate malpositions
 Excessively open sinus tarsi
Transverse-plane Angles
 Talus-first metatarsal—minus
 Talocalcaneal—minus
 Midtarsal—plus
Transverse-plane Signs
 Arrows indicate malpositions
 Bases of lesser metatarsal overlap

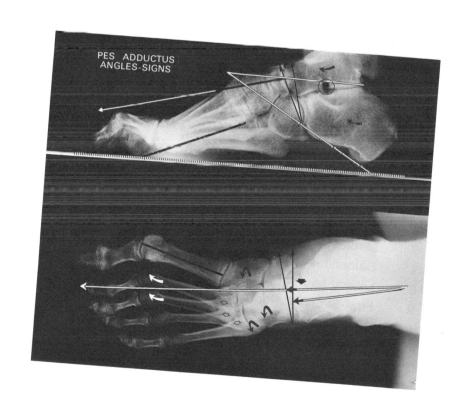

Fig. 527. Pes adductus

INDEX

INDEX

g

Gamble charting method, 402–415
Ganglion, mass, 129
Geometric illusion, 384
Giantism, pituitary, 90
Gout, 73, 75, 76
"Growing pains," differential diagnosis, 75
"Growth lines," 28, 29

h

Hallux abductus, angle, 249
        types, 250
    abductus valgus, 248–263
    adductus, 263, 264
    atypical, 257
    flexus, 263, 264
    limitus, 264–265
    valgus (see *Hallux abductus valgus*)
    varus (see *Hallux adductus*)
Hammer toe, 266, 267, 293
Hammonds' charting method, 397–399
    Posture-Poser, 376
Harris and Beath Canadian Army foot survey, 393
Heloma durum, 303–305
    molle, 305–306
Hemophilia, 83
    subperiosteal hemmorrhage, 21
Hindfoot, in pes cavus, 285
    normal, 230
    organization, 189
    special projections, 345, 346
Hyperendocrinism, 89
Hypergonadism, 93
Hyperkeratosis, basic intrinsic etiology, 302
    (see *Heloma*)
Hyperostosis, Leri's, 27
Hyperparathyroidism, 86, 92
    decreased bone density, 31
Hyperpituitarism, 89
    systemic deossification, 90
Hyperthyroidism, 85, 93
Hypertrophy, of bone, 26, 27
Hypervitaminosis, 96
    A, 96
    D, 97
Hypoendocrinism, 94

Hypogonadism, 91, 95
Hypopituitarism, 94
Hypothyroidism, 85, 94, 95
Hypovitaminosis, 96
    C, 96
    D, 97

i, j

Infections, bone, 41–51
Inflammation, traumatic, 133
Intensifying screens, 314
Involucrum, 43

Joint, articular composition, 203, 204
    axes, 173
    calcaneocuboid, special oblique projection, 345, 347
    Charcot, 83, 84, 117
    disease, 62, 81
        degenerative, 63, 64
        tuberculosis, 77
    metatarsophalangeal, 242
    midtarsal, 200, 216, 230
    organization, hindfoot, subtalar, midtarsal, 189, 198, 199
    subtalar, 192
        special projections, 345, 347, 368
    tarsometatarsal, 200, 201, 202

l

Leprosy, 48
Ligaments, 170
Line, reference, 388, 403
    table of, 389–390
Luxation, 242

m

Macroradiography, 364
Madura foot, 49, 50

V

Vein, calcified, 14
Vitamin, A, 96
      B, 86
      C, 31, 96
      D, 8, 31, 97

W

Wedge, metatarsocuneiform, 166
Weight distribution, orthodynamic, 236
Weight-supporting foot, 361–364

X

Xanthoma tuberosum multiplex, 126, 128
X-ray paper, 371, 372, 374, 375

NOTES